HEALTHY VEGAN

THE COOKBOOK

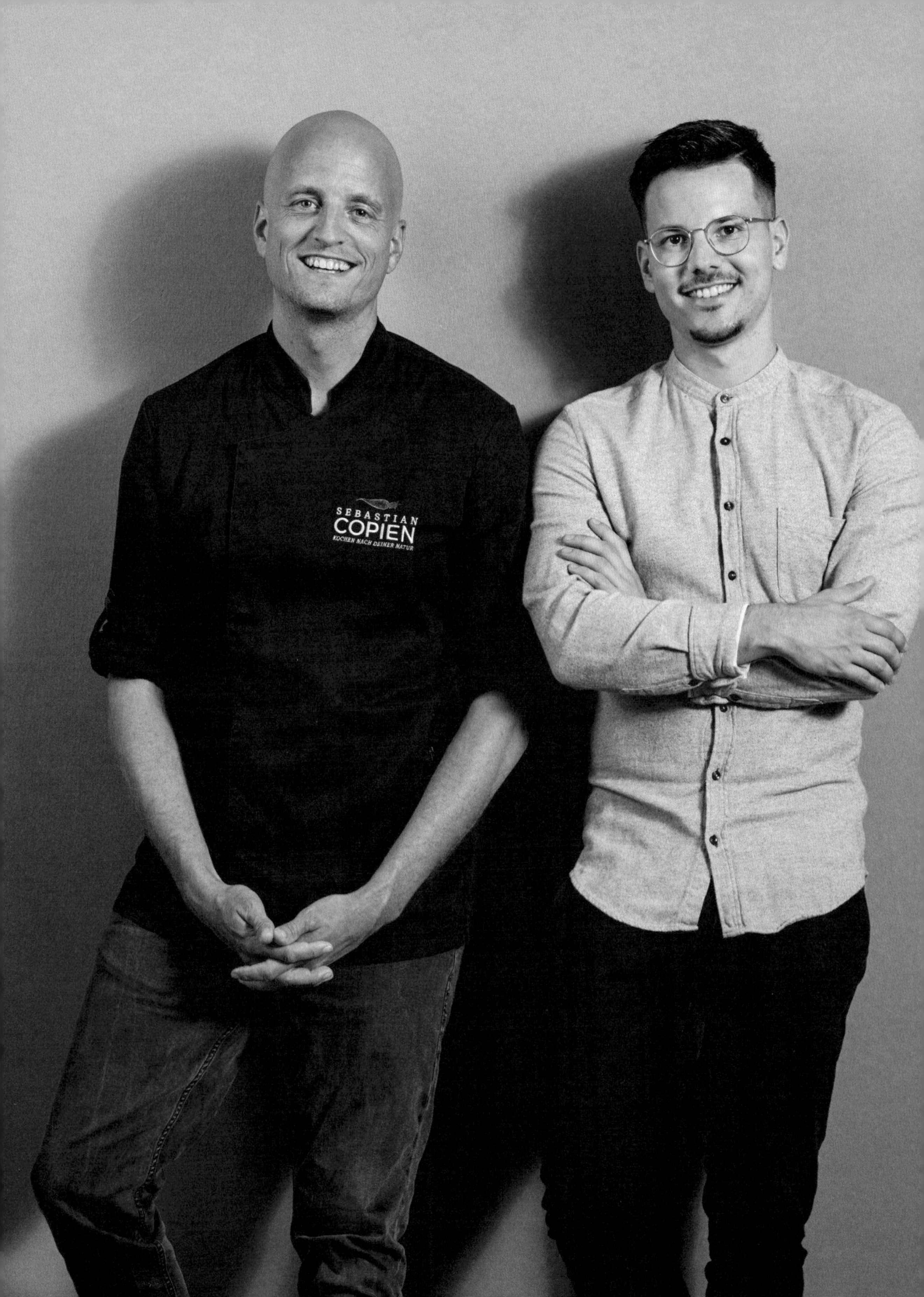
SEBASTIAN
COPIEN
KOCHEN NACH DEINER NATUR

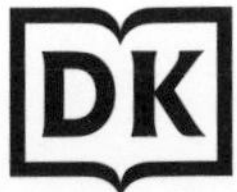

Niko Rittenau
Sebastian Copien

HEALTHY VEGAN

THE COOKBOOK

The science

This symbol shows you whether the preparation time for a recipe is short, medium, or long.

Nutritional information is provided for each recipe. ALA refers to alpha-linolenic acid, B2 to vitamin B2, and RE to retinol equivalent.

The recipes

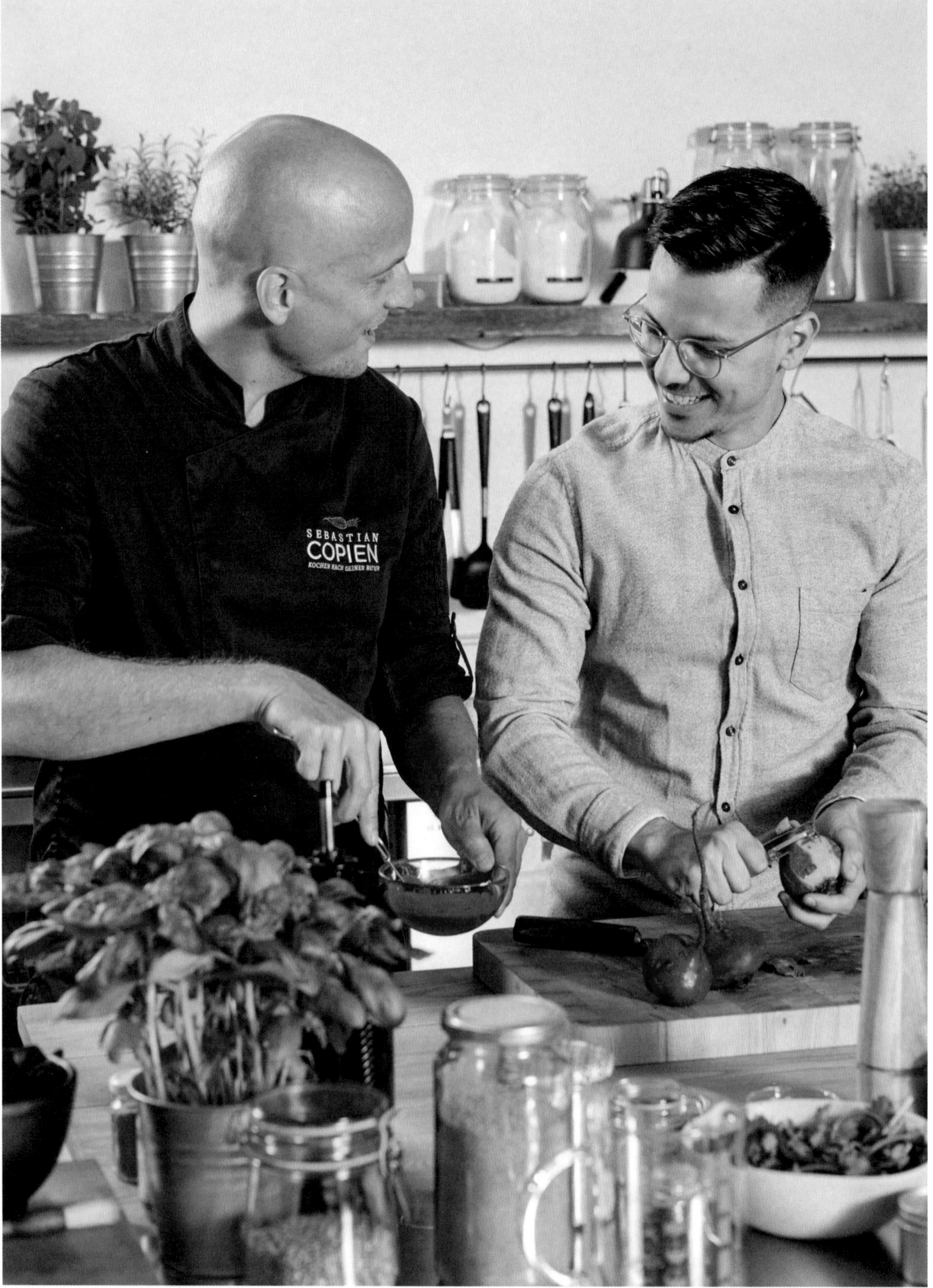
SEBASTIAN
COPIEN
KOCHEN NACH DEINER NATUR

Preface

Some people think that if you remove animal products from the menu there is not much left to eat. Meat, cheese, and other animal foods are widely regarded as intrinsic components of a "normal" diet. There are often overstated concerns about potential nutrient deficiencies on a vegan diet, but another frequent question is what on earth vegans can actually still eat. However, if you set aside your prejudice, you will find you can list a whole range of delicious recipes off the top of your head that are either already entirely plant-based or can be very easily veganised. Some national cuisines, such as Italian, Asian, and Indian, also offer plenty of completely vegan or predominantly plant-based recipes. Many people even report that changing their diet resulted in them discovering far more foods than were excluded, because modifying their eating habits prompted them to explore previously unknown or untried food products. The difficulties sometimes associated with a vegan diet are not really caused by insufficient variety in the plant-based products on offer; a much bigger problem is a lack of knowledge about the existence of these products and how to go about preparing and combining them.

This book aims to fill these gaps in your knowledge, and builds on the theoretical nutritional content from our book *Healthy Vegan* by providing cooking and nutrition tips, recipes, and detailed product expertise from a food science perspective.

With a variety of recipes for breakfast, lunch, and dinner, plus the recipe building blocks developed specifically so you can design your own delicious yet healthy plant-based dishes, this book proves vegetables can be super tasty. It is in fact often the preparation that is to blame, rather than the vegetables themselves. Over the following pages, we want to help you understand how you can devise delicious vegan menus while also ensuring your body is supplied with all the crucial nutrients.

In the first section, Niko draws on current scientific evidence to show on which food groups a vegan diet should be based, and he uses his nutritional science expertise to offer practical information about spices, oils, vinegars, and sweeteners. He also simplifies his nutritional recommendations into ten tips, which make it easy to plan and follow a wholesome and exclusively plant-based diet.

In the second part of the book, Sebastian takes readers with him into the new world of plant-based cuisine. He provides a brief theoretical introduction to help train your palate, then offers a wide variety of delicious vegan recipes that are easy to prepare for any time of day. These dishes are all designed around Niko's nutritional recommendations, so the result is the ideal vegan diet: healthy, delicious food that even non-vegans will love, and which shows how varied a plant-based diet can be.

All the best, and enjoy following the recipes!

Niko Rittenau

Sebastian Copien

Introduction

The three pillars of the vegan lifestyle

It is important for any diet that it covers our nutritional requirements in a way that is practical for everyday life, affordable, and also delicious. At the same time, we should avoid a surfeit of foods that are perceived to be unhealthy if consumed in excessive quantities. As well as looking after our own health, it is also important for our diet and lifestyle to contribute to caring for the planet and all of its living creatures. These three aims can be achieved through various dietary approaches, but the scientific literature and many popular publications have shown that a predominantly or exclusively vegan diet is one of the most effective ways of reconciling these objectives without technological innovations.

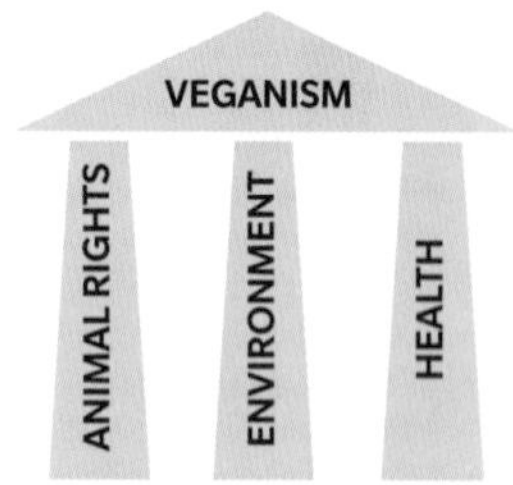

Fig. 1: The three pillars of the vegan lifestyle[1]

All the different aspects of the vegan lifestyle – animal welfare, the environment, and health – are very important, but this book concentrates primarily on the health aspects of a vegan diet.

In terms of choosing specific foods within a healthy vegan diet, we have used information from research such as the so-called Global Burden of Disease Study (GBDS) to establish the extent to which different foods impact our health. This study has been regularly updated over recent decades and the most latest version, from 2017, identifies the western diet as the third-highest (Germany,[2] Switzerland[3]) or the fourth-highest (Austria[4]) risk factor for our health. Data from the study have also allowed scientists to show which food groups within the western diet are particularly harmful or beneficial, and thus should be consumed in lower or higher quantities. Figure 2 gives an overview of these findings.

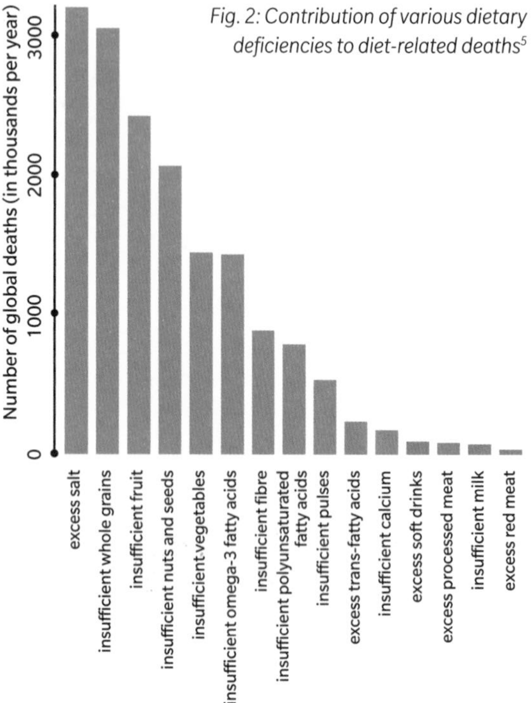

Fig. 2: Contribution of various dietary deficiencies to diet-related deaths[5]

Moving to a more plant-based diet

The GBDS results support research findings from leading cancer,[6] heart,[7] and dietary associations,[8] all of which recommend reducing the salt content in our diets. The study's findings are also in line with other recommendations from these specialist associations, suggesting that we should eat more plant-based foods and fewer animal products to stay healthy. So, with the exception of excessive salt consumption, four of the top five dietary risk factors cited by the GBDS relate to insufficient consumption of plant-based foods, such as whole grains, fruit, nuts, seeds, and vegetables.[9] If you read the ten rules issued by the German Nutrition Society (Deutsche Gesellschaft für Ernährung – DGE) about healthy food and drink, the very first rule states: "Choose mainly plant-based foods".[10] This goes on to explain further: "By following the DGE's recommendations and choosing a predominantly plant-based diet, you will put less strain on the environment and the climate than by following the average German diet. The production of plant-based foods uses fewer resources and causes lower emissions of harmful greenhouse gases than the production of animal products."[11]

In addition, the GBDS emphasizes the importance of consuming the right fatty acids in our diet, such as healthy omega-3 fatty acids. Many people automatically associate these with eating fish. However, the primary producers of omega-3 fatty acids are plants (microalgae), which are eaten by fish[12] and whose omega-3 fatty acids only accumulate in the fish as you progress along the food chain – along with certain undesired harmful substances.[13] So you do not have to eat fish to get a good supply of omega-3 fatty acids. You will find more on this subject in the section on oils (see p.28), and in Tip 4 in Niko's dietary tips (see p.60).

Calcium, sugar, and meat

A similar principle applies to reduce the risk of insufficient calcium intake. Dairy milk contains high quantities of calcium and other nutrients like protein, vitamin B12, and vitamin B2, so insufficient consumption is another risk frequently cited for plant-based diets. However, dairy milk does not have a monopoly on these nutrients and for every essential nutrient there are plenty of plant-based foods that can serve as a source.[14] For example, large quantities of calcium are contained in sesame seeds, almonds, kale, certain varieties of tofu, and there are plant-based drinks available that are fortified with the calcium-rich coralline algae, *Lithothamnion calcareum*. Even some varieties of mineral water contain enough calcium to provide an adequate supply for your body simply by meeting your daily liquid intake requirements.[15]

Another factor that should not be underestimated is the consumption of too much added sugar in various forms, a habit that is prevalent in the western world, in particular through soft drinks, which is known to increase the risk of illnesses like type 2 diabetes mellitus.[16] Bringing up the rear in the list of risk factors is the excessive consumption of processed meat and red meat, both of which are of course excluded in a vegan diet.

Niko's summary

This hierarchy of dietary risk factors is far from surprising. In the years before the GBDS study was published, extensive research had already demonstrated the connection between better health and the regular consumption of whole grains,[17] fruit, vegetables,[18] nuts and seeds,[19] and pulses.[20] And the link between excessive consumption of processed or red meat and poor health was demonstrated many years ago.[21]

All these studies and position papers show that one of the most important interventions in achieving a healthier diet is the increased consumption of plant-based foods instead of eating meat. So the following nutritional recommendations are not just the foundation for an exclusively vegan diet. The same principles apply for any omnivorous diet, which should consist of at least 75 per cent plant-based foods, according to the official healthy eating recommendations in lots of countries, including Germany,[22] Canada,[23] and the USA.[24] Non-vegans will also benefit from ensuring their diet has a greater emphasis on plant-based products.

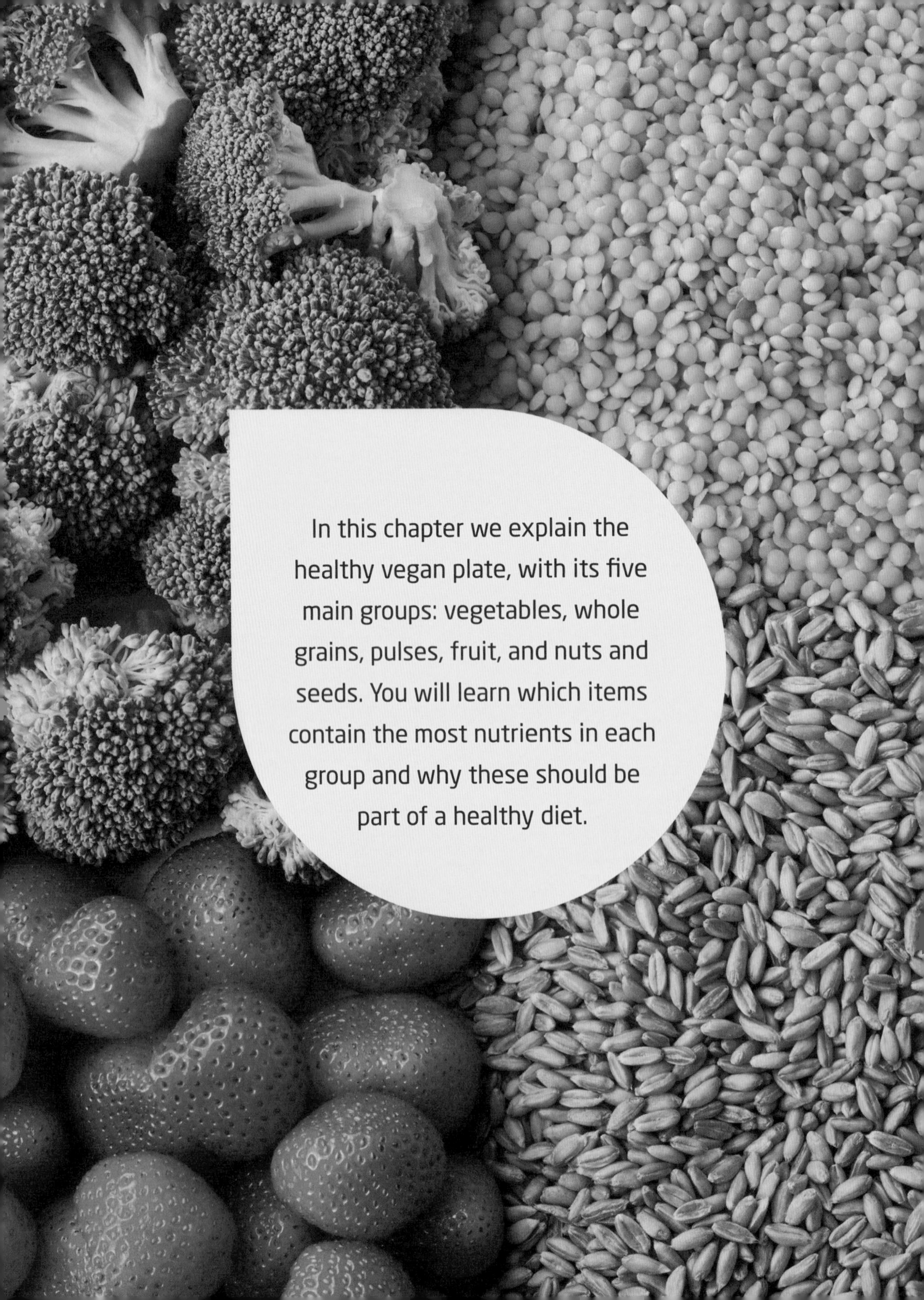

In this chapter we explain the healthy vegan plate, with its five main groups: vegetables, whole grains, pulses, fruit, and nuts and seeds. You will learn which items contain the most nutrients in each group and why these should be part of a healthy diet.

The healthy vegan plate

1. The healthy vegan plate

The healthy vegan plate is inspired by the Healthy Eating Plate of the Harvard T. H. Chan School of Public Health, and is designed to optimize the nutrient intake of people following a vegan lifestyle. It is divided into five categories: whole grains, pulses, vegetables, fruits, plus nuts and seeds. These elements also make up the basis for healthy nutrition in the WHO's Healthy Diet position paper.[25] Each group is described in detail in this book, and an overview is given below. In addition to the five main food groups, the healthy vegan plate focuses on the consumption of healthy oils (see p.28), and there is also an emphasis on adequate fluid intake (see p.69). Tip 10 (see p.75) describes how to augment a purely plant-based meal plan with appropriate nutritional supplements. This might take the form of a plant drink fortified with calcium or a carefully considered multi-vitamin that's specifically designed for the needs of people following a vegan lifestyle. We will show you how dietary supplements, used appropriately, can benefit both vegan and other diets, and that supplements themselves are not an argument against a specific dietary approach.

Whenever possible, all five main food groups should be incorporated regularly in the menu plan as part of a wholesome vegan diet. Each group contains an array of valuable ingredients with different health benefits, which in some cases cannot be obtained to the same extent by eating foods from the other groups.

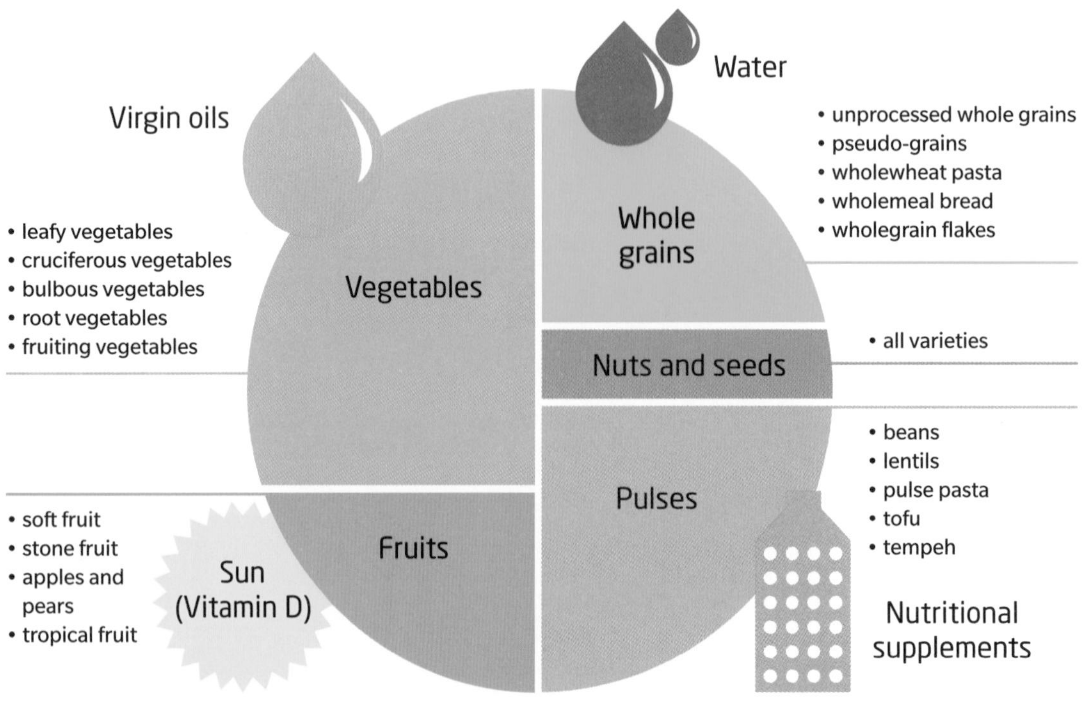

Fig. 3: The healthy vegan plate (adapted from Harvard T. H. Chan School of Public Health)[26]

1.1 Vegetables

"Eat more fruit and vegetables" is timeless advice based on robust scientific evidence.[27] In the UK, the recommendation for a healthy fruit and vegetable intake is "five-a-day", where a single portion is 80g (3oz). Some studies say that the more fruit and vegetables people eat, the lower their risk of contracting certain illnesses. In fact, research shows that as consumption rises to seven portions of fruit and vegetables a day, there is an associated steady reduction in the risk of chronic and degenerative conditions.[28, 29]

There is convincing evidence that regular consumption of vegetables lowers the risk of high blood pressure, cardiovascular disease, and stroke.[30] Not yet underpinned to the same extent by scientific research, but nonetheless still highly probable, is the claim set out in one study that suggested vegetable consumption also lowers the risk of certain cancers as well as rheumatoid arthritis, chronic obstructive pulmonary disease (COPD), asthma, osteoporosis, various eye conditions, and dementia.[31]

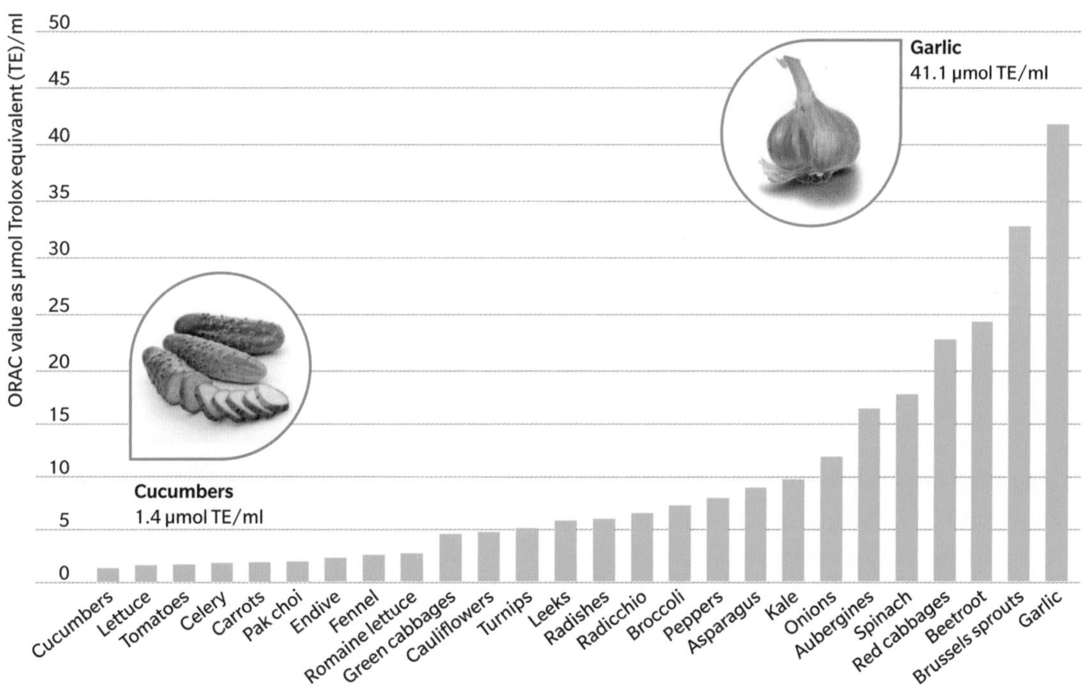

Fig. 4: Antioxidant power of selected varieties of vegetables (ORAC value in µmol Trolox equivalent (TE)/ml)[32]

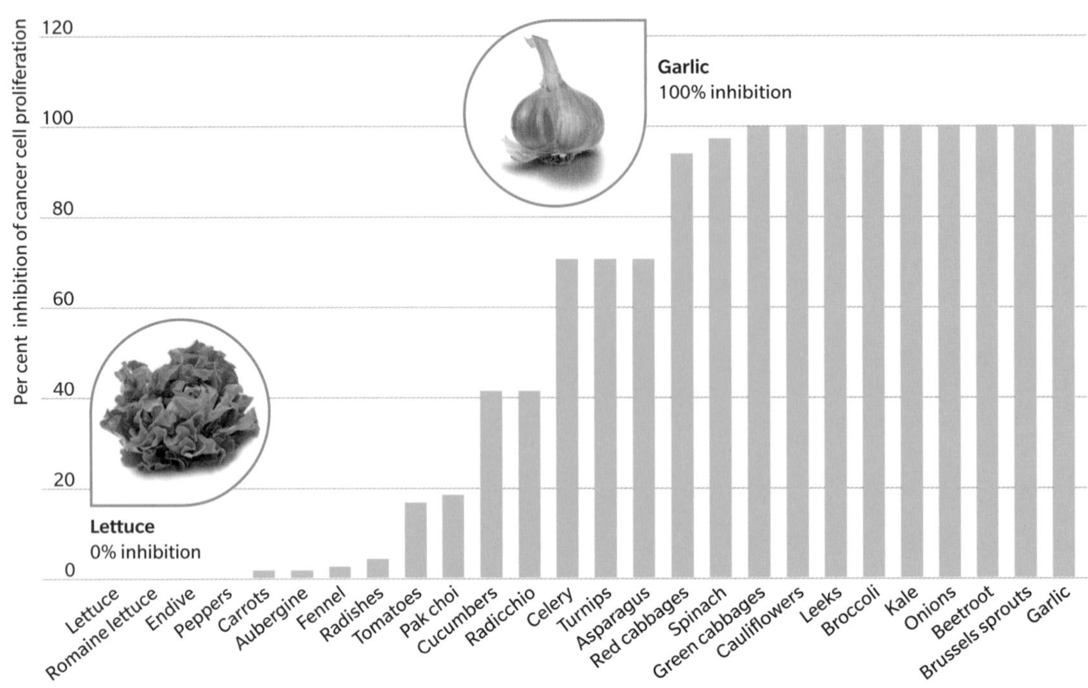

Fig. 5: Comparison of the anti-proliferative impact of vegetables (inhibition of cancer cells)[33]

Not all vegetables are equal

As shown in Figures 4 and 5, different types of vegetables vary widely in terms of their nutritional content and thus in their antioxidant effect and their potential to inhibit cancer. This is also reflected in scientific research. For example, studies that did not separate out the influence of the different vegetables consumed did not initially show any link between vegetable consumption and the risk of prostate cancer.[34] However, more detailed studies examining the effect of different types of vegetables on the risk of prostate cancer were able to demonstrate that higher consumption of cruciferous vegetables (broccoli, kale, Brussels sprouts, etc.)[35] and bulbous plants (garlic, onion, spring onions, etc.)[36] was definitely linked with a reduced incidence of prostate cancer. These differences are also shown in relation to other illnesses.[37, 38, 39] And within these groups, it is worth differentiating further to test the true potential for certain types of vegetables in reducing the risk of cancer. Not all cruciferous vegetables or bulbous plants have an equally powerful effect. A quick glance at Figure 5 reveals that kale, for example, has a more powerful cancer-inhibiting impact than red cabbages. And all these cruciferous vegetables in turn are many times more effective than pak choi, for example, even though they come from the same botanical family.[40] In terms of the antioxidant impact of bulbous plants, garlic is considerably ahead of onions and leeks.[41, 42] These findings illustrate the differences even within a single family of vegetables and suggest that many of the studies on people that have been conducted so far will not have provided accurate results regarding the preventative health benefits of eating vegetables. This is due to the failure to distinguish in detail between individual varieties of vegetables or the different ways in which they might be prepared.

All of these important differences must also be factored into specific nutritional recommendations for vegetable consumption.

It is right and proper to recommend eating more vegetables, but it would be even better to recommend particular preferred varieties. All vegetables are good, but cruciferous vegetables (cabbages, broccoli, kale, etc.), dark green leafy vegetables, and bulbous vegetables (onion, garlic, etc.) come out as the top three nutritionally beneficial varieties and should be included in your menu plan as often as possible.

Remember the following tips[43] to protect the health value of vegetables as much as possible during storage and preparation of these ingredients in cooking.

Tips on the optimum storage and preparation of vegetables

- Fresh vegetables should be stored in dark, humid conditions between 0 °C and 2 °C (32°F and 36°F)
- Vegetables that are sensitive to the cold, such as potatoes, cucumbers, aubergines, and tomatoes, etc., should be stored at a temperature between 5 °C and 10 °C (41°F and 50°F)
- Frozen vegetables should be stored in airtight containers
- When peeling and cleaning foods, only the sections that are unsuitable for consumption should be removed
- Vegetables should be washed and then chopped. They should not be immersed for long in water during washing, and they should be used and consumed quickly once they have been chopped
- Chopped vegetables for salads should be dressed immediately with vinegar or lemon juice to prevent the loss of nutrients
- Vegetables should preferably be steamed. If they are boiled, the cooking liquid should be used for sauces or soups so that the nutrients that have leached into the cooking water are not lost
- Vegetables should not be put in cold water and brought to the boil; instead, immerse them directly into boiling water to reduce the leaching out of nutrients. Vegetables should only be put into cold water if you are making stock

1.2 Whole grains

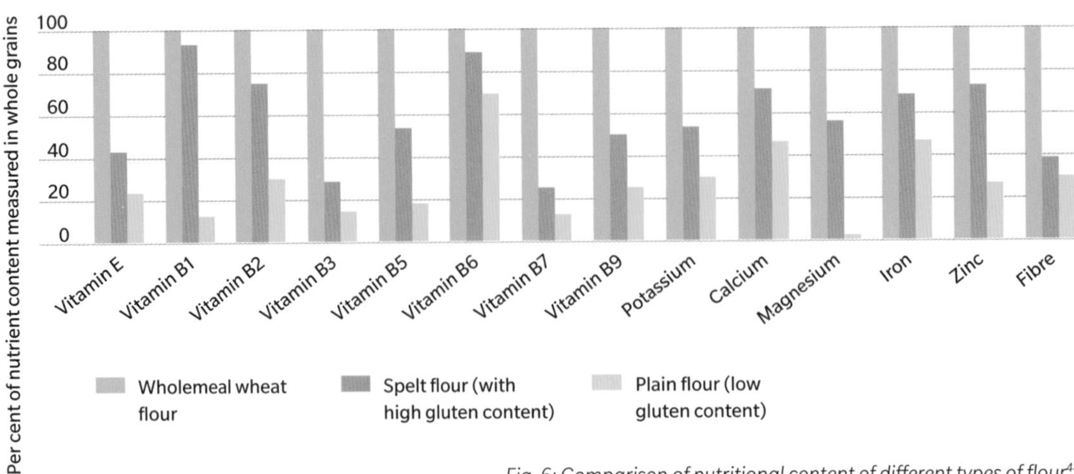

Fig. 6: Comparison of nutritional content of different types of flour[44]

Grains have always constituted a vital nutritional basis for the majority of the world's population. Globally, around half our total protein and calorie consumption comes from grains, which makes it very clear just how important they are for world nutrition.[45] Thanks to the versatility of whole grains and their excellent nutrient profile, they also play a key role on the healthy vegan plate. They might be on the menu at breakfast time in the form of oats in porridge or puffed amaranth in muesli. Wholemeal bread makes the perfect foundation for a daytime snack. And at lunch or supper time, a nutritious and filling side dish of buckwheat, rice, or quinoa or maybe wholewheat pasta, bulgur wheat, or couscous might form part of your vegan meal.

How to choose the most nutritious whole grains

Foods in the other main food groups in this chapter are rated in terms of their different antioxidant effects. For whole grains, on the other hand, the processing technique used is far more significant than which particular grain is involved. As shown in Figure 6, the nutritional value of a grain product depends to a great extent on whether it has been produced using wholemeal flour or a flour classed as type 1050 or 405. The more components of the grain kernel that are removed from the flour, the greater the loss of nutrients. That is why you should choose flour types that have as high a number as possible in their type description. This indicates a higher nutritional content; whereby wholemeal flour is always the most nutritious variety. The different numbers describe the quantity of minerals (ash) left behind when 100g (3½oz) of the relevant flour is burned.[46] The ash content is determined by the mineral content of the flour. The more components of the whole kernel that are retained in the flour, the higher the mineral content will be. So, if you burn 100g (3½oz) of a 1050-type flour, an average of about 1050mg of ash will be left, whereas for a 630-type flour, only 630mg will remain. That is why a flour with a refinement type of 1050 is nutritionally more valuable than a flour with a type value of 630, which in turn is higher in nutrients than a 405-type flour.

Healthy whole grains

Whole grains have been a part of the human diet for thousands of years. The predecessors of some of the grains that we eat now have been found in archaeological digs that date back over 100,000 years.[47] The beneficial health effects of whole grains are well documented: in the period between 2012 and 2017 alone, there were almost 100 scientific publications substantiating the positive health impact of regular wholegrain consumption.[48] These studies show influences on a wide array of health parameters, such as cholesterol levels, body weight, blood pressure, insulin sensitivity, and also certain inflammatory markers. Higher consumption of whole grains is associated with a lower risk of cardiovascular disease, type 2 diabetes, some types of cancer, as well as a reduced overall mortality rate.[49]

Processing grains and why it matters

Not all whole grains are equal. The different techniques for processing whole grains affect their health benefits in various ways. This is illustrated in Figure 7 using the so-called whole grain hierarchy by Canadian dietician Brenda Davis.

Generally speaking, the more a whole grain has been processed, the greater the loss of nutrients. So, intact whole grains sit at the tip of the whole grain hierarchy and are the healthiest wholegrain products. Intact grain kernels offer optimal protection against loss of nutrients during storage and preparation. They also have the lowest glycaemic index of all the wholegrain products, which makes them an ideal choice, particularly in nutritional therapy, for type 2 diabetes. In addition, only intact grains can be germinated, which further increases their nutritional value.[51, 52] Right at the bottom of the whole grain hierarchy are the puffed wholegrain products, which experience the greatest loss of nutrients during processing and which also cause a higher spike in blood sugar levels than intact grain kernels. All these products are better than white flour products, but the full health benefits are primarily offered by intact whole grains. However, when eaten as part of an overall healthy diet, all the items shown in the whole grain hierarchy can be eaten on a regular basis.

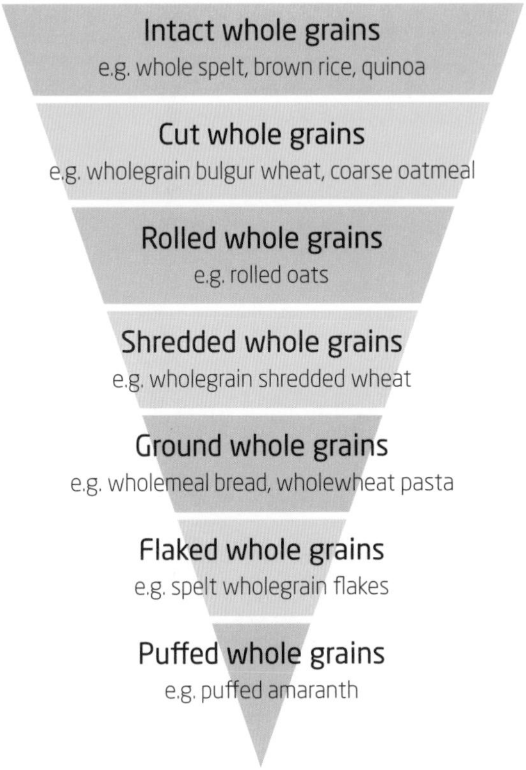

Fig. 7: Whole grain hierarchy according to Brenda Davis[50]

GLYCAEMIC INDEX

The glycaemic index is a measure that indicates a food's effect on blood sugar levels. The higher the value, the more blood sugar levels will rise after consuming this food. The wholegrain products at the tip of the hierarchy have the lowest glycaemic index, while the items at the bottom have a significantly higher rating. But even the glycaemic index for the whole grains on the lowest level of the hierarchy is significantly lower than for white flour products.

1.3 Pulses

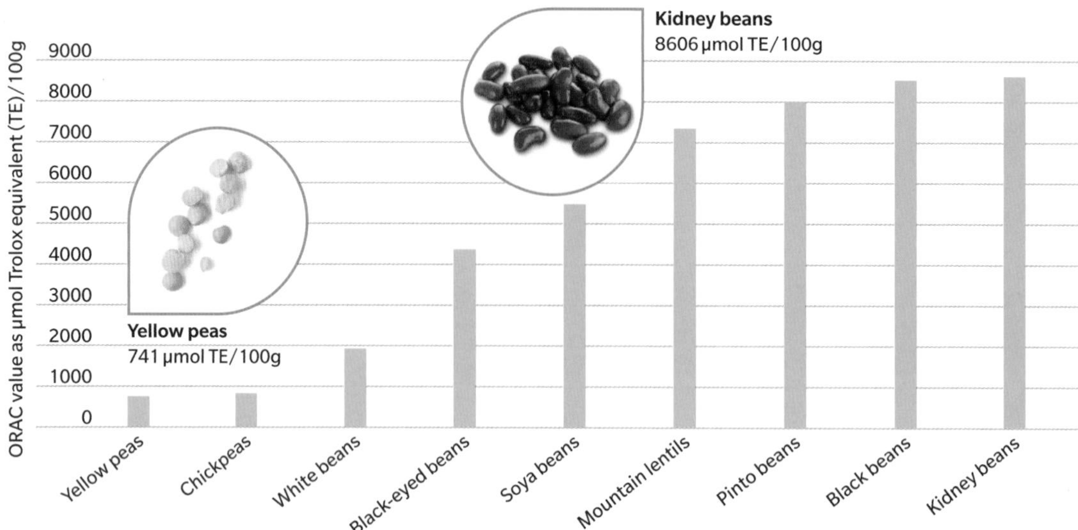

Fig. 8: Antioxidant capacity of pulses (ORAC value in µmol Trolox equivalent (TE)/100g)[53]

Pulses have been part of the human diet for about 10,000 years,[54] and products made from pulses like tofu[55] and tempeh[56] have been consumed for at least 1,000 years.

Once you start investigating pulses, you will be amazed at their health benefits and culinary potential. Pulses have an above-average fibre content of around 15–23 per cent, they are low in fat and thus contain few calories, and, depending on the variety, they contain between 25–35 per cent protein.[57] So they have long been a source of protein in the human diet.[58] Regularly eating pulses is extremely beneficial in terms of health and is associated with a reduced incidence of cardiovascular disease[59] as well as prostate[60] and colon cancer.[61]

As shown in Figure 8, the pulses with the darkest, strongest colours, such as kidney beans and black beans, have the greatest antioxidant effect measured by their ORAC value.[62] As always, however, the healthiest pulses are simply those you find tastiest because these will be the ones that you most readily include in your regular diet. In terms of the nutritional content of pulses, it does not matter whether you prepare them yourself using dried pulses or whether you use the tinned or jar varieties. If you compare the nutritional values, similar concentrations of nutrients are found in each type.[63] Of course, pulses in a jar or tin inevitably create more packaging waste and they usually have a significantly higher salt content. But if a tin of beans is tipped into a sieve and rinsed well under running water, the salt content can be reduced by an average of 40 per cent.[64]

Pulses guarantee the supply of protein

Particularly in a vegan diet, pulses play an important role as a source of protein because they contain an above-average amount of lysine. Lysine is an amino acid (a protein component) that the human body cannot create itself. If you follow a plant-based diet, you will rely on pulses

ORAC VALUE

The ORAC value (= oxygen-radical absorbing capacity) specifies the antioxidant capacity of the food. The higher this value, the better the food is at combating oxidative stress and thus preventing the occurrence of chronic degenerative illnesses.[65]

as a source of lysine to ensure an optimal supply.[66] Thanks to their high lysine content, pulses provide an ideal complement for proteins from other plant-based foods (such as grains) and they raise the so-called biological value to a level that is comparable to animal proteins. It has been recognized for decades that this mutual enhancement effect for different plant proteins does not require them to be combined in the same meal. They can be consumed over the course of an entire day and still complement each other just as well.[67]

Toxins in pulses?

There has been criticism from some groups over the consumption of pulses based on the alleged harmful effect of so-called antinutrients, such as trypsin inhibitors, lectins, and phytic acids.[68] However, these comments are not based on science, and research has shown

BIOLOGICAL VALUE

The biological value is a system for rating the quality of a food that contains protein. It indicates how effectively the body uses the dietary protein. A high biological value indicates a higher proportion of essential amino acids in relation to human requirements.[69]

that this is only a concern for raw pulses as the cooking process renders the trypsin inhibitors[70] and lectins[71] completely harmless. Phytic acid, by contrast, is relatively heat-resistant. As part of a balanced diet, though, the benefits of phytic acids – which help to regulate blood sugar levels, act as an antioxidant and can prevent cancer – far outweigh any negative impact in the form of inhibiting the absorption of minerals.[72]

Any concern about an inability to tolerate pulses also tends to be unfounded in most cases. Three experiments have shown that even at the start of their investigation fewer than half the participants experienced any kind of digestive problems from consuming pulses. And over the eight-week evaluation period, the participants' tolerance increased so much through acclimatization that ultimately about 97 per cent could digest the pulses with no issues at all.[73] The following tips could help to improve tolerance even further:

Methods to improve tolerance of pulses[74, 75, 76]

- Soaking the pulses before cooking
- Adding bicarbonate of soda to the soaking water (0.5–1g/litre)
- Allowing the pulses to sprout before cooking
- Fermenting the cooked pulses using bacteria or edible mould (e.g. in tempeh)
- Seasoning pulse dishes with spices or herbs that aid digestion, e.g. cumin, cinnamon, turmeric, ginger, dill, parsley, basil, mint, savory, anise, thyme, or fennel seeds
- Sufficient chewing and saliva production when eating
- Emphasis on easily digestible pulses like peeled mung beans (mung dal) or red lentils
- Taking alpha-galactosidase enzymes with pulse dishes

1.4 Fruit

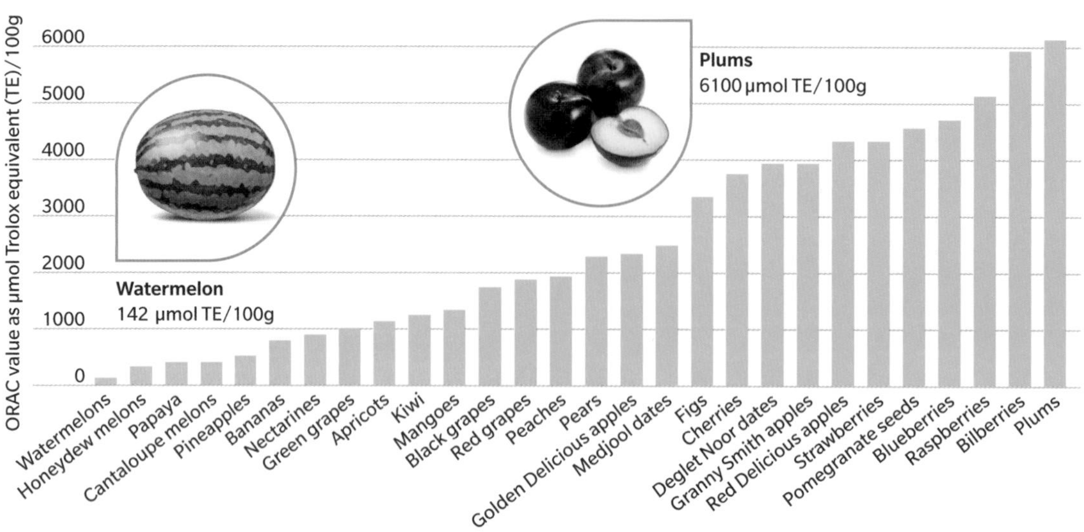

Fig. 9: Antioxidant capacity of fruit (ORAC value in µmol Trolox equivalent (TE)/100g)[77]

Fruit is an exceptionally healthy food group and should be incorporated regularly into a plant-based diet, just like the other four main food groups. The entirely justified negative press for high doses of fructose (fruit sugar) in soft drinks and syrups has wrongly also led many people to avoid fruit in the past. Regular consumption of high-sugar soft drinks and fruit juices is linked, for example, to a higher risk of illnesses such as type 2 diabetes[78, 79] and high blood pressure.[80] By contrast, however, higher consumption of fruit is associated with a lower risk of both these conditions.[81, 82] Regular consumption of fruit also lowers the risk of coronary heart disease,[83] strokes,[84] and certain types of cancer, such as breast and stomach cancer.[85] Despite the high content of (fruit) sugar, research shows very clearly that regular fruit consumption does not make you fat[86] and, in contrast to isolated fructose intake, it does not cause non-alcoholic fatty liver disease.[87]

Focus on antioxidant-rich fruits

In principle, eating all kinds of fruit is beneficial, but, as illustrated in Figure 9, certain types of fruit have a far greater antioxidant effect than others.[88] Plums are top of the list for antioxidant-rich fruit that is available in Europe. On average, plums have over forty times the antioxidant content of watermelon, which comes out bottom of this list. Other popular fruits, like bananas, provide just a seventh of the antioxidants contained in plums. As shown in Figure 9, another category of fruits also stands out – berries. These are exceptionally rich in antioxidants and so they should be included in your menu plan as often as possible. If no fresh berries are available, you can always use the frozen variety instead. Comparative studies have shown that the amount of antioxidant vitamins and secondary plant substances found in frozen fruit and vegetables is comparable to fresh fruit and vegetables that have been stored for a few days.[89, 90]

What about fructose tolerance?

Due to the sharp increase in the consumption of added fructose in mass-produced foods over recent decades, more and more people are at their limit in terms of utilizing fructose and consequently are experiencing digestive complaints. However, the issue of malabsorption of fructose is seldom caused by the fruit sugars in fruit; on the contrary, it is triggered by the far greater quantities of fructose that are added to soft drinks and sweet snacks. If you are affected by limited fructose tolerance, there are five strategies to improve absorption.

Strategies to improve fructose absorption[91]

1. Choose fruit with a glucose-fructose ratio > 1:1
2. Eat fruit in combination with glucose (e.g. breaking down starch in cereals)
3. Try to slow down digestion with the addition of fat and protein
4. Avoid fructose during and in the hours after physical activity
5. Enhance fructose absorption through regular fruit consumption

The first general principle is to focus on fruit with a balanced glucose to fructose ratio (> 1:1). Because glucose activates additional transporters for fructose in the small intestine, this improves the absorption of fructose. Suitable fruits include plums, apricots, blackberries, strawberries, grapes, and bananas.[92] Varieties of fruit with excessive fructose, such as apples and pears, and also certain concentrated juices (e.g. agave syrup), should either be avoided in this situation or made more digestible by following the tips in the illustration above.

Fruit that is rich in fructose (like apples and pears) can be combined with foods that are high in starch, such as grains, e.g. porridge served with fresh fruit. The starch that is in porridge oats is broken down into glucose as it is digested, which thus improves the absorption of fructose in the small intestine through the activation of additional transporters. This allows these foods to be better tolerated.[93]

Thirdly, fruit can be eaten with fatty foods that are rich in protein (like nuts) because the fat and protein slow down digestion. This means that less fructose enters the small intestine per unit of time, which helps take the strain off transporter capacity.[94] Fourthly, for particularly sensitive individuals, it may help to avoid consuming large quantities of fructose during and after intense physical activity because this shortens the passage of time in the small intestine, which increases the chance of the fructose transport system becoming overloaded.[95] Fifthly, you should continue eating fruit sugars in the form of fruit because, just as the number of fructose transporters in the small intestine can be reduced by avoiding fruit sugars (with the inevitable negative impact on fructose absorption), so the fructose transport activity can be stimulated by regular fructose consumption.[96]

Although some advocates of different dietary approaches continue to suggest that fruit will be better tolerated by avoiding combinations with other foods, this is not supported by any evidence from nutritional science. It is sometimes suggested that people should not combine certain foods within a meal because our digestive system cannot optimally handle several foods at the same time: this is a myth. This theory of food combining is based on a misapprehension about organic biochemical processes and also underestimates the body's capabilities.[97] In reality, the precise opposite is true and certain foods are actually more valuable for the body when consumed together.

1.5 Nuts & seeds

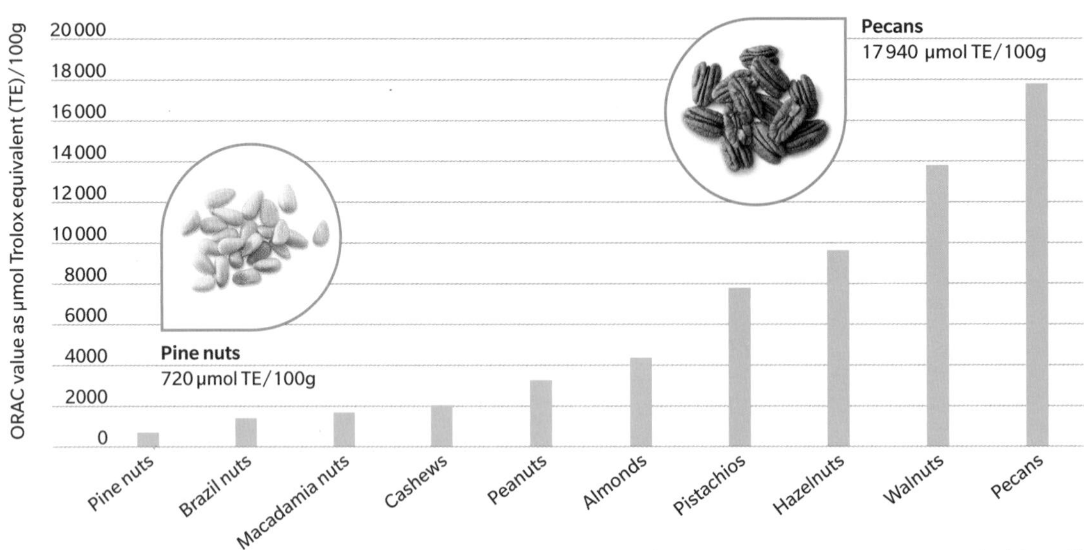

Fig. 10: Antioxidant capacity of nuts (ORAC value in µmol Trolox equivalent (TE)/100g)[98]

Nuts and seeds have been part of the human diet since Palaeolithic times.[99] They are nutritionally valuable primarily due to their high protein content and as a source of monounsaturated and polyunsaturated fatty acids. They also contain large quantities of dietary fibre and vitamins (especially niacin, vitamin B6, vitamin E, and folate), a high concentration of minerals (including copper, magnesium, potassium, and zinc), and a whole range of healthy secondary plant substances.[100]

Nuts are high in calories but are filling

Despite their healthy constituents, nuts are often avoided due to their high calorie content. However, studies have shown that people who regularly eat nuts actually eat less on average than those who seldom eat nuts.[101] This is primarily because nuts are relatively filling in a way that corresponds to their calorific value. This means they are quite unlike high-calorie junk food and soft drinks. To a great extent, the additional calories in nuts are simply offset at a different point in the day because eating nuts makes you feel full for longer.[102] In addition, unlike isolated fats (oils, margarine, etc.), not all the fat in nuts can be absorbed, so some of the fat is bonded to dietary fibre and is simply excreted without being used.[103]

The botanical definition of a nut is not necessarily synonymous with the classification of nuts in nutritional science. As shown in Figure 10, the list of nuts includes peanuts, for example, which are actually a type of legume, from a botanical perspective. However, in terms of their nutritional characteristics, peanuts are more akin to nuts and thus are included as part of this food group.[104] Figure 10 shows that pecans top the list of nuts by some margin when it comes to antioxidant properties. They are followed by walnuts, with pine nuts bringing up the rear at the bottom of the ranking.

Although walnuts can only manage second place compared to pecans in terms of antioxidants, they come out on top for their fatty acid composition, having the best ratio of omega-3 to omega-6 fatty acids of any nut.[105]

Regional superfood linseed

Among the seeds, linseed is clearly the best source of omega-3 and also contains highly effective secondary plant substances known as lignans. With the exception of a few other seeds (e.g. chia seeds), linseeds are an unrivalled source of lignans, providing between 80 to 100 times more lignans than most other foods containing this substance.[106] Regular consumption of linseed reduces the risk of high blood pressure[107] and can have a chemoprevention effect, particularly for breast[108] and prostate cancer.[109]

However, since our bodies cannot absorb the nutrients from whole linseeds and the seeds are often not sufficiently broken down during chewing, it is worth crushing linseeds before consumption. This can be done with any conventional kitchen blender. Just add whole linseeds to the blender and blitz on the highest setting for a few seconds until they have been broken up. You should ideally buy whole linseeds, as this offers optimum protection for their nutritional content, then crush them at home. Crushed linseed can then be stored for four months in a sealed container at room temperature without any deterioration in quality.[110]

You can scatter the seeds over any dish or use them as a plant-based binding agent instead of eggs. To replace one egg, stir a tablespoon of ground linseed into three tablespoons of water and let the mixture thicken.[111]

Baking with a "linseed egg" substitute like this is particularly appealing because the majority of omega-3 fatty acids[112] and lignans[113] contained in the ground linseed survive even after exposure to heat. After storing the baked item at room temperature for one week or keeping it in the freezer for two months at -25 °C (-13°F), research shows that the lignan content barely changes.[114]

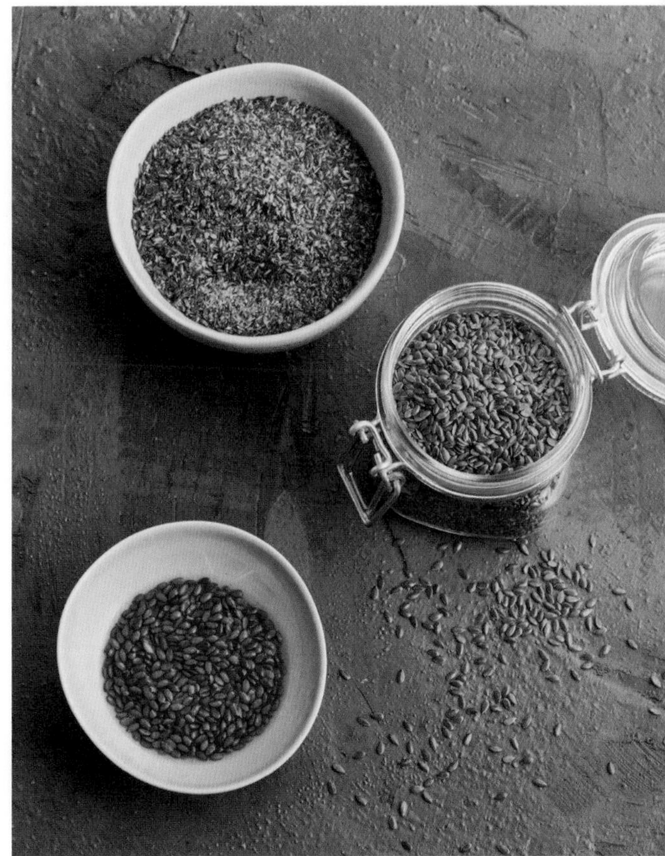

From a nutritional perspective, linseeds are always best ground as otherwise we cannot absorb lots of their valuable components.

A handful of nuts per day protects your heart

Nuts are considered to be a heart-healthy food[115, 116] and since 2003, in the USA nuts have been permitted to carry an official health claim. This is because studies show that the daily consumption of around 40g (1¼oz) of nuts (such as almonds, hazelnuts, peanuts, pecans, pine nuts, pistachios, or walnuts) as part of a low-cholesterol diet that is also low in saturated fats can reduce the risk of heart disease.[117] The British cholesterol charity,

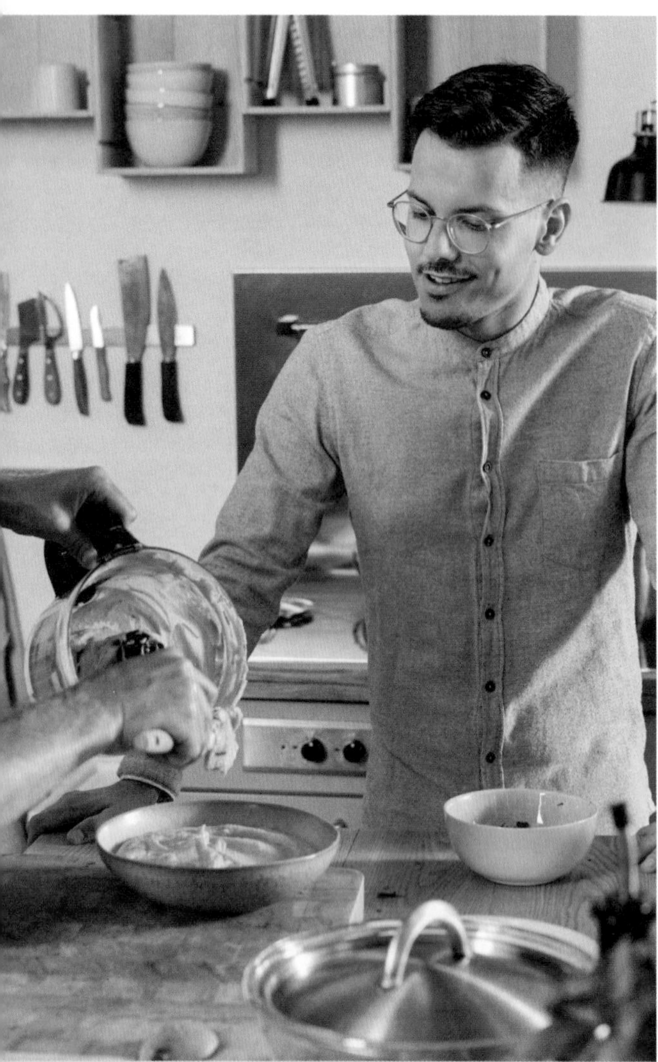

Puréed nuts and seeds make recipes creamier while also adding nutrients. Copien's lentil hummus (see p.192) gets its creamy consistency from sesame seed paste (tahini).

Heart UK, recommends the daily consumption of a handful of nuts (about 30g/1oz) to control cholesterol levels.[118]

In many online articles and books you will read that nuts and seeds should be soaked before eating to make them more digestible and to allow the body to absorb the nutrients better. Although this claim is widespread, studies show that soaked nuts are not more digestible and cannot be distinguished from those that are unsoaked in other parameters such as their phytic acid content.[119, 120] Consequently, nuts do not need to be "activated" (soaked) before eating. However, in some of our recipes we do recommend soaking walnuts beforehand, as this helps to reduce their bitter flavour.

Don't worry about toxins in nuts

During cultivation and processing, or if stored incorrectly (in excessively moist/warm conditions), some foods can be susceptible to mould, and this is particularly true for nuts and grains. The most significant fungus is *Aspergillus flavus,* which produces very harmful aflatoxins.[121] These are colourless, odourless, and tasteless[122] and are not adequately eliminated by common preparation techniques such as boiling, frying, or baking.[123] In the past, nuts were occasionally found on sale with higher levels of aflatoxins that exceeded the permitted statutory limits.[124] However, thanks to more stringent controls and greater awareness among producers, aflatoxin levels in nuts have fallen sharply over the last decade and nowadays you do not need to worry about this issue.[125, 126] There is also a trick you can use to protect against aflatoxins: by consuming dark green leafy vegetables at the same time as nuts, the absorption of carcinogenic aflatoxins can be greatly reduced because the chlorophyll that is contained in the leafy greens forms an indigestible substance with the aflatoxins. This has the effect that these are absorbed in far smaller quantities into the bloodstream via the small intestine.[127] To ensure you get the maximum benefit from eating nuts, you should remember the following points:

Notes on the optimum storage and preparation of nuts[128]

- It is better to buy whole nuts rather than ground because they are less susceptible to spoiling
- Ground nuts and seeds, in particular, should be stored in a well-sealed container in the fridge. For longer storage periods, it is advisable to freeze them in an airtight container
- Nuts that taste or smell unpleasant should never be eaten
- Buy nuts and oily seeds as locally as possible. You can get hazelnuts and walnuts grown in the UK and almonds from Europe
- When buying nuts, always try to get good-quality, organic nuts, and preferably fairtrade
- If possible, nuts should be eaten as part of a recipe. The fat contained in nuts allows certain nutrients in other ingredients to be absorbed more readily, and the chlorophyll in dark green vegetables can potentially further reduce the absorption of any remaining tiny quantities of aflatoxins in the nuts

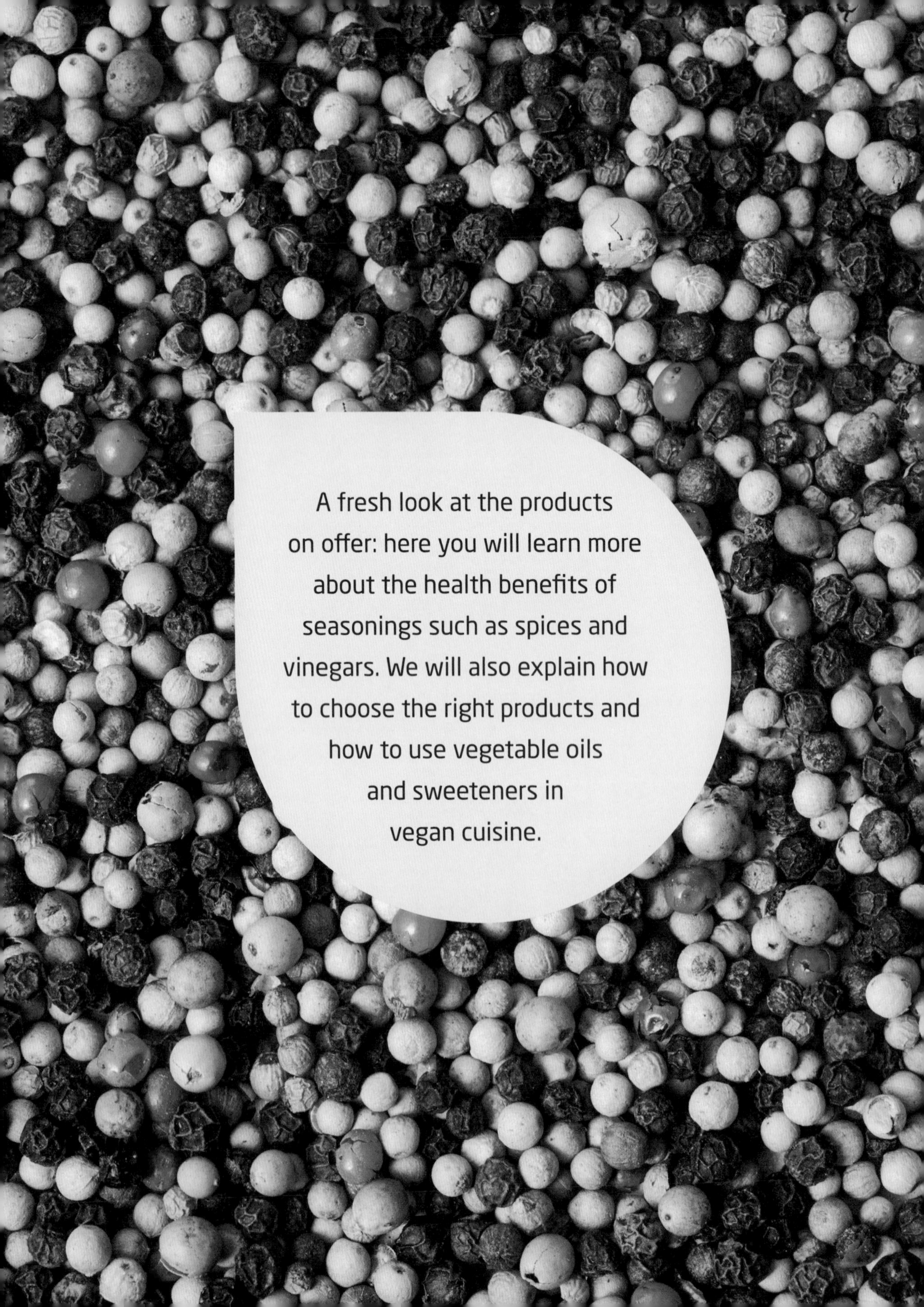

A fresh look at the products on offer: here you will learn more about the health benefits of seasonings such as spices and vinegars. We will also explain how to choose the right products and how to use vegetable oils and sweeteners in vegan cuisine.

Product expertise

2. Oils, vinegars, seasonings, and sweeteners from a nutritional science perspective

These products are "worth their salt", as the saying goes. Vinegars, oils, spices, and herbs all function as flavouring agents. You can read here how we rate these items from a health perspective, how you can use them, and what alternatives are available.

2.1 Edible oils

The earliest culinary use of edible oils like olive oil is thought to have been over 5,000 years ago on the island of Crete.[129] When talking about edible oils nowadays, it is important to specify precisely what kind of oil is involved. There are enormous differences between the various processing methods, both in terms of the quality of the flavour and the oil's health benefits.[130] For example, a cold pressed extra virgin olive oil that is produced using mature, carefully processed olives is worlds apart from a refined frying oil made from olives. This chapter will demonstrate why it is important to avoid such refined oils as far as possible, and to instead use high-quality, organically produced, virgin oils. There are also big differences between the various kinds of virgin oils, due to their fatty acid composition.

Fatty acid composition and effect

The main distinction that we make about fatty acids is between saturated, monounsaturated, and polyunsaturated fatty acids and, in the latter case, between omega-6 and omega-3 fatty acids. Even within this group, fatty acids may have very different effects depending on their respective chemical compositions. Dietary fats (lipids) consist primarily of triglycerides, which in turn are made up of a glycerol molecule that is bound

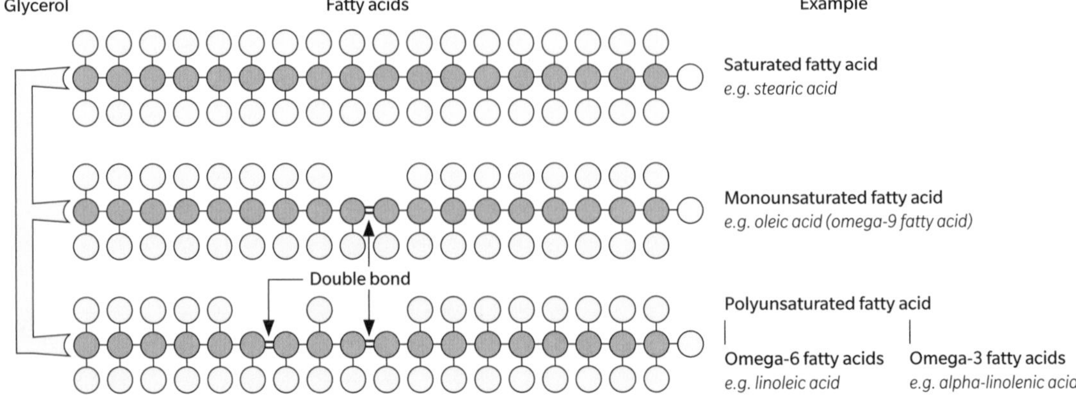

Fig. 11: Chemical structure of a triglyceride[131]

TYPE OF OIL	SHELF LIFE AFTER INITIAL OPENING	STORAGE CONDITIONS
Oils rich in omega-3 *(e.g. linseed, hemp, chia oil)*	**4 weeks**	**in the fridge**
Oils rich in omega-6 *(e.g. sunflower, corn, safflower oil)*	**3 months**	**in the fridge**
Oils rich in omega-9 *(e.g. olive, avocado, macadamia oil)*	**9 months**	**in the cupboard (away from light)**
Oils rich in saturated fatty acids *(e.g. cocoa butter, coconut, palm oil)*	**see best-before date on the label**	**in the cupboard (away from light)**

Tab. 1: Shelf life for different cooking oils based on their fatty acid composition[132]

to three fatty acid molecules – as is illustrated in Figure 11.

The term saturated fatty acid is used when every carbon atom in the chain of fatty acids is bound to two hydrogen atoms. If two adjacent carbon atoms in a fatty acid chain are only attached on one side to a hydrogen atom, the result is a gap in the chain. At this point, the carbon atoms are then connected to each other with a double bond (see Figure 11). If there is only one double bond in the fatty acid's carbon chain, this is called a monounsaturated fatty acid. If there are two, three, or more double bonds in the fatty acid, this is called a polyunsaturated fatty acid.[133] The location at which the first double bond occurs in the fatty acid chain determines whether it is classified as an omega-3 fatty acid (first double bond after the third carbon atom), an omega-6 fatty acid (first double bond after the sixth carbon atom), or an omega-9 fatty acid (first double bond after the ninth carbon atom).[134]

Broadly speaking, double bonds make a fatty acid more sensitive to oxygen and heat. The more double bonds that a fatty acid has, the more reactive and sensitive it is in the kitchen and the shorter the shelf life of the relevant oil. But a glycerol molecule can also be attached to three identical or three different fatty acids. This is what produces the large number of different kinds of fats.

Table 1 shows the shelf life for selected vegetable oils after opening.

The best-before date on the label for cooking oils applies to the unopened bottle and is not applicable once the oil has been opened. Only oils with a very high proportion of saturated fatty acids are so insensitive that the best-before date on the label still applies after opening. For all other oils, the shelf life is significantly shorter once open (see Table 1).

Edible oils in the kitchen

While oils that mainly consist of saturated or monounsaturated fatty acids can indeed be used for frying, sautéing, and roasting, oils with a high proportion of polyunsaturated fatty acids should only be used for cold dishes.

The number of saturated and unsaturated fatty acids also determines the consistency of an oil. The more saturated fatty acids that an oil contains, the firmer the fat will be at room temperature. And the more monounsaturated and polyunsaturated fatty acids it contains, the more liquid it will be, even in the fridge.[135] Olive oil consists mainly of monounsaturated fatty acids and, although it does not solidify in the fridge, it will coagulate slightly and thicken at cooler temperatures. This does not affect the quality and will be resolved as soon as the oil is stored at room temperature again. Figure 12 gives an overview of the fatty acid composition of common cooking oils.

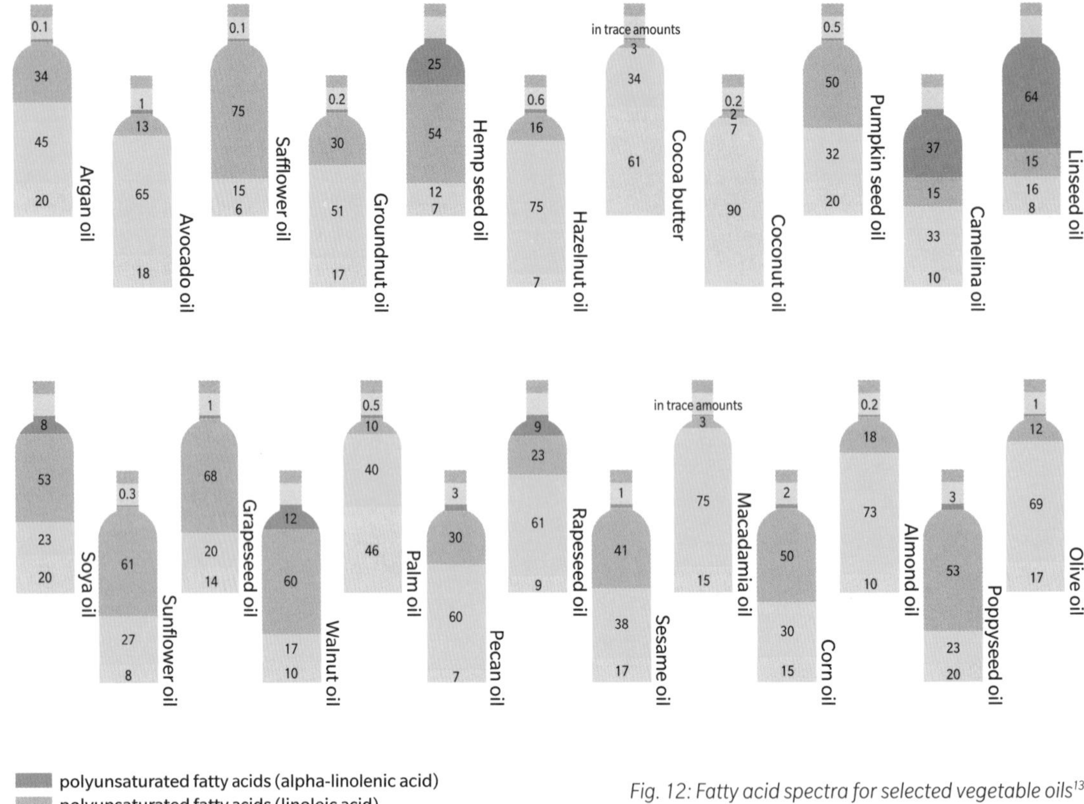

Fig. 12: Fatty acid spectra for selected vegetable oils[136] (The percentages are specified as average values and, therefore, do not add up to 100 per cent.)

Virgin and refined oils

Apart from the composition of fatty acids in different oils, you can also categorize them into cold pressed (virgin) oils and refined oils based on how they have been processed. Our recommendation for all cooking methods (cold dishes, sautéing, roasting, etc.) is to use high-quality, organic, virgin oils with the appropriate fatty acid composition for the desired application. Compared to refined oils, these retain lots of valuable components (fat-soluble vitamins and secondary plant substances).[137] Table 2 lists the most important differences between these two methods for producing oils.

COLD PRESSED (VIRGIN) COOKING OILS	REFINED COOKING OILS
aromatic	flavourless
intense colour	almost colourless
rich in valuable substances	low levels of valuable substances
spoil quickly	keep for longer periods
can contain harmful substances if low in quality	even if low in quality, harmful substances are removed by refining

Tab. 2: Characteristics of virgin and refined cooking oils[138]

Once they have been pressed, virgin oils can only be filtered. This means their fatty acid structure is not altered in any way and the characteristic taste of the original food product is retained.[139] Refined oils, on the other hand, are usually produced from oils that have been extracted using solvents. These oils then undergo degumming, deacidification, bleaching, and deodorization to create the almost colourless, flavourless oils you see on the supermarket shelves. Refined oils are also low in nutrients. Although refined oils have a longer shelf life and, depending on the variety, are more stable when exposed to heat, these advantages are to the detriment of the oil's quality and health benefits. Apart from the price, there are few reasons for consumers to purchase refined oils.

Since extra virgin olive oil is also suitable for sautéing and roasting, no other oils are needed for the recipes in this book. All the other virgin oils are also excellent products and can easily be used instead. For reasons of simplicity, we have limited the ingredient lists in the recipes to extra virgin olive oil to make it easier to organize your shopping and cook these dishes at home. When buying virgin oils, you should always seek out the highest-quality products, because the fact that they have not been refined means that possible contaminants, such as heavy metals, pesticides, and mycotoxins are not removed from the oil. However, if the crop has been cultivated in good conditions and if the raw materials have been harvested, stored, and processed with care, these substances will not be found in the oil in the first place.

The taste and smell of an oil will be impaired long before a rancid oil is harmful to your health. So you can rely on your senses and only use oils as long as they smell and taste pleasant.[140]

The following tips are important when buying and storing oils:[141]

- Look out for organic quality
- For olive oil, only buy the extra virgin variety
- High-quality olive oils with a high polyphenol content have an intense, fruity, sharp flavour
- Always buy oils in dark bottles (not in plastic or metal containers)
- If possible, these bottles should also be packed in a cardboard box to provide the oil with optimal protection
- Look for oils in tall, narrow bottles, because the oil in these containers has less contact with oxygen
- Try to buy oil in small quantities to avoid long storage periods
- Only open the oil when you are actually ready to use it for the first time, and make a note of the date to remind you of the best-before date starting from this point
- When you first open the oil, smell it to ensure it is in good condition and make a mental note of what the oil smelled like. This will let you check the quality of the oil by smelling it again over the coming weeks

The correct temperature when cooking with oils
Depending on the chosen oil, the correct roasting temperature is between 130 and 140 °C (266 and 284°F). For frying, the temperature is between 160 and 170 °C (325°F and 338°F).[142] If an oil is heated too much, some of the fatty acids will gradually break down and this creates toxic decomposition products, which it is essential to avoid. You can use an infrared thermometer to keep an eye on temperature changes in the oil in the pan.

A term often used in connection with cooking temperature is the smoke point. The smoke point is the lowest temperature at which you can see the first clear signs of smoke developing above a heated cooking fat or oil. This temperature depends in part on the proportion of free fatty acids in the oil and is also influenced by the oil's fatty acid profile and the proportion of secondary plant substances. The higher the proportion of free fatty acids and polyunsaturated fatty acids, the lower the smoke point. An oil that has already been heated several times (e.g. for frying) will have higher levels of free fatty acids than fresh oil. Virgin oils generally have a higher proportion of free fatty acids than refined oils (because these are removed during the refining process). However, particularly when they are fresh and have been produced to a high-quality standard, virgin oils may also have very low levels of free fatty acids, comparable with those found in refined oils. If the olives are damaged during pressing, for example, or if they are stored for too long before pressing, the proportion of free fatty acids rises.[143] This is not necessarily reflected in the flavour. Under EU legislation, extra virgin olive oil must have a free fatty acid content no higher than 0.8 per cent, while a basic virgin oil can contain up to 2 per cent.[144] Oils should never exceed their smoke point when being heated. Table 3 contains a detailed list.

As can be seen from Table 3, oils with a high proportion of polyunsaturated fatty acids, such as linseed oil and hemp seed oil, are not suitable for heating. These oils should only be used for cold dishes, such as making salad dressings, or for adding to warm dishes after they have been cooked. The table confirms that refined vegetable oils have a significantly higher smoke point than their virgin counterparts; however, cold pressed oils such as extra virgin olive oil are still sufficiently heat resistant to be used for cooking. Even the so-called "high oleic" varieties of vegetable oils are also suitable for heating in their virgin form. For example, while many kinds of virgin sunflower oil have a high proportion of polyunsaturated omega-6 fatty acids and can only be heated to around 100–120 °C (212–248°F), high-oleic virgin sunflower oils, by contrast, have a high proportion of monounsaturated omega-9 fatty

EDIBLE OIL	SMOKE POINT IN °C
Avocado oil	250–270
Coconut oil (refined)	220–240
Coconut oil (cold pressed)	170–190
Corn oil (refined)	220–240
Corn oil (cold pressed)	150–170
Grapeseed oil (refined)	220–240
Grapeseed oil (cold pressed)	120–140
Groundnut oil (refined)	220–240
Groundnut oil (cold pressed)	130–150
Hemp oil (cold pressed)	100–120
Linseed oil (cold pressed)	100–110
Olive oil (refined)	220–240
Olive oil (cold pressed, extra virgin)	190–210
Olive oil (cold pressed, virgin)	170–190
Rapeseed oil (refined)	200–220
Rapeseed oil (cold pressed)	120–140
Safflower oil (refined)	230–250
Safflower oil (cold pressed)	120–140
Sesame oil (refined)	210–230
Sesame oil (cold pressed)	160–180
Soya oil (refined)	220–240
Soya oil (cold pressed)	150–170
Sunflower oil (refined)	220–240
Sunflower oil; high oleic (cold pressed)	160–180
Sunflower oil (cold pressed)	100–120
Walnut oil (cold pressed)	120–140

Tab. 3: Smoke points of selected vegetable oils[145, 146, 147, 148]

acids and can be heated to between 160 and 180 °C (320 and 350°F). If an oil is heated too strongly, harmful substances can develop, and the oil should no longer be used. Below is a list of features that occur if an oil has been heated for too long and thus is no longer suitable for consumption:

Characteristics of cooking oil that has been heated too much[149]

- The oil begins to smoke strongly
- The original colour of the oil becomes noticeably darker
- The oil begins to foam
- The oil becomes thicker and more viscous
- The oil smells rancid and acrid

Versatile olive oil

In countries like Greece, Spain, and Italy almost every dish is prepared with (extra) virgin olive oil.[150] Hippocrates called olive oil the "great healer" and Homer referred to it as "liquid gold".[151] But olive oils are often given confusing labels that make it very difficult to assess their quality. If an olive oil is not specifically designated "virgin", for example if it is simply advertised as "pure olive oil" or "olive oil", it is highly likely to be a refined olive oil, to which, at best, a certain amount of virgin olive oil may have been added to improve its flavour. Contrary to widespread belief, olive oil (irrespective of its type) is sufficiently heat-resistant for use in roasting at temperatures up to 180°C (350°F).[152, 153] It also retains most of its valuable, healthy components during cooking at these temperatures.[154] Thanks to the high proportion of antioxidants in extra virgin olive oil, the formation of potentially toxic substances such as acrylamide is also minimized during baking and frying.[155]

Depending on the variety, olive oil contains between 55 and 83 per cent monounsaturated omega-9 fatty acids, called oleic acids. Compared to the polyunsaturated omega-6 fatty acids, called linoleic acids (the dominant fatty acid in sunflower oil, for example), oleic acids are 50 times less susceptible to oxidation and thus they are significantly less sensitive during storage and processing.[156] Research has also shown that replacing saturated fatty acids with monounsaturated fatty acids (as is found predominantly in olive oil) can lower "bad" LDL cholesterol without noticeably lowering "good" HDL cholesterol.[157] Polyunsaturated fatty acids, such as the alpha-linolenic acid in linseed oil, were also shown to have a beneficial impact on cholesterol levels, even if they are not used as a replacement for saturated fatty acids.[158] Extra virgin olive oil is also considered to be good for your heart[159, 160, 161] and the secondary plant substances it contains, such as oleuropein[162] and oleocanthal,[163] have an additional antioxidant and anti-inflammatory impact. If vegetables like aubergine, squash, tomatoes, or potatoes are prepared in high-quality olive oil, this significantly increases their antioxidant capacity when compared to these ingredients in raw form.[164]

Extra virgin olive oils can also inhibit the rise in blood sugar levels when consumed at the same time as high-glycaemic index foods such as white bread.[165] So it makes sense from a nutritional science perspective that olive oil is served alongside white bread in Mediterranean countries. It is also unsurprising that regular consumption of extra virgin olive oil is associated with lower insulin resistance (and thus with a lower risk of type 2 diabetes).[166]

2.2 Vinegar

Vinegar is one of the oldest ingredients for seasoning in the world. Thousands of years ago, the Babylonians, Egyptians, Persians, Greeks, and Romans were already using vinegar to season their dishes and to preserve foods. Sometimes they even drank it, heavily diluted, as a refreshing beverage.[167] The earliest evidence of the use of vinegar goes back roughly 10,000 years.[168] Vinegar is produced by fermenting an alcoholic liquid like wine or cider with the help of oxygen. Once the alcohol has fermented, the raw vinegar is decanted into a vat, where it is left to mature for up to a year. Finally, it is filtered and usually reduced to an acidity level of around 5 per cent.[169]

The use of vinegar as a therapeutic product also has a long tradition and its use in medical applications goes back many thousands of years.[170] Vinegar has an antioxidant effect, it regulates blood sugar levels, lowers cholesterol, reduces blood pressure, and has an antimicrobial impact, too.[171]

Vinegar keeps blood sugar levels in check

Thanks to its ability to regulate blood sugar levels, vinegar was widely used in popular medicine well before the development of pharmaceutical products to treat diabetes.[172] After the consumption of high-glycaemic foods (such as white flour and sugar), vinegar regulates blood sugar levels[173] by helping the body's cells absorb sugar from the bloodstream more effectively.[174] This effect is particularly interesting for individuals with pre-diabetes or similar metabolic issues, because these illnesses cause the insulin sensitivity of cells to be restricted and this can be improved by consuming vinegar with meals.[175]

Figure 13 illustrates the positive effect of vinegar on blood sugar and insulin levels after eating (bagel with butter and orange juice). There is a much shallower rise and fall in both levels when 20ml of vinegar (1.3 tablespoons) is taken at the same time compared to eating the same meal without vinegar.

Bagel with butter and orange juice

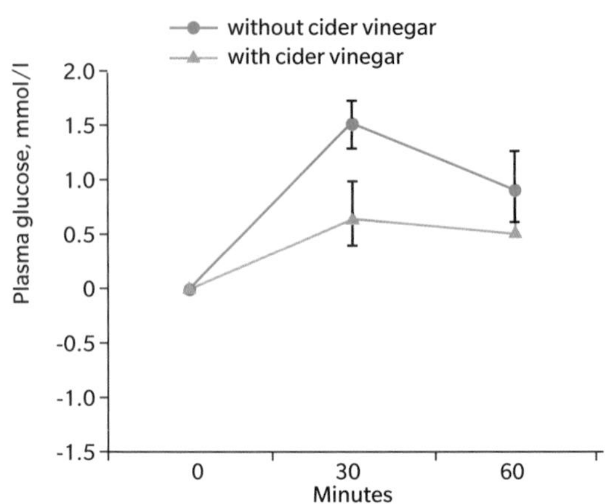

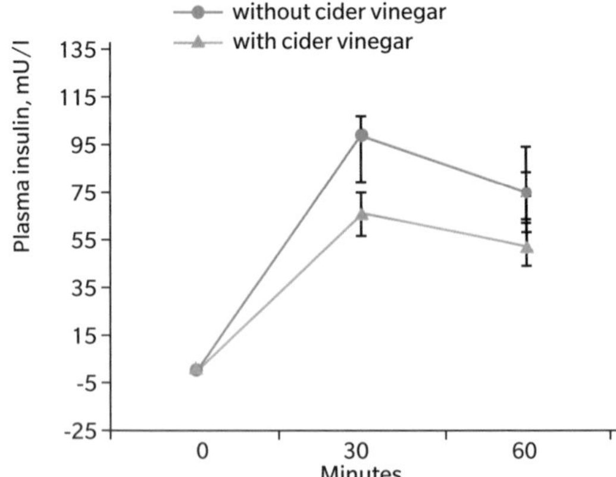

Fig. 13: Rise in blood sugar and insulin after a meal, with and without vinegar[176]

Perhaps it is no coincidence that vinegar is often included in traditional dishes that would otherwise cause a steep rise in blood sugar levels after consumption. For example, the white rice in sushi is always prepared with rice vinegar, which reduces the rise in blood sugar levels after consumption by about one-third.[177] And studies have found that the addition of cucumbers pickled in vinegar (instead of fresh cucumbers) could reduce the rise in blood sugar after eating white bread by around one-third.[178] If you are eating high-glycaemic foods, such as rice, white flour products, and potatoes, it makes sense to include vinegar at the same time. Another good example is potato salad, where the preparation method offers a double benefit. Allowing the potatoes to cool down lowers their glycaemic index (see p.17) because some of the starch in the potatoes is converted into so-called resistant (indigestible) starch. And by adding vinegar, the rise in blood sugar levels can be further inhibited.[179] A study has shown that the addition of 1 tablespoon of vinegar to two meals per day (2 tablespoons in total per day) not only reduced the spike in blood sugar levels after eating a meal, but also had a greater impact on the fasting blood sugar levels of people with a high risk of type 2 diabetes than the diabetes medication metformin.[180] A daily intake of 2 tablespoons of vinegar was also linked with a moderate reduction in the so-called "long-term" sugar value (HbA1c), which offers a good indication of blood sugar levels over the previous two to three months.[181, 182] The addition of vinegar in these amounts also boosts satiety and so can help support weight loss.[183] In a test phase lasting eight weeks, participants taking added vinegar were also shown to have significantly improved blood lipid scores (cholesterol and triglyceride).[184]

An intake of as little as 2 teaspoons (10g) of vinegar per day has been shown to have a positive effect on blood sugar regulation after high-glycaemic meals.[185]

Taking 2 tablespoons of vinegar (30ml) with a meal has been shown in studies lasting several weeks to have no side-effects and thus to be a safe intervention,[186] and even if you consume 2 tablespoons of vinegar with each of your three main meals (3 x 30ml/1fl oz = 90ml/3fl oz) to help stabilize your blood sugar and insulin levels, a four-week experiment showed no negative side-effects.[187] More than this amount should not be consumed in the medium to long term. While the impact of vinegar on regulating blood sugar and blood fat levels has been well researched and is backed up with evidence, most of the other alleged human health benefits for vinegar lack supporting data. We certainly do not advocate more extensive use of vinegar. For example, while the use of vinegar to remove head lice might not be dangerous (as long as the vinegar does not come into contact with the eyes),[188] it is nonetheless ineffective.[189] And the use of vinegar to tackle discolouration of teeth is also not advised. It is true that vinegar is a highly effective method for removing stains,[190] however, it can also cause demineralization of the teeth thanks to its acidity and thus is not recommended because the adverse effects outweigh any potential benefits.[191, 192]

In our book we exclusively use cider vinegar. This is because we want to make your shopping as simple as possible. We do not want you to have to buy too many different ingredients to follow our recipes. Other types of vinegar are also invaluable and beneficial to your health. A wide range of different vinegars is available, and any high-quality vinegar can easily be substituted (as long as the flavour works for the relevant dish). Close attention should be paid to quality when it comes to vinegars. For example, a "pure" or "genuine" wine vinegar can only be produced 100% from red or white wine. These varieties should not be confused with cheaper wine vinegars, which usually consist of a blend of roughly 80 per cent spirit vinegar with 20 per cent genuine wine vinegar.[193] Cider vinegar, on the other hand, is obtained from fermented, naturally cloudy apple juice. In contrast to most varieties of vinegar, which are matured in vats for about a year, special gourmet vinegars like high-quality balsamic vinegar (made from grape must) are usually laid down for at least four years and sometimes as long as 40 years.[194] This long storage period allows their exceptional flavour to develop and the result is a really special culinary product.

2.3 Herbs and spices

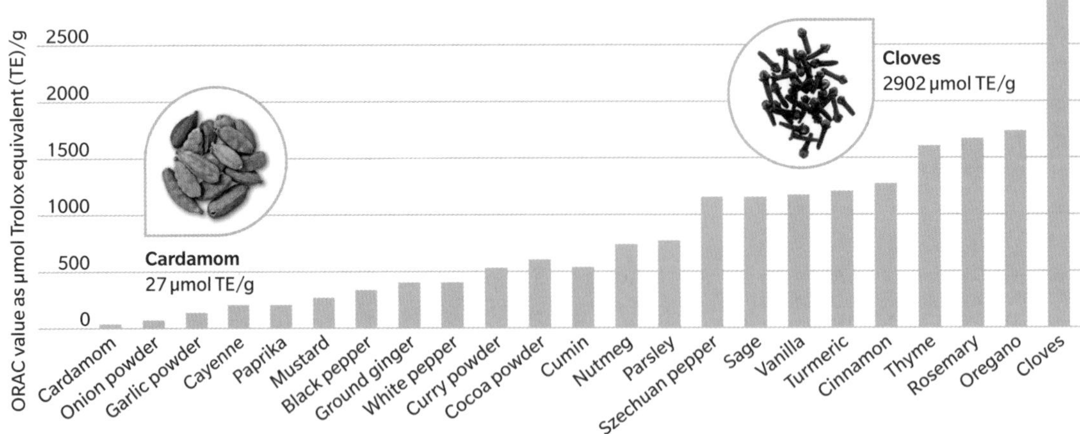

Fig. 14: Antioxidant capacity of spices and dried herbs (ORAC value as µmol Trolox equivalent (TE)/g)[195]

The use of herbs and spices to enhance food is no recent phenomenon; this technique was already being used over 7,000 years ago in the Neolithic period.[196] Fresh, dried, or frozen herbs and a huge variety of spices can be used to improve meals, both from a culinary and a health perspective. Many of these ingredients have antioxidant or anti-inflammatory properties and can stimulate your appetite and aid digestion.[197] Figure 14 ranks the various dried herbs and spices based on their antioxidant capacity, showing which you should focus particular attention on for everyday consumption.

Figure 15 uses three sample dishes to demonstrate that even small quantities of herbs and spices can contribute significantly to the antioxidant effect of a meal. The recipes in this book use ingredients that possess powerful antioxidant properties. Although their antioxidant content might not rise to the same extent as some of the examples in Figure 15, the amount is nonetheless significant.

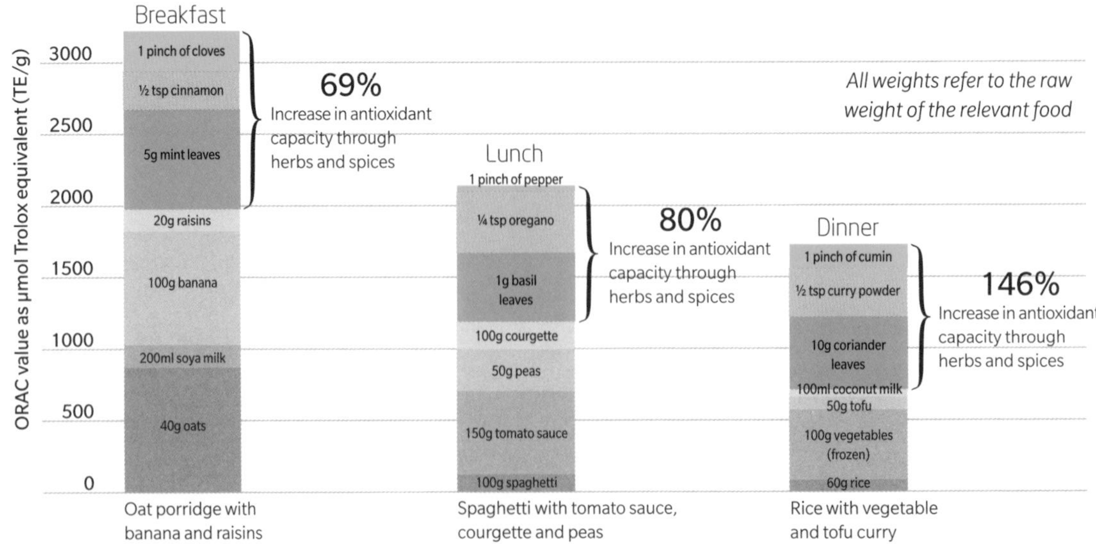

Fig. 15: Increased antioxidant capacity of selected dishes through the addition of herbs and spices (based on the ORAC value as µmol Trolox equivalent (TE)/g) [198]

Product expertise: spices

In the following sections, we provide information on making the right choices when buying and using the most common spices:[199, 200, 201, 202, 203]

Ginger: In cooking, we use the woody root (rhizome) of the roughly 1m- (3ft-) high ginger plant. The root is shaped a bit like antlers. Its flesh is pale yellow and should be plump and juicy. Knotty, dried ginger is lacking in quality. Fresh ginger root can be kept in the fridge for several weeks if wrapped in kitchen paper and stored in an airtight box. Grated ginger can also be frozen in ice-cube-sized portions and will then keep for up to six months. Ginger can be beneficial for migraines,[204] menstrual pain,[205] and nausea.[206]

Organic ginger with a firm, smooth skin does not necessarily have to be peeled. To peel ginger as sparingly as possible, you can scrape off the skin using a spoon with a sharp edge. Ginger adds a fresh, sharp touch to a dish and its wonderful flavour means it can be used in lots of recipes. You can sauté ginger with onion in the pan, or just add it to your food at the end in the form of juice or finely grated. Sautéing intensifies its flavour. However, if it is cooked for too long, ginger will lose its freshness. Some people find the taste of ginger overly intense if the pieces are too large. That is why it is best to grate it finely or use a garlic press to squeeze it into the food (this will only work for fresh ginger) or chop it very finely.

Cumin: Cumin refers to the dried seeds from a plant in the Apiaceae family (formerly known as umbellifers). The seeds are similar in appearance to caraway but are slightly paler and have a more bitter flavour. The whole seeds will keep for many years without deteriorating in quality if stored in dry, airtight conditions away from light. Once ground, they rapidly lose their aroma. Due to cumin's powerful flavour, it should always be measured carefully. It has antioxidant properties and it can regulate blood sugar levels[207] as well as improve blood lipid scores (cholesterol and triglyceride).[208] Freshly ground cumin should ideally be sautéed at the start of cooking along with other spices, such as turmeric, coriander, ginger, and fresh chillies. This allows its flavour to develop fully.

Turmeric: Turmeric is also known as Indian saffron due to its brilliant yellow colour. In cooking, we primarily use the root (rhizome) of the roughly 1m- (3ft-) high turmeric plant. The root has a fleshy interior with an intense yellow colour and should be plump and juicy. Fresh turmeric can be kept in the fridge for several weeks if wrapped in kitchen paper and stored in an airtight container. Ground turmeric should be kept dry and away from the light in an airtight container and only stored for a short period as it loses its taste and smell rapidly. Provided it is protected from light, the colour of this spice will virtually never fade, which means this visual cue is not a good indicator of freshness. Studies show that turmeric can alleviate the symptoms of many inflammatory illnesses, such as arthritis, Crohn's disease, irritable bowel syndrome, and many others.[209] The average daily intake of turmeric in India consists of a ¼ teaspoon of ground turmeric (0.7g).[210] This quantity should also be included in your daily vegan diet. If using fresh turmeric, this is roughly equivalent to ½cm (¼in) of the root. In order to optimize the bioavailability of the secondary plant substance curcumin in turmeric and to increase the concentration of curcumin in the blood as much as possible, we always recommend consuming turmeric with some dietary fat[211] (oils, nuts, seeds, avocado, olives, etc.) and black pepper.[212] Amongst all the different kinds of pepper, black pepper has the highest quantity of the secondary plant substance piperine, which significantly increases the concentration of curcumin in the blood, thus enhancing its potential health benefits.[213] Turmeric is a popular colouring agent used in food. But it is important to exercise caution because too much turmeric will first turn the

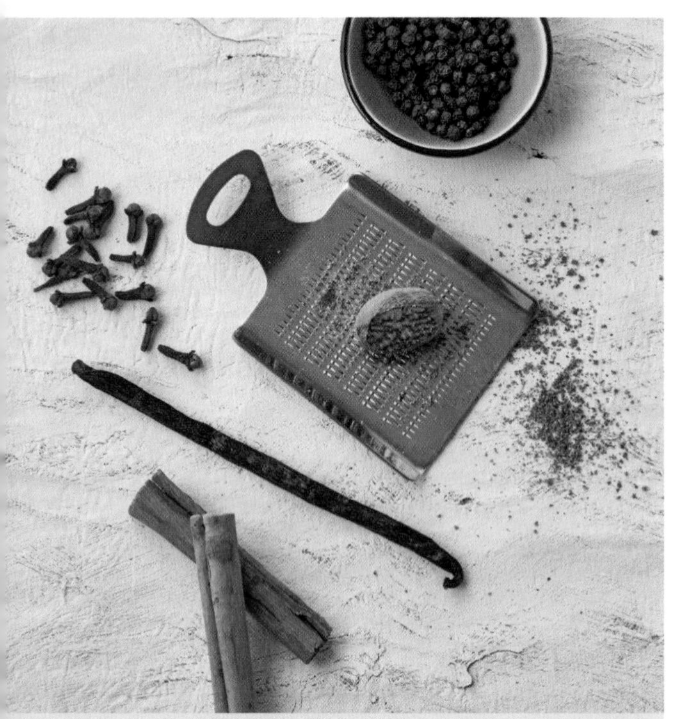

Not only do spices add the finishing touch to a recipe, they also contribute lots of healthy substances.

colour pale green then rust brown, and the flavour can easily become too dominant. It is best to gently fry the turmeric at the start with the other heat-resistant spices and never add it as a seasoning at the end. Turmeric can also work beautifully if added in moderation to Mediterranean dishes.

Nutmeg: In cooking, we use the dried kernels from the nutmeg tree as well as the nutmeg's seed covering, or aril, which is known as mace. If stored whole, nutmeg will keep for a long time. Once ground, however, it rapidly loses its flavour. Nutmeg has antioxidant properties, and it also stimulates the digestive system and acts as an analgesic[214] and mood enhancer.[215] But you need to be careful with the quantity: just 2–4 teaspoons of grated nutmeg can be fatal.[216, 217] However, the spice has such a strong taste there is no danger of you consuming this amount unintentionally in one go. Due to its intense flavour, nutmeg should be used sparingly to season your food. Grate whole nutmeg immediately before use with a nutmeg grater or zester, adding it directly to the food once it has finished cooking, as the flavour dissipates rapidly. Mace can also easily be ground using a coffee grinder kept for the purpose. Nutmeg is a classic ingredient in lots of savoury dishes and stews. It goes beautifully in mashed potato, dumplings, and lots of other dishes and adds a touch of lightness. As with all spices, the quality is crucial. Mace has a slightly more delicate, floral flavour than nutmeg itself.

Cloves: These are the dried flower buds of the clove tree. There is a simple way to test the quality of cloves by just placing them in water. Good-quality cloves will float vertically, while those of lower quality will float horizontally on the water because they contain fewer essential oils.[218] High-quality cloves feel oleaginous and will release some essential oils if pressed with a fingernail. If stored away from light, moisture, and oxygen, whole cloves will keep for around two years. When ground, on the other hand, they rapidly lose their aroma. Among the most common spices, cloves have the highest proportion of antioxidants.[219] Cloves have powerful anti-inflammatory and blood-clotting properties[220] in addition to having an antiviral and antimicrobial effect.[221] They have an intense flavour and so should be used sparingly. In addition to their floral aroma, they have a distinctly astringent note. Ground cloves can be toasted and cooked as part of the dish or added as seasoning at the end. They work well in savoury dishes such as cabbage recipes (e.g. red cabbage, sauerkraut) but also in sweet recipes such as spice cakes, plum jam, and baked apples.

Paprika: A spice made from the dried, ground conical fruit of the plant *Capsicum annuum*. The smell and the taste of paprika depends strongly on the variety. In particular, the secondary plant substance capsaicin has a major influence on the aroma and spiciness of the relevant powder. This substance is primarily found in the seeds and membrane of the pepper. The more of these spicy components that are ground up with the milder flesh of the fruit, the less bright red but the hotter the paprika will be. The most frequent varieties are regular paprika (fiery red colour and mild, fruity flavour), sweet paprika (dark red colour, slightly spicy flavour with a sweet and fruity element), hot paprika (yellowy-red colour and a spicy taste), and smoked paprika.[222] Smoked foods such as salmon often contain high concentrations of harmful, polycyclic, aromatic hydrocarbons. In higher concentrations, these are suspected to cause cell damage and have a carcinogenic effect.[223] However, as studies have shown, this is not the case for smoked ground paprika[224] or liquid smoke,[225] so both these spices can be used in cooking. Ground paprika should be stored so it is protected against air, light, and moisture and it must be used quickly as it rapidly loses its colour, intensity, and aroma. Ground paprika lowers blood lipids and blood pressure[226] as well as having an anti-inflammatory effect[227] and it is always a good choice if you are trying to introduce umami, spice, and savoury flavours to a recipe. The spicy, sweet, and sometimes hot flavour will enhance any stew or oven-roasted vegetable dish. Smoked paprika is always a great option if you want to evoke the taste of meat. If you roast ground paprika it develops a wonderful spicy aroma – but take care, because too much heat can make the paprika bitter.

Pepper: Obtained from the dried or preserved fruit of the pepper plant, it is sold as black, white, green, or red pepper. The different colours and flavours depend on the ripeness of the berries and how they are processed. Green pepper is produced using unripe, green, unpeeled peppercorns. Red pepper is made from the fully ripe peppercorn fruit. Black pepper is made by allowing the unripe, green fruit to dry slowly, turning black in the process. White pepper is produced using the fully ripe red peppercorns, which are soaked for several days before the red skin is removed from the flesh of the fruit, which is then dried. Black pepper contains the greatest quantity of the secondary plant substance piperine and has the strongest taste. Red pepper is fairly hot, but with an added fruity note. White pepper is less aromatic and slightly milder than black pepper. Green pepper is milder, fresher, and very aromatic. Whole peppercorns keep for a long time but once ground, they quickly lose their flavour. Peppercorns preserved in brine should be stored in the fridge once opened and used quickly. Pepper promotes the absorption of lots of secondary plant substances and micronutrients as well as having antioxidant, anti-inflammatory, and chemopreventive properties.[228] Pepper is best freshly ground in a pepper mill and only added to the food once it has finished cooking. As a universal spice, pepper can be combined with all the other common spices and so can be added to almost any dish. Pepper ensures a great pungent flavour in food and can be added in liberal quantities. The peppery flavour unfolds best if the ground or whole pepper is cooked slightly. So, for example, you could add whole peppercorns to a soup that cooks for 30 minutes, because the long cooking time will allow them to soften and they can be eaten with the soup like pickled peppercorns.

Vanilla: It is a spice made from the fermented pods of various kinds of orchid. The pods are 14–20cm (5½–8in) long, glossy, blackish brown in colour, flexible, and (for Bourbon vanilla) coated in white vanilla crystals. Inside they contain tiny, glossy, dark brown seeds in a black, fragrant, fruity pulp. Three types of vanilla are found on sale: Bourbon vanilla, Mexican vanilla, and Tahitian vanilla. The latter has a more intense flavour, but the other varieties are also popular. The intact vanilla pods can be stored for a few years and will keep their flavour as long as they are kept dry in an airtight container, away from light. Vanilla extract, on the other hand, should be stored in the fridge and used quickly. Research has shown that vanillin, a bioactive substance found in vanilla, also has an antioxidant effect and can help prevent cancer.[229] Since the flavour components in vanilla are lost when exposed to heat, this spice should only be added at the end of the cooking process, wherever possible. Vanilla in all its forms acts as a flavour enhancer, whether it is used in savoury or sweet dishes. The discreet addition of vanilla to spicy dishes helps harmonize the flavour of all the ingredients and adds a really special touch. Once again, care should be used with this seasoning and there can be great differences in the flavour depending on the quality. To make the most of the vanilla pod once you have scraped out the seeds, just add it to a tub of salt – rather than to the usual pot of sugar. This allows its aroma to be delicately incorporated into a wide range of dishes.

Cinnamon: This spice consists of the dried bark that comes from various kinds of cinnamon tree. A basic distinction is made between two varieties: Cassia cinnamon (Chinese cinnamon) and Ceylon cinnamon (Sri Lankan or true cinnamon). Ceylon and Cassia cinnamon taste quite different. Cinnamon is said to help regulate blood sugar levels, although this characteristic only applies to the Cassia cinnamon varieties, which contain coumarin. It should be noted that coumarin is toxic in higher doses. Having said that, someone who weighs 70kg (154lb) could consume ½ teaspoon of Cassia cinnamon per day without exceeding the average limit for coumarin. Nonetheless, to be on the safe side, we advise mainly using Ceylon cinnamon. Children, in particular, can easily exceed the limit for coumarin in their daily consumption (0.1mg/kg body weight) with an average content of 3mg per g of Cassia cinnamon.[230] Ceylon cinnamon does not regulate blood sugar levels, but it does avoid the potentially toxic effect of Cassia cinnamon. Ceylon cinnamon is still an exceptionally healthy spice. It inhibits bacteria and fungi, aids in tissue repair, protects the heart, and reduces the risk of cancer.[231] Whole cinnamon sticks can be stored for up to four years in airtight, dark, dry conditions. Ground cinnamon, however, rapidly loses its flavour. In drinks or dishes with plenty of liquid, you can add whole or broken cinnamon sticks (in a spherical spice infuser). For all other uses, ground cinnamon is preferable. Cinnamon is a miracle worker in the kitchen – although many people associate its flavour with sweet dishes and Christmas recipes, it tastes just as good in plenty of savoury dishes. A slow-cooked stew, e.g. with tomatoes, also tastes quite different if seasoned with ground cinnamon rather than a cinnamon stick. A dash of cinnamon in a vegan chilli or Bolognese really works wonders and, if added in moderation, it improves pretty much any food.

General tips on herbs and spices

When buying, storing, and preparing herbs and spices, there are several tips you should remember. If you stick to the following principles, you can bring the health benefits and culinary value of the original raw ingredient to the final dish:[232, 233, 234, 235, 236]

- Never chop herbs when wet because this can result in the loss of water-soluble flavourings
- Always chop herbs immediately before they are going to be used
- Only add heat-sensitive herbs such as basil, chervil, and borage just before the end of the cooking time
- Herbs such as rosemary, marjoram, tarragon, thyme, sage, and bay will only release their full flavour when exposed to heat, so these should be allowed to cook with the food for at least 15 minutes
- Add herbs to salad dressings at least 10 minutes before serving
- For dishes that are not heated, add any spices 20–30 minutes before consumption to allow their flavour to develop
- Spices that are not chopped, such as whole cloves, juniper berries, or caraway seeds, will only release their flavour gradually. For this reason, they should be added at the beginning of a recipe
- Ground spices like pepper and cloves should only be added towards the end of the cooking period
- Whenever possible, spices should be bought whole and freshly ground at home
- Each spice should be ground in a separate mill to avoid the different spicy aromas intermingling
- Spices with hard stalks or leathery leaves (such as bay leaves, rosemary, or thyme) should be cooked whole with the relevant dish and removed before serving
- Smaller or roughly chopped spices can be cooked in a spice infuser (like a tea strainer) or spice sachet
- Always store dried herbs and spices in dry, airtight, dark conditions

2.4 Sugar and alternative sweeteners

People love sweet things. This predilection has not come about by chance but was of crucial importance during human evolution. A sweet flavour usually indicates that a food is non-toxic[237] and packed with energy.[238] Human breast milk also contains a large proportion of sugar in the form of lactose to encourage the baby to drink and ensure it gets sufficient nutrients.[239] None of this was a problem as long as sugar was not excessively available in isolated form. But nowadays, where soft drinks, sweets, and other sugary foods are available on every corner and at any time of day, this preference for sweet things is proving to be disastrous. The production of crystalline sugar (sucrose) from sugar cane goes back to around 700 CE and granulated sugar has been created from sugar beet since the early nineteenth century.[240] The industrial production of sugar in the UK began in around 1912, but it has been a hugely popular sweetener since the mid-eighteenth century. In Germany, industrial production began in around 1850, which caused the price to fall dramatically in Europe and sugar consumption gradually began to rise. Figure 16 shows this increase; from less than 5kg (11lb) per person per year in the period after 1850 to the current consumption of almost 35kg (78lb) of sugar per person per year.

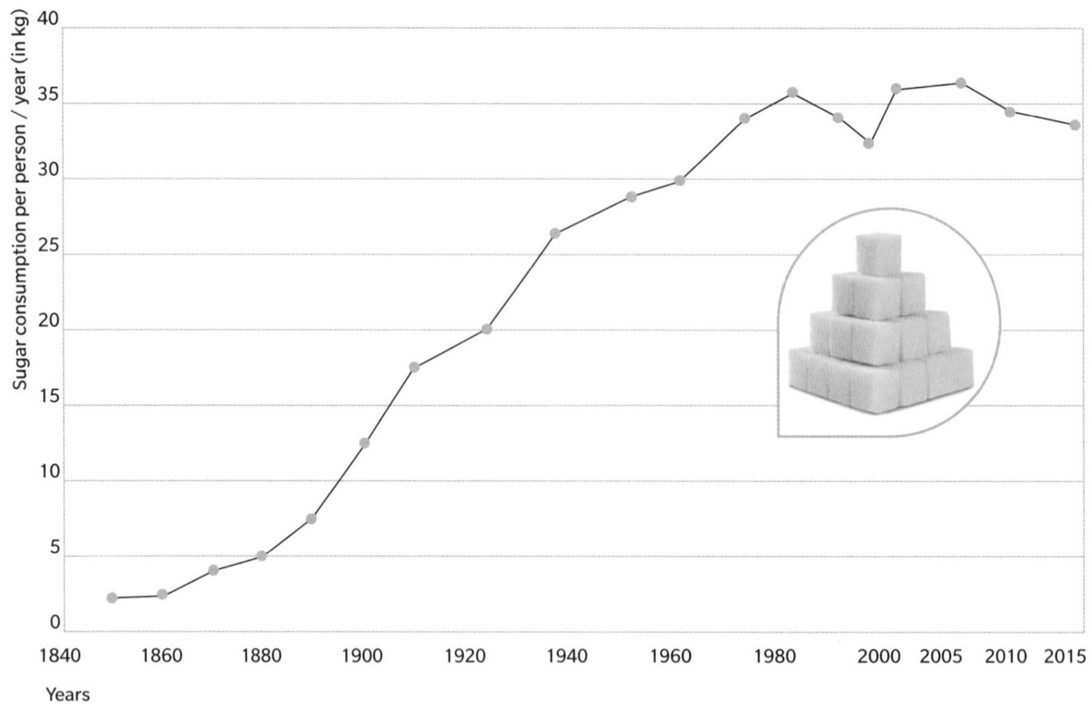

Fig. 16: Changing consumption of household sugar in Germany from 1850 to 2015 in kg/person per year[241, 242]

The different types of sugar

When people talk about sugar, granulated sugar, sugar cubes, or household sugar they are generally referring to the disaccharide sucrose. This in turn consists of one molecule of fructose (fruit sugar) and one molecule of glucose (grape sugar). So if you consume large quantities of sugar (sucrose) you are automatically consuming large quantities of fructose and glucose. That is why the average person eating a western-style diet gets a large amount of fructose, not by eating fruit, but from soft drinks, sweet treats, and other industrially processed foods.[243] Fructose is about 1.6 times sweeter than household sugar[244] and is more soluble than other sugars. This makes it a popular choice as a sweetener in food manufacturing. Corn syrup containing fructose (HFCS, high-fructose corn syrup) is also found in lots of soft drinks and sweet foods. Standard HFCS varieties have a fructose content of around 55 per cent, and you can find some varieties with a fructose content of 90 per cent.[245] This means on average it does not have significantly more fructose than household sugar, which consists about fifty-fifty of fructose and glucose. By contrast, other sweeteners, such as agave syrup, consist predominantly of fructose.[246] Excessive sugar consumption does not just involve a surplus of empty calories, it also increases the risk of a whole range of chronic degenerative illnesses.[247] Grape sugar (glucose) causes blood sugar levels to rise rapidly and significantly after consumption.[248] This in turn causes long-term oxidative stress[249] and increases the risk of type 2 diabetes[250, 251] and cardiovascular disease.[252, 253] Fructose might have a comparatively low glycaemic index, but an excess of isolated fructose (not fruit!)[254] is associated with the development and rapid progression of illnesses such as non-alcoholic fatty liver disease[255] and metabolic syndrome.[256] Whether it is fructose or glucose – it is important to drastically reduce added sugar of all kinds. The World Health Organization (WHO) advice is to limit the consumption of added sugar to less than 10 per cent of your daily calorie intake.[257] For example, for a calorie intake of 2000 kcal per day, this means about 50g (2oz) of sugar. To stay within these guidelines, annual sugar consumption must be less than 18kg (40lb) per person. This is about half the amount currently being consumed in countries like the UK and Germany.[258] Other publications from specialist bodies recommend a stricter reduction to no more than 5 per cent of your energy intake.[259] So it makes sense to find healthier ways of incorporating sweet tastes in recipes to minimize the amount of sugar being served. The following strategies will help:

Train your palate

In a similar manner to salt (see p.66), your taste buds can get used to sweeter or less sweet flavours, and it is possible to wean yourself off sugar. By gradually adding less sugar, your tastes will adapt over time until you perceive foods that

Techniques for reducing household sugar

- Train your palate
- Fresh fruit as a sweetener
- Dried fruit as a sweetener
- Date sugar as a sweetener
- Erythritol as a sweetener

contain sugar to be much sweeter than before.[260] In a study, test subjects who followed a reduced-sugar diet for three months rated the taste of dishes to be 40 per cent sweeter than the control group who did not follow the reduced-sugar regime.[261] This shows that you can derive the same enjoyment from less sugar.

Fresh fruit

As discussed in the subsection on fruit as one of the five main food groups (from p20), fruit is extremely healthy and makes a great substitute for sugar if a recipe allows this. For example, bananas make a good substitute for eggs in cakes because they are sweet and help bind the ingredients. Half a mashed ripe banana can be used instead of one egg. Because the flavour of the banana is retained after baking, this binding agent is particularly suitable for recipes where the banana flavour blends well with the other ingredients, for example, the banana and oat cookies on p.236. Frozen bananas make an ideal sweetener for healthy ice cream recipes (see p.235). Alternatively, you can use 60g (2oz) of unsweetened apple purée or apple sauce plus 1 teaspoon of oil instead of one egg in your baking. Apple purée does not have as strong a flavour in the finished product as banana and it also ensures a wonderfully moist texture.

Dried fruit

Dried fruits such as dates make an excellent, nutritious sugar substitute. For example, the peanut balls with peach (see p.232) get their sweetness in part from dates. Dates can be puréed with a pinch of salt and some lemon and water to make a store cupboard date paste (see p.97), which can replace conventional sugar to add sweetness to recipes like the apple whole grain pancakes (see p.228). Due to their sticky consistency, dried fruits have a reputation for being worse for tooth decay than traditional refined sugar. However, studies have refuted this. It is thought that antioxidants contained in the fruit inhibit the bacteria in the oral cavity that would otherwise cause tooth decay.[262, 263]

Date sugar

Date sugar, also known as date powder, is made from whole dates. After harvesting, these are washed, heated using steam, dried, then finely ground.[264] Date sugar must not be confused with date syrup, which is not a nutritious ingredient. This sweetener is made by boiling down the dates with water, then pressing, filtering, and condensing the mixture to create a syrup. As a result, all the fibre is lost. Date sugar, on the other hand, is high in fibre. The wholesome nature of this ingredient is also reflected in its antioxidant content. Date sugar comes out well ahead of other options when it comes to antioxidant capacity, as shown in Figure 17 below.

Erythritol

Erythritol belongs to the family of so-called sugar alcohols. It has about 60–80 per cent of the sweetness of sucrose.[266] Sugar alcohols, also known as polyols, are not dependent on insulin

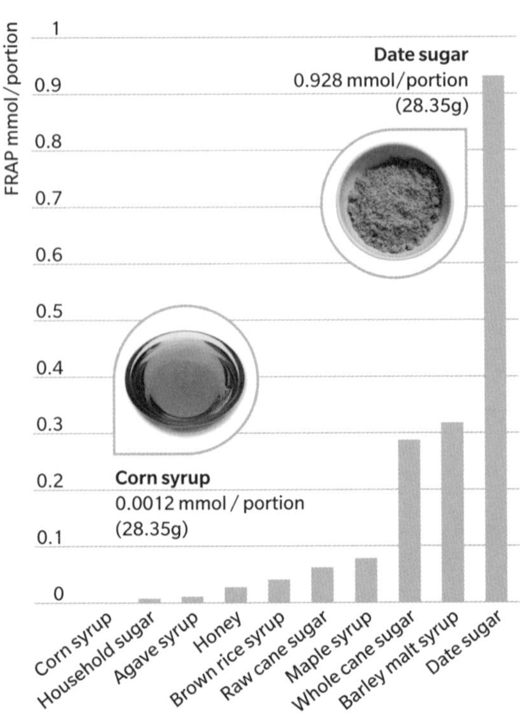

Fig. 17: Antioxidant content for selected sugar alternatives shown as ferric reducing abilty of plasma (FRAP) in mmol/portion[265]

to be metabolized, which means there is no rise in insulin levels following their consumption (unlike sugars such as glucose).[267] However, in large quantities, sugar alcohols can have a laxative effect. But the body can be trained to tolerate these substances better through increased exposure.[268] Erythritol occurs in small quantities in foods such as watermelons, peaches, grapes, and so on, but for mass production it is obtained by fermenting corn or wheat.[269] Among all the alternative sweeteners, erythritol seems to occupy a special position. Unlike sugar, erythritol (E968)[270] does not cause tooth decay [271] and it acts as an antioxidant.[272] Unlike other sweeteners, erythritol is also almost completely reabsorbed in the small intestine and is excreted unchanged in urine.[273] The reason this is so important is that the absorption in the small intestine means the erythritol is usually very well tolerated, whereas other sweeteners often have a laxative effect.[274] Other sweeteners are not absorbed in the small intestine and so are transferred to the large intestine.[275] As a result, sweeteners such as aspartame (E951), saccharin (E954), sucralose (E955),[276] and acesulfame K (E950)[277] can potentially have an unwelcome effect on intestinal flora (and can possibly impair glucose tolerance) in a way not seen for erythritol. In the past, sweeteners like aspartame have also been suspected in rare cases of triggering fibromyalgia,[278] migraines,[279] and high blood pressure[280] and causing negative effects on cognitive ability and mood (particularly if consumed in large quantities).[281] Even though aspartame and other sweeteners are approved for use as food additives in limited quantities, they cannot be regarded as entirely unproblematic for general human consumption.[282, 283]

In addition to erythritol, tests have shown positive effects for the sugar alcohol xylitol. Xylitol seems to protect against tooth decay,[284] it is well tolerated and again avoids the negative effects on intestinal flora associated with other alternative sweeteners.[285] In fact, xylitol seems to have a prebiotic potential with a positive impact on the composition of the intestinal flora.[286]

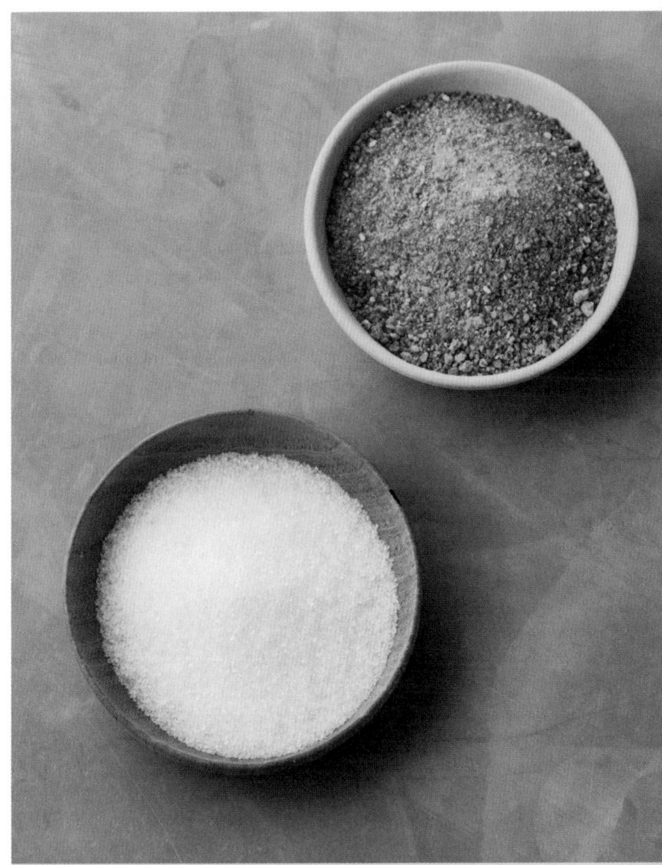

Erythritol and date sugar are good alternatives for traditional household sugar.

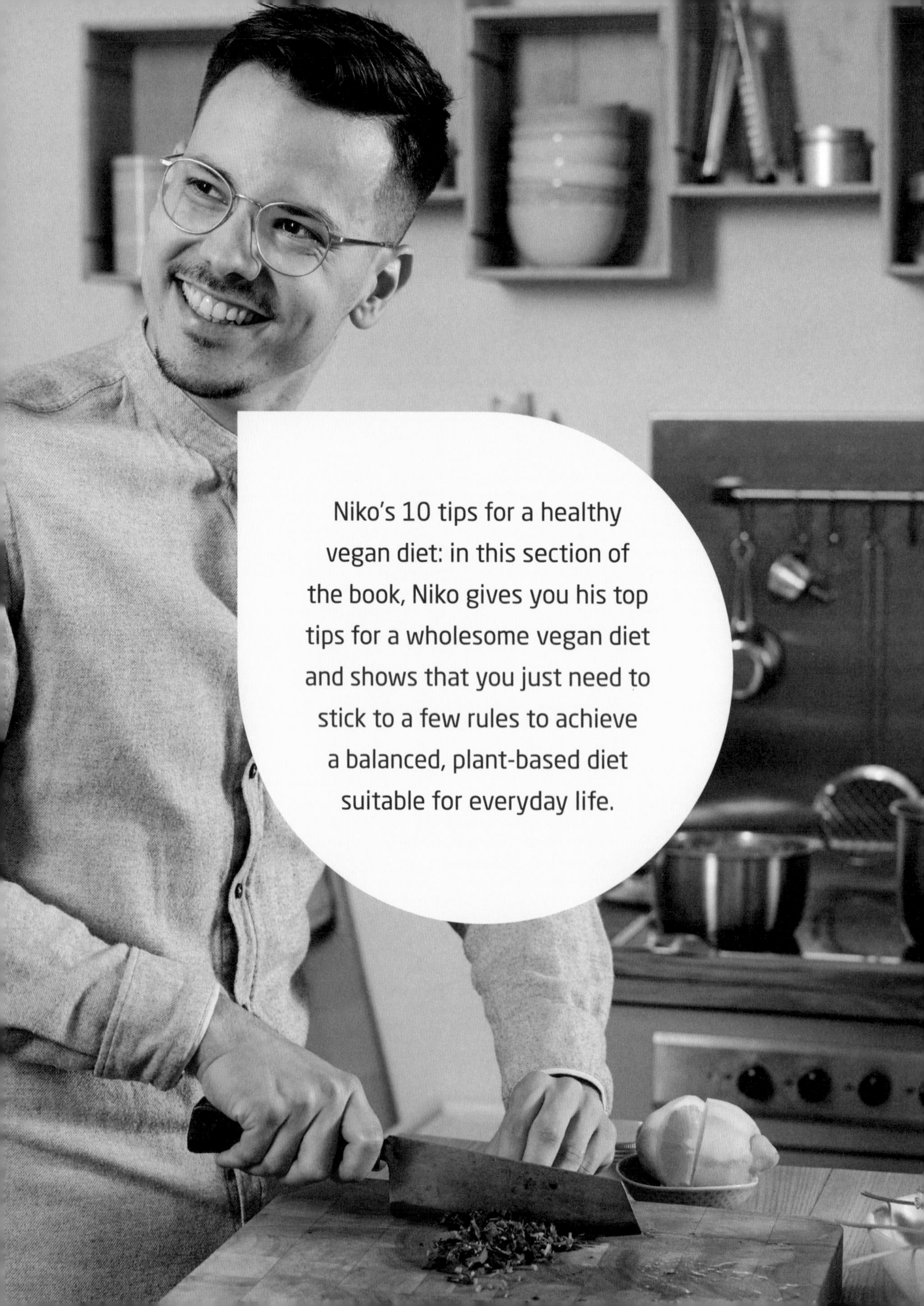

Niko's 10 tips for a healthy vegan diet: in this section of the book, Niko gives you his top tips for a wholesome vegan diet and shows that you just need to stick to a few rules to achieve a balanced, plant-based diet suitable for everyday life.

Nutritional tips

3. Niko's 10 tips for a healthy vegan diet

The nutritional issues that surround healthy eating in general and a healthy vegan diet in particular can be complex, not to mention confusing. Theoretical knowledge about the correct dietary approach is only half the story, so to help you apply the most important scientific findings about a wholesome plant-based diet to your everyday life, the following section contains ten tips for successfully integrating the key aspects of a healthy vegan diet in your daily routine.

Niko's 10 tips for a healthy vegan diet

1. There are no healthy/unhealthy foods
2. Food choices, not macronutrient ratio
3. One eye on calories
4. Don't demonize fat
5. Optimizing mineral absorption
6. Eat the rainbow
7. Be clever with salt
8. Don't forget to drink
9. Count hours instead of calories
10. Don't be afraid of food supplements

Niko's recommendations

These ten tips have been put together with a focus on the vegan diet, but they can easily be applied to other diets with a few simple modifications. In addition to these ten specific tips, general healthy eating principles still apply, of course. For example, everyone should find their own choice of foods to suit their personal needs. Eating should take place in a calm environment, only when you are genuinely hungry, and you should always chew your food well to produce plenty of saliva. Eating should bring pleasure and enhance our lives. So, your specific diet should only be as restrictive as required, and it should be easy to incorporate in your daily routine. While good-quality food can be expensive, with a few adjustments, a well-balanced vegan diet can be designed to suit any budget.

The daily vegan diet should be made up of the five main food groups – vegetables, whole grains, pulses, fruits, nuts and seeds – and should also include plenty of healthy spices and herbs. The choice of foods should ideally be as regional and seasonal as possible and include plenty of variety to ensure maximum enjoyment. Whenever possible, shop for organic, fair-trade food and develop a feel for good quality as well as paying attention to the various quality seals.

Optimal supply of all nutrients

A vegan diet is well-balanced if it provides you with the ideal quantity of all essential (vital for life) and semi-essential nutrients as part of your personal calorie intake. At the same time, any substances that are potentially harmful to your health in larger quantities (for instance, salt [sodium chloride], saturated fatty acids, trans-fatty acids, sugar, etc.) should be kept to a minimum in your menu plan. However, you do not need to perform painstaking calculations to meet the nutritional recommendations every single day. A better way to approach this is to try to cover all your nutritional requirements on average over the course of each week. To start with, you may need to do some calculations and you might pay closer attention to the ingredients in specific foods, but over time you will develop a feel for which foods cover which proportion of your specific nutritional requirements.

Nutritional information on recipes

To help you develop these instincts, all the recipes in this book provide nutritional details for the macronutrients (carbohydrate, fat, protein), fibre, total calories, and salt content per portion. In addition, each recipe specifies the quantity of potentially critical nutrients, such as iron, zinc, calcium, iodine, vitamin B2, vitamin A (or retinol equivalent), lysine, and alpha-linolenic acid. Since the soil in many parts of Europe is low in selenium, plant-based foods in these areas do not provide any appreciable quantity of this nutrient. For this reason, we have not listed selenium values separately. The Vegan Society suggest that people following a vegan diet can take a selenium supplement (see Tip 10, p.75). To put the nutritional information in the recipes in the right context, below you will find the recommended intake for the most relevant, essential nutrients within a vegan diet. These have been adapted from the German Nutrition Society reference values, which have been modified in part based on recommendations for people following a vegan diet and in part (vitamin D and selenium) based on the most up-to-date scientific findings. Any other vital nutrients that are not mentioned will be automatically provided as part of a varied vegan diet containing sufficient calories, and thus do not require special attention.

Daily nutrient intake for adults as per the German Nutrition Society, adapted for a vegan diet[287]

Protein: 0.9g /kg body weight

Fibre: ≥ 30g

Alpha-linolenic acid (ALA): ≥ 1% of nutritional energy

Vitamin A: 1mg retinol equivalent

Vitamin D: 40 to 60IU/kg body weight

Vitamin B2 (riboflavin): 1.4mg (men) or 1.1mg (women)

Vitamin B12 (cobalamin): 6µg / ≥ 100µg

Calcium: 1000mg

Iron: 10mg (men) or 15mg (women)

Iodine: 200µg

Zinc: 16mg (men) or 10mg (women)

Selenium: 1 to 2µg/kg body weight

Recommended protein intake

The recommended daily protein intake is calculated with reference to a person's normal weight (BMI < 25kg / m^2). To compensate for the fact that proteins from plants are sometimes slightly less digestible, the DGE recommendation for protein in a mixed diet has been adjusted to 0.9g protein per kg body weight.[288] Overweight or obese people should use their theoretical optimal weight to calculate their personal protein requirement because a higher proportion of body fat does not increase the protein requirement, unlike a higher proportion of muscle mass. Protein can be obtained by eating protein-rich foods such as pulses, whole grains, nuts, and seeds. For higher protein requirements (e.g. for athletes) there is nothing against using a high-quality vegan protein powder. This should be checked for heavy metals and other harmful substances and should be formulated based on pulses (such as peas) combined with other sources of protein.

Plenty of fibre

Irrespective of how much carbohydrate your diet contains, you should always make sure you stick to the minimum dietary fibre intake of 30g (1oz) per day. The figure of 30g (1oz) should be regarded as the minimum and it can certainly be beneficial to consume far more than this as part of a wholesome vegan diet. All nutritious plant-based foods contain smaller or larger quantities of dietary fibre.

Omega-3 fatty acids without fish

The recommended intake of the omega-3 fatty acid alpha-linolenic acid (ALA) has been increased to 1 per cent of the total calorie intake in order to improve the chance of the body synthesizing sufficient quantities of the long-chain omega-3 fatty acids eicosapentaenoic acid (EPA) and docosahexaenoic acid (DHA) from ALA, which in a mixed diet would already be supplied in that form via fish such as salmon.[289] For around 9 kcal per g fat, this would work out as roughly 2g ALA for a calorie intake of 2,000 kcal. This quantity should be covered through plant-based sources of omega-3 such as linseed, hemp seeds, chia seeds, walnuts, and their relevant oils. In some cases, it makes sense to supply additional ready-made EPA and DHA from microalgae oils (see Tip 10, p.77).

Source vitamin A from plants

If you regularly include foods in your menu that are rich in beta-carotene, e.g. carrots, sweet potatoes, and squash, you can easily cover the recommended intake of 1mg retinol equivalent (RE) per day. As explained in Tip 4 (see p.60), it is very important for these beta-carotene-rich foods to be eaten along with a plant-based source of fat to optimize beta-carotene absorption.[290]

Sun or supplements for vitamin D

Exposing the skin to sunlight prompts the body to produce vitamin D. If you seldom go outdoors, you run the risk of experiencing a vitamin D deficiency. If this happens, it will be necessary to take a vitamin D supplement. The recommended intake is 40 to 60 IU per kg body weight for individuals with a normal weight.[291] Overweight people (BMI > 25 kg/m^2) should take one and a half times this quantity and those who are obese should take double the daily dose.[292]

Vital B vitamins

According to Public Health England, the recommended daily intake of vitamin B2 is 1.3mg for men and 1.1mg for women, and the same figures can be applied for those on a vegan diet. Vitamin B2 can be provided from foods such as mushrooms, almonds, and yeast flake seasoning.

The recommended B12 intake is very dependent on the intervals at which it is consumed, due to the body's limited ability to absorb B12 in any time period. If vitamin B12 is supplied via fortified foods at several points in the day, a total intake of around 4 to 6µg per day will suffice.[293] On the other hand, if it is only consumed once a day, a dose of 100µg or more is recommended.[294] The reasons for these differing intake levels are explained in detail in Tip 10 (see p.75).

Sufficient minerals

The recommended quantity of 1000mg calcium per day can easily be covered through foods rich in calcium (like sesame seeds, chia seeds, and almonds), plant-based drinks that have been fortified with calcium, and mineral water that is rich in calcium. Public Health England recommends a daily intake of 8.7mg iron for men and 14.8mg iron for women up to the age of 50, which can easily be covered in most cases by eating plant-based foods that are rich in iron (such as pumpkin seeds, sesame seeds, and linseed) as part of a varied, nutrient-rich diet. Most foods that contain lots of iron are also rich in zinc, so the recommended daily intake of 9.5mg for men and 7mg for women can easily be achieved in a well-planned vegan diet. The recommended iodine intake of 200µg per day can be ensured by using iodine-rich seaweed such as nori or wakame in precisely measured doses (1–3g/0.04–1oz of dried seaweed such as wakame, dulse, or nori is enough to cover the daily iodine requirement[295, 296] and too much iodine can damage the thyroid) or by using iodized table salt or taking an iodine supplement.

While it is true that Brazil nuts are very rich in selenium, there is enormous variation between individual nuts[297] and, for instance, because the soil in most European countries is very low in selenium,[298] plant-based foods that are locally grown there contain only very small quantities of this element. For this reason, we currently recommend that if you are living in a country with low selenium levels in the soil, you should take a dietary supplement to cover the daily requirement of 1 to 2µg/kg body weight[299, 300] until the soil has been successfully enriched with selenium, following the model implemented in Finland.[301] Unless animal feed is fortified appropriately, even animal products would not contain optimal quantities of selenium due to the lack of this element in many European soils.[302] This is why animal products for consumption are effectively supplemented with selenium via the animal itself. Our previous book *Healthy Vegan* includes detailed tables listing the best sources for all the vital nutrients. In Tip 5, optimizing mineral absorption (see p.62), we describe ways to greatly improve the intake of minerals by consuming other nutrients at the same time to help you achieve an optimal supply.

Tip 1: There are no healthy/unhealthy foods

Nutritious unprocessed plant-based foods

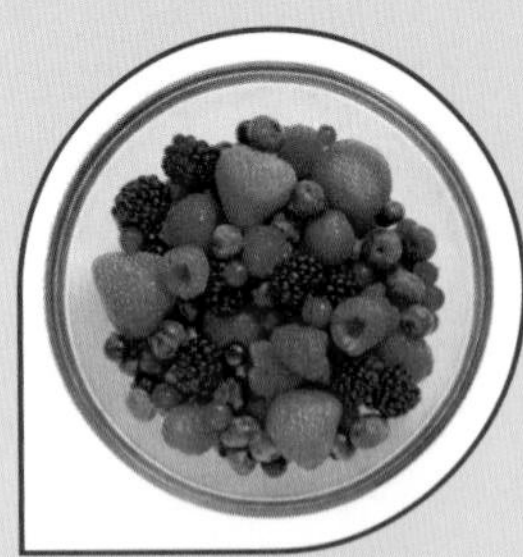

- Fresh fruit
- Fresh vegetables
- Intact whole grains
- Dried pulses and beans
- Nuts
- Seeds
- Herbs
- Microgreens
- Shoots

Nutritious processed foods

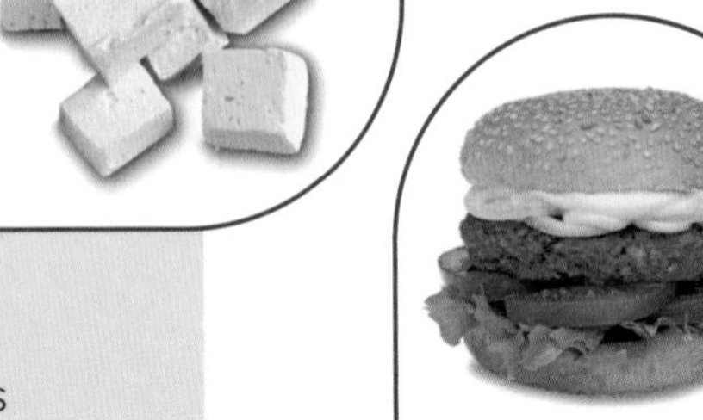

- Wholewheat pasta
- Wholemeal bread
- Tinned pulses
- Tinned tomatoes
- Frozen vegetables
- Frozen fruit
- Tofu
- Tempeh
- Plant-based drinks
- Plant-based yogurt
- Miso
- Spices
- Nut butters
- Dried fruit
- Fermented vegetables

Low-nutrient processed foods

- White flour products
- Sweet treats
- Soft drinks
- Junk food
- Alcohol

90% | 10%

Fig. 18: Modified illustration of Dr Fuhrman's 90–10 rule[303]

There are no unhealthy foods. Nor indeed are there healthy foods. For example, one piece of cake per week as part of an overall nutritious, healthy diet will not do you any harm. Equally, one apple per week within a poorly balanced, unhealthy diet will not contribute any great health benefits in terms of your overall nutrition. There are, however, healthy and unhealthy diets and lifestyles. It is extremely important to recognize this. Firstly, because it is the only reasonable scientific perspective on diet and, secondly, because it gives us the necessary leeway to treat ourselves occasionally without feeling guilty, focusing instead on the bigger overall picture. The world's largest specialist nutrition association, the Academy of Nutrition and Dietetics (AND), refers to this as the Total Diet Approach, designed to reduce the exaggerated focus on "good" and "bad" foods, instead emphasizing the importance of people's overall diet.[304] The advantage of this kind of strategy is shown by a survey indicating that almost two-thirds of respondents were more interested in finding out what kinds of nutritious foods they should be eating more of than they were in hearing about prohibited foods.[305] Further research revealed that over three-quarters of respondents said their main reason for not wanting to eat more healthily was a reluctance to completely give up certain foods.[306] Such a drastic approach is not even necessary, but the widespread "all or nothing" mindset means that lots of people have a false impression of what a healthy diet looks like and would be surprised to discover that it can include a certain number of less nutritious but utterly delicious items. In principle, any food can be part of a healthy diet provided it is eaten in moderation. Studies also show that not everyone responds in the same way to food. For example, different people have different blood sugar levels after eating identical food.[307] That is why a much more individual approach is essential and any sweeping generalizations made about nutritional recommendations should be avoided.

Rules that are too strict are demotivating

There is also evidence to show that excessively rigid eating guidelines and strict black-and-white thinking can easily cause us to feel unsettled, helpless, and anxious about our diet and there comes a point where people are likely to just ignore nutritional recommendations.[308] But it is important not to get the wrong impression about the Total Diet approach. Of course, our strategy is still focused on drastically reducing foods with unhealthy fatty acid profiles, added sugar, large quantities of salt, alcohol, and empty calories. And for ethical reasons, we recommend an entirely plant-based diet. At the same time, this approach leaves room for personal preferences and is sufficiently flexible to be implemented as a long-term dietary strategy. In addition, ingredients such as salt and sugar can help make valuable nutritious foods more palatable and, therefore, more popular. For example, if the flavour of vegetables is enhanced using Stefan Marquard's technique[309] – seasoning with a mix of five parts salt and one part sugar – this is an example where an ingredient that is low in nutrients and harmful in larger quantities can actually help make healthy foods, like vegetables, more delicious so you are happy to eat more of them. In this case, the benefits clearly outweigh any potential drawbacks.

A little of what you fancy

Figure 18 picks up this concept and illustrates it following the 90–10 rule devised by nutritionist Dr Joel Fuhrman as part of his Nutritarian Diet. We have adapted this therapeutic concept to make it less rigid, creating a more generally applicable approach for you to follow. This allows about 10 per cent of your intake to consist of any plant-based foods at all. Our focus is on the remaining 90 per cent, which should consist of wholesome, minimally processed and unprocessed, nutritious, plant-based foods. The list of minimally processed, wholesome, plant-based foods includes items in the five main food groups in the vegan diet plus fresh herbs, shoots, and microgreens. Nutritious processed foods include all fermented foods, frozen vegetables, dried fruit, wholegrain products such as bread and pasta, soya products such as tofu and tempeh, spices, dried herbs, and lots of other items. As already shown in the sections covering the five main food groups, different foods interact with each other. So, products that are low in nutrients should ideally be combined with more nutritious foods to partially offset their harmful effects.

The following combinations will reduce blood sugar spikes following consumption of white flour:

- Combine white flour products with pulses
- Combine white flour products with vinegar
- Combine white flour products and foods that are high in sugar with berries
- Combine white flour products with plenty of vegetables and spices

Pulses have such a positive impact on blood sugar levels they not only help to regulate blood glucose for the meal in which they are eaten, they can also affect the following meal – even if a whole night has passed between these meals.[310] They can also reduce the spike in blood sugar levels after the simultaneous consumption of white flour. Consequently, pulses should ideally be included in your diet on a daily basis. Similar blood-sugar-regulating effects have been demonstrated following the consumption of white flour in combination with vinegar, [311] as described in detail in the section on vinegar (see from p.34). This explains why sushi, for example, does not trigger such a severe rise in blood sugar levels despite the fact it is made from white rice; the effect of the rice is mitigated by the addition of vinegar.[312] Thanks to their secondary plant substances, berries also have a stabilizing effect on blood sugar levels if they are eaten with foods that are high in sugar.[313] In addition, some secondary plant substances in vegetables and spices act as antioxidants and can regulate blood glucose, which means they can also curb an excessive blood sugar spike after eating white flour products and potentially inhibit the associated oxidative stress.[314]

So, if the question is whether white rice is "good" or "bad", the counterquestion should be "how is it being eaten?" If served as a side dish with other "bad" foods, such as a breaded escalope, the white rice will be more detrimental than if served as part of a meal packed with "good" foods, such as a vegetable curry with pulses and fresh herbs. Other crucial factors on the effect of a foodstuff include time of day,[315] eating patterns,[316] and physical activity levels.[317] This is why we need to talk about a healthy diet as part of an overall healthy lifestyle.

Tip 2: Food choices, not macronutrient ratio

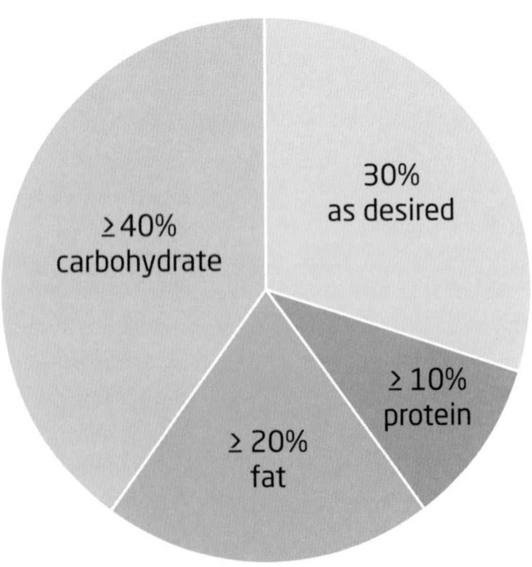

Fig. 19: Sample model for macronutrient distribution

People have been fixated for decades with the question of whether a high-carb/low-fat or a low-carb/high-fat approach is better for our health. There really is no correct answer to this question because we do not simply eat macronutrients like carbohydrates and fats. Our diet includes different kinds of macronutrients, not all of which have the same effect on the body. A food should always be considered as a total package, in which the nutritional value is not determined by its individual components but by their collective impact. These components may have compensatory or synergistic properties. An even more important consideration is the overall composition of the different foods within a dish or even the total dishes consumed over the course of a day, as described in detail in Tip 1 (see p.52). There are lots of foods that are rich in carbohydrates – from wholemeal bread and fresh fruit to white bread and cakes. Fat can also mean all sorts of possible items. Margarine, deep-frying fat, linseed oil, and extra virgin olive oil are all fats, but they could hardly be more different in terms of their health value. That is why a healthy vegan diet should not be aiming for a specific macronutrient ratio; instead, the emphasis should be on choosing high-quality, nutritious foods.

None of the three macronutrients is inherently bad, and a certain quantity of all three should be incorporated in your menu plan. Nutritional bodies agree there is no single optimal ratio between the three macronutrients fat, protein, and carbohydrate.[318] The precise proportion of macronutrients on someone's plate will be influenced by their particular personal preferences, their state of health,[319] and their sporting objectives.[320]

Protein percentage

There are, however, minimum thresholds for all three macronutrients that apply to the vast majority of people. For example, protein should make up at least 10 per cent of your nutritional energy intake. Studies have shown that a minimum so-called protein-energy ratio of 10 per cent, i.e. the proportion of protein compared to the overall nutritional energy intake, can adequately cover protein requirements as part of a vegan diet.[321] So the minimum threshold is set at this value. In many cases, it is advisable for people following a vegan diet to get a slightly higher protein intake of around 15 per cent of their overall calories to compensate for the fact that plant-based proteins are slightly less digestible due to their high fibre content.[322, 323] Particularly for participants in power sports, a protein intake of 20 per cent might even be recommended, as long as it involves healthy protein-rich foods. Whether you opt for 10, 15, or 20 per cent or some other figure in this range, this is nowhere near as important as the specific choice of protein sources. As long as pulses, whole grains, and other plant-based sources of protein are regularly included in your menu plan and you consume enough calories overall, you will ensure an adequate supply of protein and the potentially critical amino acids for your body.

Fat percentage

Contrary to the claims of strict low-fat advocates, the aim should be to consume a minimum of 20 per cent fat in relation to your overall energy intake. This is because the latest nutritional research shows clearly that the fat phobia of recent decades is not only unfounded but that high-quality fats play a crucial role within an overall healthy diet.[324] Ultimately, the absolute quantity of fat is less crucial than the issue of whether certain healthy high-fat foods, such as nuts and seeds, are included in your diet in sufficient quantities and whether there is an adequate supply of (semi-)essential fatty acids. Even high-quality unrefined vegetable oils can (optionally) form part of a healthy vegan diet. If you incorporate appropriate quantities of all these healthy fats in your menu plan, you will not fall much below the 20 per cent fat proportion and, in many cases, a value between 20–40 per cent fat will be obtained.

Carbohydrate percentage

A lower limit of 40 per cent of your nutritional energy has been identified for carbohydrate intake. If carbohydrate consumption falls below 40 per cent of your nutritional energy, in most cases this means there is an inadequate supply of valuable grain products, fresh fruit, and vegetables. If high-quality, nutritious sources of carbohydrate are chosen, the proportion of carbohydrate can happily be even higher than 40 per cent. In fact, even 50 or 60 per cent is conceivable, provided these larger quantities of carbohydrate are not consumed at the expense of essential fatty acids and amino acids.

Summary

In conclusion, there are a whole range of macronutrient relationships involved in choosing the right foods, and no single macronutrient should be excessively restricted. Irrespective of the specific macronutrient arrangement you ultimately choose, it is important to ensure the minimum intake of the following nutrients in each case:

Minimum intake for selected nutrients:

≥ 30g fibre/day

≥ 30mg lysine per kg body weight/day

≥ 1 per cent of energy from alpha-linolenic acid/day

The selected carbohydrate intake level must ensure the EFSA (European Food Safety Authority) recommended minimum intake of 30g (1oz) dietary fibre is guaranteed.[325] With regard to protein intake, irrespective of the absolute quantity consumed, it is vital to adhere to the WHO (World Health Organization) stipulation of 30mg of the essential amino acid lysine per kg body weight.[326] Regardless of how much fat is consumed in total, people following a vegan diet should double the recommended minimum intake for the essential omega-3 fatty acid alpha-linolenic acid and ensure that at least 1 per cent of their total energy intake is in the form of this fatty acid.[327] For a female weighing 60kg (132lb) with moderate activity levels, this equates to a recommended intake of around 2g ALA per day. If these values are achieved through the relevant minimum macronutrient intakes shown in Figure 19, the remaining 30 per cent of macronutrients can be distributed in whatever way desired. If it becomes clear that the chosen macronutrient arrangement results in insufficient fibre (carbohydrate), lysine (protein), or ALA (fat), the intake of the deficient macronutrient should be increased based on the best sources for the relevant substance. To get a feel for this, the quantities of fibre, lysine, and ALA are specified alongside the three macronutrients for each recipe in this book.

Tip 3: One eye on calories

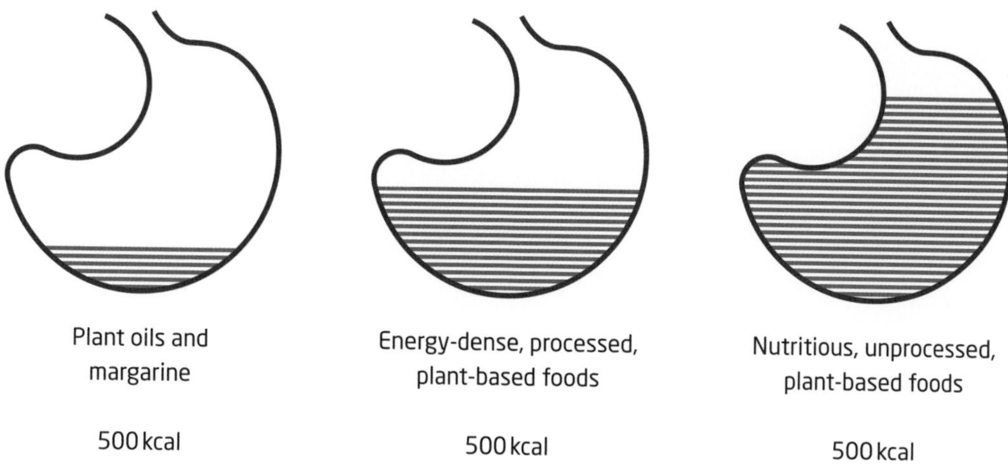

Fig. 20: Comparative illustration of the energy density of different foods[328]

Keeping one eye on calories means ensuring that a well-planned vegan diet provides the organism with the nutritional energy it needs, without supplying too much or too little. To achieve this, there is no need to painstakingly calculate total calories, but it is worth developing a feel for roughly how much energy a meal is providing. For this reason, calorie information is included for every recipe in this book. The key message here is that it is not the quantity of food that makes us overweight or underweight: the main contributing factor is the energy content of the food. So it is not particularly useful to simply reduce portion sizes when you are trying to lose weight, or to increase them to put on weight. What you need to do is alter the energy density. Regardless of whatever weight goal you are pursuing, you should not need to experience constant hunger or feel permanently obliged to eat more than you want to.

A great benefit of wholesome vegan food is that you can eat until you are full without having to count calories. This feeling of satiety is influenced by a combination of different factors. The immediate feeling of being full during and directly after a meal is primarily down to the volume of the food consumed (detected by mechanoreceptors in the stomach) and the nutrient density of the digested food (measured by chemoreceptors in the stomach and small intestine).[329] Since wholesome plant-based foods have a high water content and a high proportion of dietary fibre while also being low in fat (with the exception of nuts, seeds, etc.), these foods have a lower total energy density when compared to many processed plant and animal products. However, thanks to their greater volume, these wholesome plant-based foods are more filling than other foods with an equivalent calorie content. As well as the concentration of macronutrients (especially carbohydrates and proteins), the micronutrient content (vitamins and minerals) also influences this sense of satiety. Research shows that a nutrient-dense diet can reduce the feeling of hunger.[330] Both these mechanisms explain why a nutritious diet based predominantly on plant-based foods is so successful for weight loss even without enforcing any calorie restrictions.[331] In studies of this kind, many participants were found to automatically limit their calorie intake, even without being asked to do so, simply because they felt more full due to the large volume of food and greater nutrient density of their meals.

Insufficient calorie intake is not healthy

The positive aspect of a plant-based diet just described allows many overweight people to achieve their ideal weight without going hungry and helps people whose weight is normal to maintain their desired weight. On the other hand, it can have an adverse effect for people who eat infrequently and in very small portions or who follow a highly restrictive vegan diet. It is possible for people to fall into a long-term calorie deficit without being aware this is happening. Some very specific vegan diets advocate an extremely low-fat approach with a very high proportion of raw foods, and this can result in feeling satiated despite a low-calorie intake. This is another reason why it is important to keep an eye on calories.

For example, if you work out the volume of 500 kcal of different foods, you can see from Figure 20 that the same number of calories can equate to very different volumes depending on the relevant food product. For 500 kcal, it is possible to eat slightly over 50g (1¾oz) of vegetable oil, around 80g (3oz) of almonds, 200g (7oz) of wholemeal bread, almost 400g (14oz) of cooked young soya beans (edamame), just over 500g (1lb 2oz) bananas, or an entire 1.8kg (4lb) of rocket.[332] As you can see, although the quantity of calories for all these foods is identical, they vary greatly in volume and the degree to which they will make you feel full.

You can eat very large portions of fruit and vegetables and you will consume far fewer calories than if you ate the same weight of grains or pulses, or even nuts, seeds, and oils. Because our bodies are often able to get less energy from raw plant-based foods than from the same foods once they are cooked,[333] this unintended calorie restriction can be particularly pronounced if a large quantity of raw food is included in your diet, and this can result in unwanted weight loss. Apart from the lower energy yield, there is also an overall lower energy content in lots of raw vegan dishes compared to their cooked equivalents, which makes an even bigger contribution to unwanted calorie reduction, as illustrated in Table 4. Three pasta dishes are listed, which each have significantly different calorific density for similar nutritional volumes:

Meat Bolognese with spaghetti	Calories per portion	Low-calorie vegan tomato sauce with spaghetti	Calories per portion	Calorie-rich vegan Bolognese with spaghetti	Calories per portion
80g wholewheat spaghetti *(uncooked weight)*	287 kcal	300g courgette spaghetti *(uncooked weight)*	63 kcal	80g wholewheat spaghetti *(uncooked weight)*	287 kcal
200g Bolognese sauce	222 kcal	200g Tuscan sauce	66 kcal	200g Bolognese sauce	222 kcal
20g Parmesan	75 kcal	5g yeast flakes	17 kcal	20g vegan Parmesan *(15g cashews / 5g yeast flakes)*	106 kcal
Total calories	**584 kcal**	**Total calories**	**146 kcal**	**Total calories**	**569 kcal**
Macronutrients	**per portion**	**Macronutrients**	**per portion**	**Macronutrients**	**per portion**
Carbohydrate	71g	Carbohydrate	17g	Carbohydrate	78g
Fat	19g	Fat	3g	Fat	15g
Protein	27g	Protein	10g	Protein	23g

Tab. 4: Comparison of calories, carbohydrate, fat, and protein content in different pasta dishes[334]

On the far left, in the orange column, a pasta dish with meat Bolognese and Parmesan is listed, which provides 584 calories per portion. In the middle, in blue, there is a low-calorie vegan version of this dish, in which the wholewheat spaghetti is replaced by courgette spaghetti, and the meaty Bolognese replaced by tomato sauce. Yeast flakes have been used instead of Parmesan. This dish might make you feel similarly full in the short term; however, it offers just 146 kcal per portion, which is barely a quarter of the calories in the non-vegetarian version. The third recipe, in the green column, consists of an energy-dense plant-based alternative to the meat-based pasta dish. Here, a soya Bolognese with a cashew and Parmesan topping has been selected to be served with the wholewheat pasta. This provides 569 kcal per portion, which is almost the same energy density as in the meat dish. This simplified example should show how important it is in a vegan diet to find recipes that are not just a good plant-based alternative in terms of their taste and their vitamin and mineral content. The food should also offer a similar calorie content – particularly if you want to maintain or even increase your weight. Table 4 also shows that a vegan option containing adequate calories can come close to the meat equivalent in terms of its carbohydrate, fat, and protein content, and the low-calorie courgette pasta version supplies significantly less of all three of these macronutrients. To get an overall feel for which foods are rich in energy, Figure 21 shows the calorie density per 100g (3½oz) of different plant-based foods:

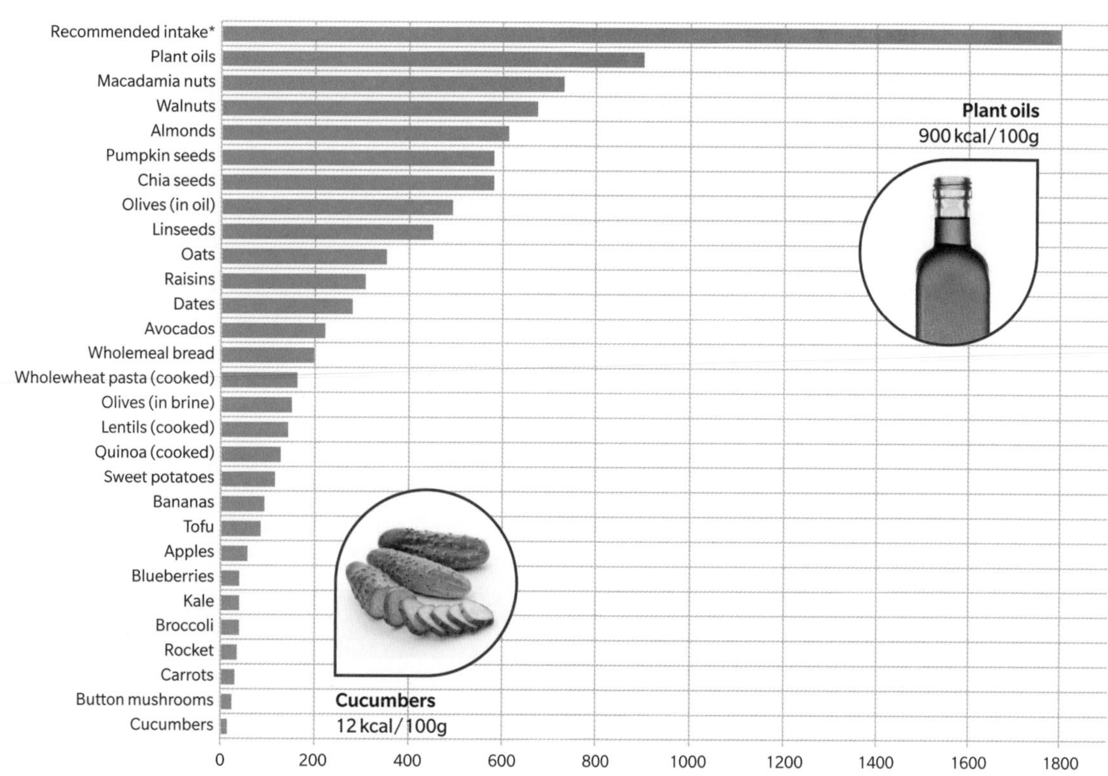

Fig. 21: Calorie content of selected plant-based foods[335]

Tip 4: Don't demonize fat

As early as the 1990s, pioneers such as Dr Dean Ornish[336] and Dr Caldwell Esselstyn[337] were able to demonstrate that a low-fat and predominantly or entirely plant-based diet was therapeutically effective in combating heart disease. And in the last decade, nutritionists such as Dr Neal Barnard[338] and Dr John McDougall[339] achieved similarly positive results in the treatment of type 2 diabetes with a low-fat, plant-based diet. As recently as 2013, in the German Nutrition Society's 10 rules published in "Healthy eating and drinking", rule number 5 stated: "Minimize fat and fatty foods".[340] In the updated edition from 2017, however, this rule has been replaced by the edict "Use healthy fats", and thus no longer recommends a strict fat reduction.[341] This development reflects the general trend in the latest nutritional science findings, suggesting that fat per se does not need to be reduced. Instead, suboptimal fatty acids should be limited, and the focus should be shifted to an adequate supply of good sources of fat. This paradigm shift is long overdue because research findings over recent years have shown that the fat content in food is not the sole indicator for the incidence of illness and obesity.

The quality of the fat is what matters

In controlled experiments lasting a year or longer, varying the fat content in food by 18–40 per cent did not influence the development of body fat.[342] This clearly suggests the fat phobia of recent decades is antiquated. However, the fundamental categorization of fatty acids has not changed at all. In line with all the leading heart,[343] health,[344] and nutrition associations,[345] Public Health England continues to recommend reducing your intake of saturated fats (usually from animal products and exotic oils) and trans fats (mostly from industrially hydrogenated plant fats), and increasing your intake of monounsaturated (e.g. olive and rapeseed oil) and polyunsaturated fats (e.g. linseed, hemp, and chia seeds).[346] Even former advocates of a strict low-fat diet, such as Dr Dean Ornish, now endorse the consumption of nuts thanks to the abundance of convincing data on their health benefits.[347]

Focus on essential fatty acids

A plant-based diet that is too low in fat also carries the risk of failing to provide the minimum intake of essential (vital for survival) fatty acids. These fatty acids include both the polyunsaturated fatty acids linoleic acid (omega-6) and alpha-linolenic acid (omega-3).[348] However, the typical western (vegan) diet with a normal fat content provides an excess of linoleic acid.[349] For this reason, we recommend using fewer oils that are rich in omega-6 (like sunflower oil, safflower oil, and corn oil) as these provide lots of linoleic acid. On the other hand, you should incorporate more foods containing omega-3 into your menu plan because even with a diet that has sufficient fat overall, an adequate supply of this substance is not automatically guaranteed.

The quantity of alpha-linolenic acid (ALA) in a vegan diet should be at least 1 per cent of the total calorie intake.[350] For a 60kg (132lb) female with moderate activity levels and an approximate calorie requirement of 1800 kcal, this gives a recommended intake of around 2g ALA per day. The quantity of linoleic acid should be at least 2.5 per cent and no more than 5 per cent of your daily calorie intake (5–10g for 1800 kcal).[351] The aim is to achieve a ratio of omega-3 and omega-6 fatty acids of 1:5 or less.[352] An intake of linoleic acid up to 10 per cent is also workable, provided the quantity of ALA is increased to 2 per cent to compensate, so the 1-to-5 ratio is preserved.[353] This relationship between the fatty acids is significant because it is the only way the body will be able to generate its own long-chain omega-3 fatty acids eicosapentaenoic acid (EPA) and docosahexaenoic acid (DHA) from the short-chain omega-3 fatty acid ALA.[354] And these long-chain fatty acids are important for our cognitive capacities and for the health of our blood vessels.[355] In our recipes, you will find details of how much ALA is contained in each dish.

The impact of insufficient fat intake

Apart from the potential shortage of vital fatty acids in a low-fat vegan diet, there is also the disadvantage that a low-fat approach greatly reduces the rate of absorption for a whole range of nutrients. This effect is illustrated in Figure 22, which shows the example of differing absorption rates for the secondary plant substances beta-carotene and lycopene from salads with different fat content.

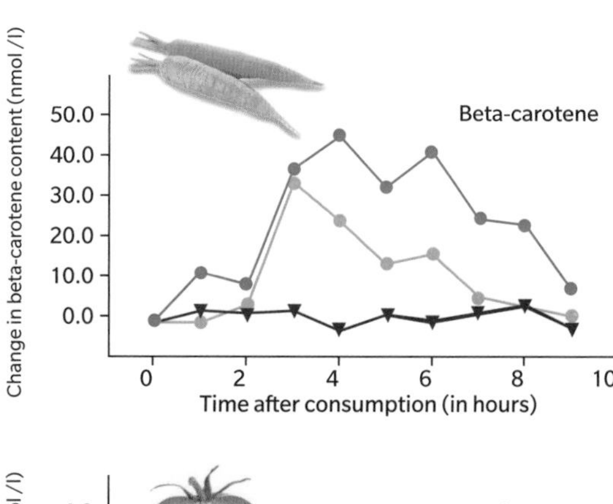

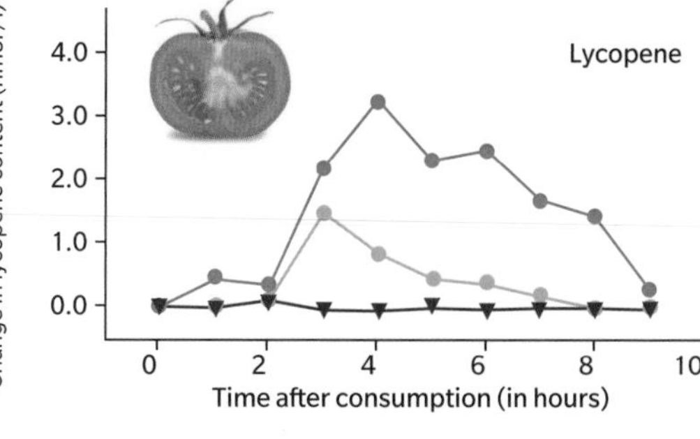

Fat-free salad dressing (0g oil) ▼
Reduced-fat salad dressing (6g oil) ●
High-fat salad dressing (28g oil) ●

Fig. 22: Absorption rate of beta-carotene and lycopene from test meals with varying fat content[356]

With a fat-free salad dressing containing 0g of oil, these two secondary plant substances are barely absorbed at all, whereas with a fat-reduced dressing that contains 6g (⅕oz) of fat, the rate of absorption clearly rises. And the absorption is even higher with a high-fat dressing containing 28g (1oz) of fat.[357] In addition to the effect on these two secondary plant substances, the same increase in absorption through fat can be seen for other substances, such as the curcumin in turmeric.[358]

Dietary fat increases the absorption capacity for several other nutrients, and these are listed below.

Fat increases the absorption of:

- Secondary plant substances (curcumin, beta-carotene, lycopene, etc.)[359]
- Fat-soluble vitamins (vitamins A,[360] D,[361] E,[362] and K[363])
- Long-chain omega-3 fatty acids (EPA and DHA)[364]

Knowledge about this enhanced absorption of certain substances is hugely important. For one thing, it is a further argument against a strict low-fat diet and, for another, it explains why it is so important for nutritional supplements, such as capsules with EPA/DHA from microalgae oil or drops with vitamin D, to be taken with meals. Otherwise, these substances cannot be absorbed as well by our bodies. The tiny quantity of oil contained in vitamin D drops or microalgae oil capsules is not enough to optimize the absorption rate.

Tip 5: Optimizing mineral absorption

The Vegan Society names a total of five minerals as potentially critical in a purely vegan diet. These are iron, calcium, zinc, iodine, and selenium.[365] This is in line with the German Nutrition Society, which offers ten tips that emphasize improving the absorption rate for these nutrients to ensure you get an optimal supply. This is because, in addition to the quantity provided, it is primarily the percentage absorption rate that determines how good or bad the ultimate supply turns out to be.

Reduce phytic acid

Ensuring phytic acid levels are kept low is particularly important as part of a vegan diet because the absorption of so many minerals (such as iron, zinc, and calcium) is inhibited through phytic acid from plant-based foods such as whole grains, pulses, nuts, and seeds.[366] However, there are ways to reduce levels of phytic acid and there are a range of substances that promote absorption, thus offsetting the inhibiting effect of the phytic acid.

It should also be noted that phytic acid itself does also have several positive impacts in the diet, in addition to its absorption-limiting characteristic. Phytic acid has anticarcinogenic, antioxidant, immunomodulating, cholesterol lowering, and blood-glucose-regulating effects.[367] While it is true that phytic acid can contribute to deficiencies in poorer countries where there is a suboptimal supply of minerals, this is far less significant within a balanced vegan diet in many European countries.[368]

Nonetheless, if you still want to reduce the proportion of phytic acid in your diet, there are many cooking techniques that will help. Depending on the food, techniques such as soaking, sprouting, fermenting, and any kind of heating, can ensure that the phytic acid content is reduced. By soaking your grains or pulses then allowing them to sprout, you will activate the enzyme phytase, which breaks down phytic acid. The heat involved in cooking or baking reduces phytic acid directly.[369] These methods are particularly effective in combination. So, you can soak pulses and whole grains overnight before cooking, or you can leave them to sprout to further reduce the phytic acid, and finally, you can expose them to heat during cooking. In fermented foods, a large proportion of the phytic acid they contain is broken down during the fermentation process, so sourdough breads, tempeh, fermented tofu, etc. are also excellent sources of minerals.

Selenium and iodine

Both the potentially critical minerals selenium and iodine generally have excellent bioavailability from plant-based foods and supplements, so in this section we will not be discussing any issues about their absorption. They should simply be consumed in sufficient quantities, but do not overdo it as there is a fine margin between an optimal supply and excess.

Iron, calcium, and zinc

However, when it comes to iron, calcium, and zinc it is extremely important to optimize their absorption as they are highly susceptible to substances that promote or inhibit absorption. For iron, a wide variety of measures are available that can promote absorption.

Improved iron absorption through:

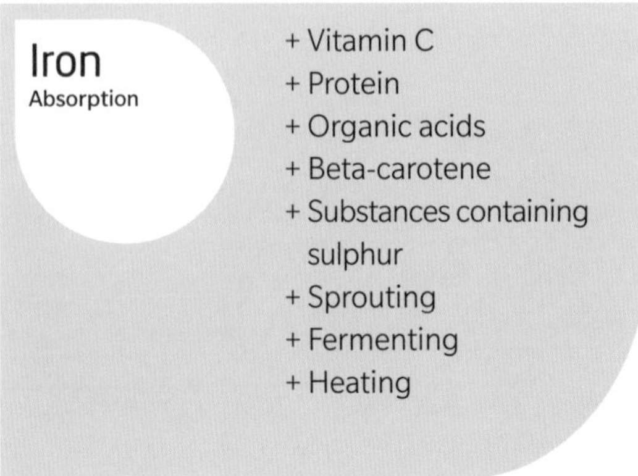

Vitamin C is probably the most promising factor in terms of iron uptake because it is so effective at facilitating absorption and is also available in large quantities in plenty of plant-based foods. In one study, it was shown that a dose of just over 60mg of vitamin C could almost triple the iron absorption.[370] This amount is roughly what would be found, for example, in 40g (1½oz) of red pepper.[371] Vitamin C's capacity to increase absorption applies both to vitamin C in food and in nutritional supplements if these are taken at the same time as a meal containing iron.[372] Dietary protein (both animal and vegetal) also has a beneficial impact on iron absorption.[373] Organic acids, such as citric acid (in fruit such as raspberries, kiwis, strawberries, and oranges, and in vegetables such as tomatoes and peppers),[374] malic acid (in rhubarb, apricots, cherries, plums, blackberries, and blueberries),[375] and lactic acid (from fermented foods like sauerkraut) have also been shown to have a positive impact on iron absorption.[376] The use of soy sauce instead of salt can increase iron uptake because it contains organic acids produced by the fermentation process.[377] Beta-carotene has also proven to be highly effective in increasing iron absorption, enabling a doubling or tripling of the iron uptake depending on the quantity supplied, and thus offsetting the inhibiting effects of phytic acid and polyphenols.[378, 379] The simultaneous consumption of sulphurous substances from bulbous plants like leeks, garlic, spring onions, and chives can also increase iron absorption.[380]

Improved calcium absorption through:

Calcium
Absorption

+ Vitamin D
+ Protein
+ Organic acids
+ Prebiotics
+ Sprouting
+ Fermenting
+ Heating

Calcium, on the other hand, does not profit from precisely the same absorption-enhancing substances as iron. The role of vitamin C in calcium absorption is inconsistent and not yet fully understood.[381, 382] However, vitamin D has a very powerful beneficial impact on calcium uptake and it is the most significant factor for improving absorption.[383] As with iron, calcium absorption is enhanced by dietary protein[384] and organic acids.[385] The simultaneous consumption of certain kinds of prebiotic dietary fibre – for example, inulin from ingredients including leeks, asparagus, onions, wheat, garlic, chicory, oats, soya, and Jerusalem artichoke[386] – can also promote calcium uptake.[387, 388]

Improved zinc absorption through:

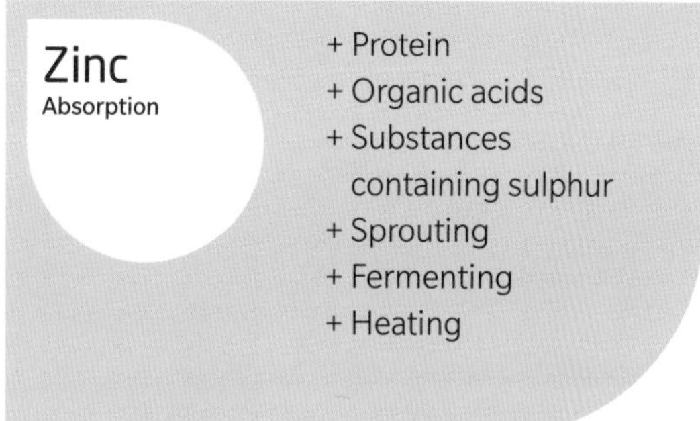

Dietary protein also promotes the rate of absorption for zinc, as do organic acids, such as citric acid.[389] The addition of sulphurous substances from onions and garlic also improves absorption.[390] Unlike calcium, there is less clear evidence of any improvement in zinc absorption for prebiotic dietary fibre such as inulin.[391] Tests looking at the effect of vitamin C on zinc have also failed to demonstrate the kind of powerful increases in absorption found for iron.[392] As for the other minerals described, culinary techniques such as sprouting, fermenting, and any kind of heating also indirectly promote absorption because they reduce (to varying degrees) the concentration of phytic acid in food, which inhibits mineral absorption.[393]

Tip 6: Eat the rainbow

Lycopene (e.g. red peppers, tomatoes, strawberries)
Beta-carotene (e.g. carrots, sweet potatoes, squash)
Curcumin (e.g. turmeric)
Chlorophyll (e.g. spinach, kale, rocket)
Cyanidin (e.g. blueberries, blackberries, red cabbage)

Fig. 23: Illustration of selected secondary plant substances in fruit and vegetables[394]

Secondary plant substances
Found in vegetables, fruit, pulses, nuts, and wholegrain products, secondary plant substances give these plant-based foods their smell and colour.[395] Figure 23 lists some of the best-known secondary plant substances by colour with examples of their sources in the human diet. Eating these substances regularly helps lower the risk of a large number of chronic degenerative illnesses, such as heart disease, cancer, type 2 diabetes, high blood pressure, and many more.[396] The term "secondary plant substance" was first used about 100 years ago by the plant physiologist and Nobel Prize winner Albrecht Kossel.[397] As the name suggests, only plant-based foods contain secondary plant substances. The term "secondary" here refers to the fact that these substances do not belong to the primary plant substances that are responsible for providing energy (fat, carbohydrate, protein);[398] however, their importance for the health of the organism is in no way secondary.

Secondary plant substances are created by the plant as a defence mechanism against pests and pathogens, to produce colour and as attractants.[399] The precise number of secondary plant substances is still not fully known today. It is estimated there are around 100,000 in the plant world, 5,000 to 10,000 of which are in human food.[400] In white cabbage alone, 49 different plant substances and their metabolic end products have been identified so far.[401] Over time, humans have learned which secondary plant substances are toxic and which have health benefits. To a certain extent, we have co-evolved alongside plants.[402] Over the course of evolution, the human body has adapted to the consumption of secondary plant substances through a predominantly plant-based diet, developing metabolic pathways to make the most effective use of these nutritional components.[403]

Positive effects
As shown in Figure 24, secondary plant substances have wide-ranging positive effects and most of the additional health benefits offered by plant-based foods can be traced back to these substances.

For example, anthocyanin[405] from blueberries, red cabbage, etc. and curcumin from turmeric[406] (both of which belong to the group of polyphenols) have anticarcinogenic,

Secondary plant substances	Positive health effects								
	AC	AM	AO	AT	IM	AI	BPR	CL	BSR
Carotenoids (e.g. beta-carotene, lycopene)	●		●		●			●	
Phytosterols (e.g. beta-sitosterol)	●							●	
Saponins (e.g. asparagoside)	●	●			●			●	
Glucosinolates (e.g. sulphoraphane)	●	●						●	
Polyphenols (e.g. anthocyanin, curcumin)	●	●	●	●	●	●	●		●
Protease inhibitors (e.g. trypsin inhibitors)	●		●						●
Monoterpenes (e.g. menthol)	●	●						●	
Phytoestrogens (isoflavones)	●		●		●				
Sulphides (e.g. allicin)	●	●	●	●	●	●	●	●	

AC = anticarcinogenic AM = antimicrobial AO = antioxidant AT = antithrombotic IM = immunomodulating AI = anti-inflammatory BPR = blood pressure regulating CL = cholesterol lowering BSR = blood sugar regulating

Fig. 24: Health effects of secondary plant substances[404]

antimicrobial, antioxidant, antithrombotic, immunomodulating, blood-pressure-regulating, anti-inflammatory, and blood-sugar-regulating effects.[407] The carotenoids lycopene[408] and beta-carotene[409] both have anticarcinogenic, antioxidant, and immunomodulating properties and also help to lower cholesterol.[410] As already described in Tip 4 (see p.60), many of the secondary plant substances, such as beta-carotene, lycopene, curcumin, etc. are significantly better absorbed by the body if the foods containing these substances are eaten along with a source of fat, such as nuts, seeds, or vegetable oils.[411]

Chlorophyll (just like phytic acid) cannot be categorized in any of the groups specified in Figure 24, but it is also one of the secondary plant substances.[412] Chlorophyll acts as an antioxidant and can help inhibit cancer.[413] It can even bind potentially carcinogenic substances, such as aflatoxins from mouldy food, thus drastically reducing their absorption and negative impact.[414]

Eat colourfully

To enjoy all these positive health effects, you should eat as colourful a range of foods as possible. You can see with your own eyes which foods are particularly rich in secondary plant substances. As a rule, the darker and stronger the colour, the richer the food will be in secondary plant substances. If you have a choice between two different foods (e.g. between white and black quinoa, or white and purple cauliflower), you should always choose the one with the strongest colour.

Tip 7: Be clever with salt

Reducing salt has been a controversial topic of discussion for years in the media, and it would be easy to get the impression that there is no consensus as to whether increased salt consumption is harmful to your health. This could not be further from the case. Large-scale, high-quality reviews have shown that reducing salt intake can significantly lower blood pressure[415] and thus reduce the associated risk of cardiovascular disease.[416, 417] In addition, the risk of stomach cancer goes up with increasing salt intake.[418] Leading nutrition,[419, 420] cancer,[421, 422] and heart[423, 424] associations also make the following statement: salt (sodium chloride) consumption in western countries is too high and should be limited to a daily maximum of 5g (1 tsp) salt (2000mg sodium)[425] for healthy individuals and 3g (½tsp) salt (1200mg sodium) for people with high blood pressure.[426, 427, 428] Despite this advice, the average amount of salt consumed by adults in the UK is 10g (0.35oz) per day for men and 7.1g (0.25oz) for women, which is on average 43 per cent higher than the recommended maximum.[429]

As mentioned at the start of this book, the most comprehensive study to date that has looked at people's lifestyles and the development of different diseases is the Global Burden of Disease Study, which established that poor diet in western countries is almost always among the top three risk factors for illness and premature death. The study also identified that excessive salt consumption is the greatest risk factor within this overall pattern of poor nutrition.[430]

Reducing salt

The good news, however, is that you can still make delicious food even with recipes that are lower in salt. This book will show you how. When it comes to your sensitivity to salt, a similar process applies as for sugar: over time you can make big changes to adapt your palate.

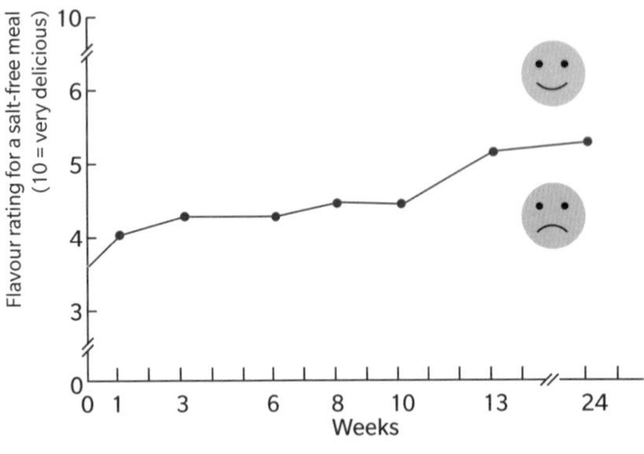

Fig. 25: Change in sense of taste for salt-free meals in a salt-reduced diet[431]

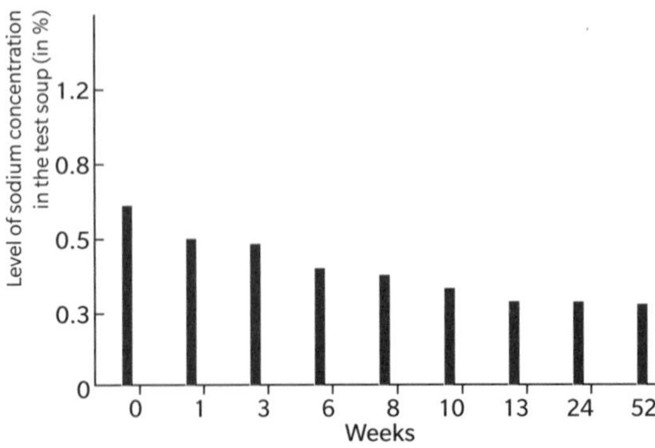

Fig. 26: Voluntary reduction of salt to achieve tasty meals in a salt-reduced diet[432]

Just as you can get used to eating foods that are high in salt, you can also wean your taste buds off this predisposition. Figure 25 shows how a group of test subjects responded to a salt-reduced diet over the course of several weeks and how they began to like the same salt-free soup more and more over a 24-week period while on a salt-reduced menu plan. This can be explained because their taste buds became more sensitive to the taste of salt over this period.[433] In a separate test, when this group was asked to season a salt-free soup to their own liking so it tasted as good as possible, a significant increase in their sensitivity to salt can be seen between the start and end of the 24-week study period (see Figure 26). The amount of salt added to achieve the same positive taste experience was reduced by over a half between the first and last week of the test period. And more than half a year after the experiment had ended, when participants were asked again to season an unsalted test soup to their own liking, the group members added a similar reduced quantity of salt as they did at the end of the original test period. This suggests a long-term adjustment in sensitivity to the taste of salt and a sustained change in behaviour.[434]

Aromatic alternatives

Deliberately reducing salt also brings other benefits. It lets us seek out tasty alternatives that are healthy and packed with flavour; ingredients that we might not otherwise use to the same extent. Fresh and dried herbs, spice mixes, vinegar, etc. will become central components in your cooking, adding more flavour while simultaneously improving the nutritional value. Apart from simply reducing the amount of salt, there are a range of suggestions on how to eat less salt while creating food with an exceptional flavour and on how to avoid the long-term negative effects despite a high salt intake. The following list summarizes these options.

Training your palate to get used to eating less salt, as just described, is undoubtedly one of the most effective ways of reducing your salt intake.

Strategy number two is to use a low-sodium salt product (available in health food shops, online, and in well-stocked supermarkets). These

Reducing the negative effect of salt:

- Get used to less salt
- Use low-sodium salt
- Salt food on your plate, not in the pan
- Use salt-free spice mixes
- Use miso paste instead of salt
- Consume plenty of potassium, secondary plant substances, and fibre

products replace some of the sodium with potassium. The result is that low-sodium salts contain about 50 per cent less sodium than conventional salt.[435] If you suffer from a potassium imbalance or have any kind of renal insufficiency, you should consult your doctor before using a low-sodium salt product.[436]

Salt is also perceived more intensely if our tongue comes into direct contact with the salt on the surface of a food than if it is incorporated within a dish. That is why it is best to salt food at the table rather than in the pan. You can get a saltier taste with a smaller quantity of salt.

Strategy number four is to use salt-free spice mixes containing dried vegetables and herbs, which can deliver fantastic flavours without any salt at all. You can make your own or buy ready-made products.[437]

By using miso paste instead of salt, you can add a lovely umami flavour to your food as well as compensating for the negative effects of high salt intake. Although miso paste is high in salt,

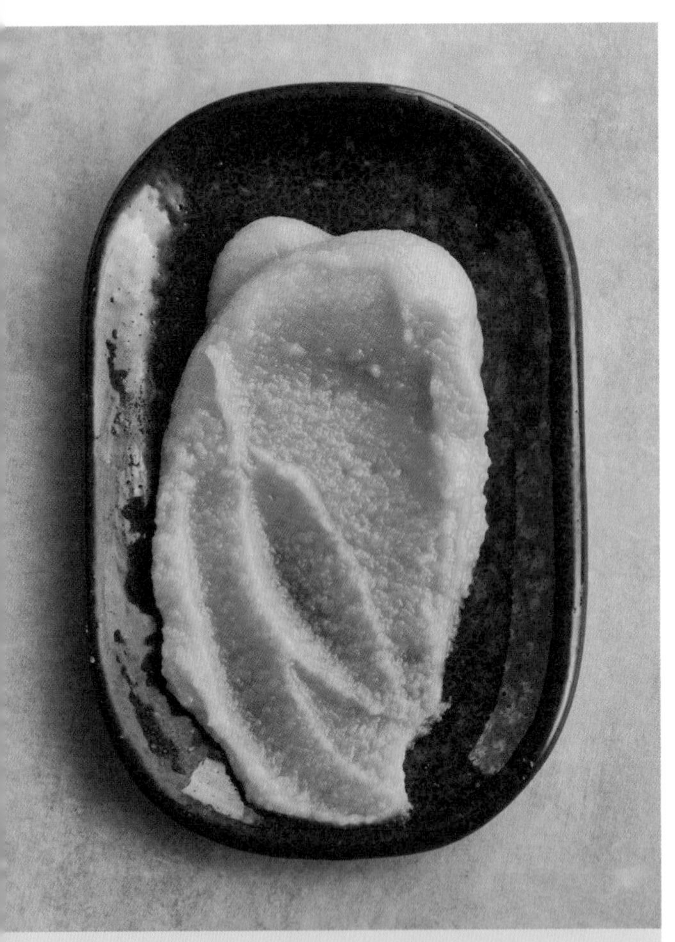

Miso pastes contain secondary plant substances and thus do not have the same negative impact on our health as salt, even if eaten in larger quantities.

increased miso consumption does not have the negative effects associated with increased salt consumption in terms of the risk of stomach cancer[438] and high blood pressure.[439]

Last but not least, a predominantly plant-based diet is itself a protective factor against the negative effects of excessive salt consumption, so vegans can treat the thresholds for salt intake a bit more liberally than meat eaters. Thanks to the wide array of plant-based foods that they eat, vegans often get above-average quantities of potassium,[440] secondary plant substances,[441] and dietary fibre.[442] This provides three significant compensatory components in larger quantities than feature in the standard western diet. All three of these can help reduce the negative impact of salt on blood pressure, vascular health, and the risk of cancer. However, this by no means offers vegans a free licence to consume unlimited quantities of salt.

Tip 8: Don't forget to drink

An adult's body consists roughly of 50 to 60 per cent water; for an average baby this can even be as high as 70 per cent.[443] It has been shown that the human body can go for up to 40 days (depending on external circumstances) without food during a hunger strike or extended period of fasting.[444] Being deprived of fluid, on the other hand, becomes life-threatening after just two to four days (again, depending on the external circumstances).[445]

Our health, well-being, and physical performance are heavily dependent on the supply of fluids. Even small fluctuations in hydration levels can have an appreciable impact. That is why it is important not to drink just when you feel thirsty but to make it a habit to take on sufficient fluids over the course of the day and particularly in the morning, immediately after you get up. Just a 1 per cent loss of fluid in the body results in a significant feeling of thirst. If you fail to respond to this feeling, a fluid loss of 2 per cent or more can cause you to feel unwell, and from 4 per cent nausea may set in. From 5 per cent your ability to concentrate deteriorates, from 8 per cent dizziness may occur, and from 9 per cent mental confusion may arise.[446] Just a slightly reduced fluid intake results in increased fatigue, lower alertness, and impaired performance.[447] A large-scale study has shown that people who drink five or more glasses of water per day have about half the risk of dying from heart disease than a group who drank just two glasses or less.[448] The recommended daily intake of fluids is approximately 35ml (1fl oz) liquid per kg (2¼lb) body weight.[449] Breastfeeding mothers should drink an additional 500–700ml (16–25fl oz) to compensate for the milk that their body is producing.[450] About a third of this total amount is covered by the water contained in your food and the remaining two-thirds should be supplied through drinks, as illustrated in Figure 27.

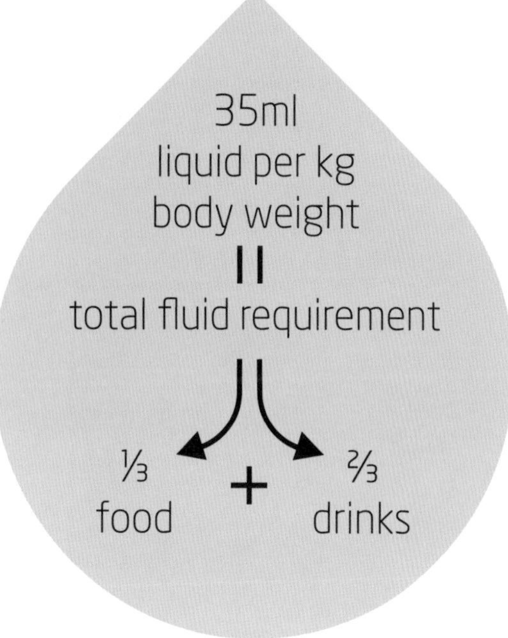

Fig. 27: Total daily fluid requirement for humans[451]

Accordingly, a 60kg (132lb) person would have a daily fluid requirement of 2.1 litres (3½ pints). Since an average of about one-third (700ml/25fl oz) of this amount is provided by the water contained in food, this leaves 1.4 litres (2½ pints) to be supplied in the form of drinks. The less liquid contained in your food, the more you will need to drink to compensate. Lots of plant-based foods have a water content between 70 per cent (banana, avocado) up to and even over 90 per cent (strawberries, spinach, cucumber, tomatoes), while others have a far lower water content, such as cooked pasta and pulses with about 60 per cent, and nuts and seeds with less than 10 per cent.[452] The actual quantity of water required is also influenced by other factors, which makes it impossible to specify a precise recommended intake. For example, the more salt and protein you eat, the more water will be needed because both these substances increase water excretion.[453] This increased water excretion caused by salt is also the reason why someone on an island surrounded by sea water will still die of thirst, unless they have another source of water available. Due to its high salt concentration, drinking 500ml (16fl oz) of sea water would result in around 800ml (1¼ pints) of water being eliminated from the body, thus removing 300ml (10fl oz) more water than it supplies.[454] The quantity of food available also plays a role in the specific fluid requirements. The less a person eats, the more they should drink, because an average of about 200–300ml (7–10fl oz) of so-called oxidation water is produced when metabolizing nutrients, which is absent when fasting. This missing fluid must then be supplied through drinks instead.[455] Careful estimates suggest that the long-term, safe upper limit for daily fluid intake for adults is around 10 litres (17½ pints).[456]

As shown in Figure 28, most of this daily fluid intake should consist of water. You really do not need to drink anything else unless you find it

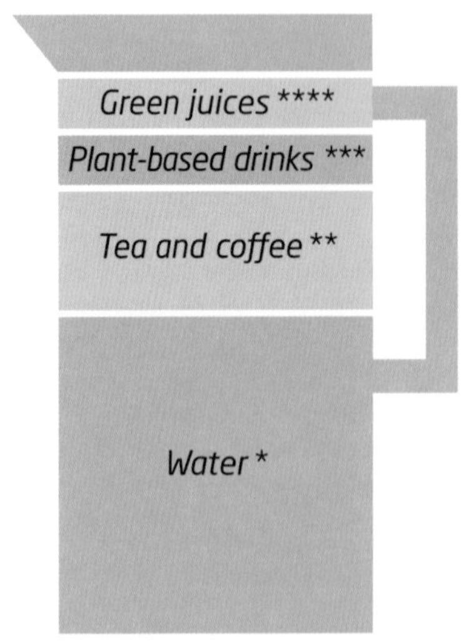

* incl. infused water, ** no added sugar,
*** enriched with calcium, **** with low proportion of fruit

Fig. 28: Suitable drinks to cover the fluid requirement[457]

boring to drink water all the time. If you want to add a bit of flavour to your water, you can make your own so-called infused water by adding your choice of herbs, fruit, and vegetables to the water overnight. This allows the water to absorb some of the flavour of the infused ingredients.[458]

The second category of recommended drinks is unsweetened teas and coffee. Tea is just as low in calories as water (provided you do not add sugar) and it provides a whole array of beneficial nutrients. Green tea is best of all because it has been shown to lower cholesterol[459] and blood pressure[460] as well as having a stabilizing effect on blood sugar levels.[461] For this reason alone, it is worth drinking one or more cups of tea every day. The best kind of tea is a finely ground tea powder like matcha, because here you consume the whole tea leaf along with all its ingredients. Contrary to its earlier poor reputation, coffee served without cow's milk and sugar is a harmless[462] and sometimes healthy[463] drink, which you can drink in moderation even on a daily basis.

The third category of drinks that can happily form part of your daily fluid intake consists of plant-based drinks enriched with calcium. If we take an enriched soya milk as an example, not only does it provide the same quantity of calcium as cow's milk, with a calcium content of 120mg/100g, it also has the same quantity of protein at about 3.5g protein/100g.[464] Unfortunately, the EU rules on organic production prohibit the enrichment of plant-based drinks with important vitamins, such as B12[465], but conventionally produced varieties can ensure the supply of some of this vitamin through B12 supplementation.

In addition, freshly pressed green juices can (but do not have to) be included in your daily menu plan. As we learned when choosing teas, the motto of "the more the better" does not necessarily apply here either. This is because some herbs and leafy vegetables have very high concentrations of specific substances (such as oxalic acids) that can be harmful if consumed in excessive quantities. Variety and the right balance are crucial.[466] When selecting green juices, the focus should be on juicing vegetables, leafy greens and herbs, only adding as much fruit juice as required to create a good flavour. By juicing fruit, you can easily produce very large quantities of concentrated (fruit) sugar.

Just as we described for food, specific drinks are not intrinsically healthy or unhealthy; what matters most is whether your overall drink consumption is healthy or unhealthy as part of an overall healthy or unhealthy diet. Nonetheless, you should avoid processed soft drinks if possible. And the earlier fallacy that a bit of alcohol could be healthy has been clearly refuted by recent research, so alcohol consumption should be kept to an absolute minimum.[467, 468]

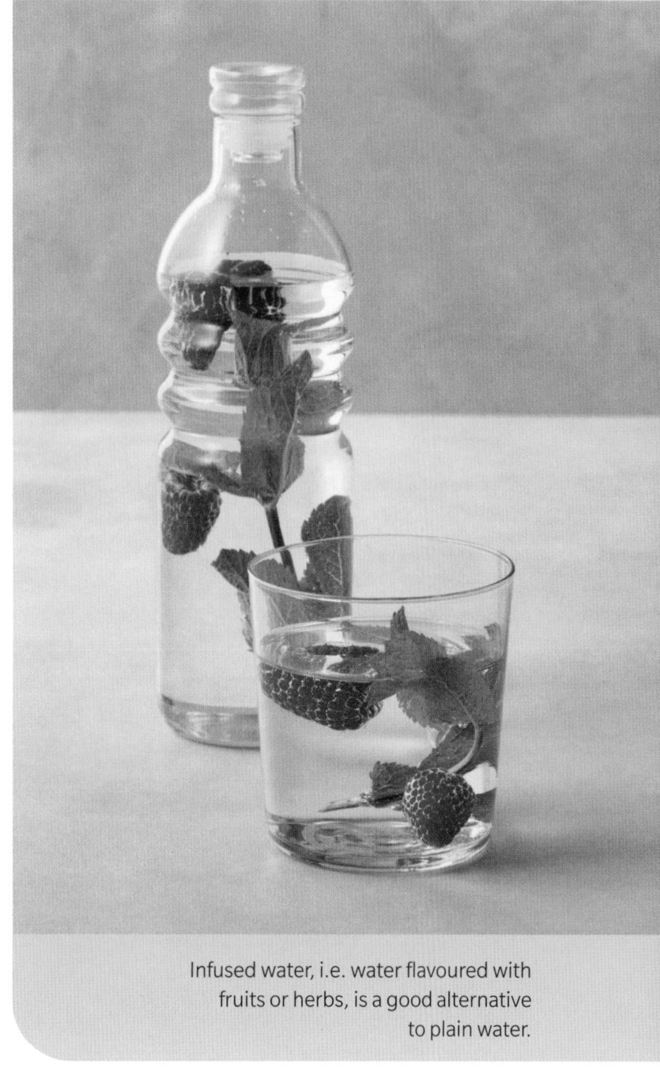

Infused water, i.e. water flavoured with fruits or herbs, is a good alternative to plain water.

Tip 9: Count hours instead of calories

Our health is affected by what we eat, what we do not eat, how much we eat, and how we eat, and for some time evidence has been building to show that when we eat (and when we do not eat) also has an influence.[469, 470] It seems that a calorie is not simply a calorie; the effect it has on our body can depend on the time of day that we consume it. The terms intermittent fasting (IF) or interval fasting describe a nutritional pattern rather than a specific diet. This approach can be implemented as part of any type of diet. It simply describes a nutritional strategy where you identify a particular time window for consuming food and avoid taking in calories during the remaining period.[471] For example, you could select one day per week to be a fasting day, while eating on the remaining six days. Depending on whether you want to lose weight or maintain weight, the missing calories on the fasting day can either be offset on other days to stabilize your weight, or the fasting day could create an overall calorie deficit for the week, which will promote weight loss. A form of intermittent fasting that is particularly practical for everyday life is so-called time-restricted feeding (TRF), where you eat every day but only within a feeding window that lasts several hours, with nothing being consumed for the rest of the day.[472]

How time-restricted feeding works

Unlike classic fasting, strategies like TRF can be used by adults of any age, including over longer periods of time. It can be an effective component in nutritional therapy for overweight people and for people suffering from high blood pressure, type 2 diabetes and metabolic syndrome.[473] However, it is extremely important for anyone suffering from a primary disease of any kind to consult their doctor before changing their diet. Different approaches are available to determine the length and time of the feeding window in TRF. Figure 29 shows an example of a 10-hour eating phase (10/14) with a 14-hour fasting phase.[474, 475, 476] Choosing the length of the feeding window, and thus the degree of restriction, depends primarily on whether you are aiming to maintain your normal weight and stay healthy or whether you are seeking to lose excess weight. There is no hard-and-fast rule about the number of meals you should consume within the feeding window, but on average in a 10-hour feeding window you

10-hour feeding window

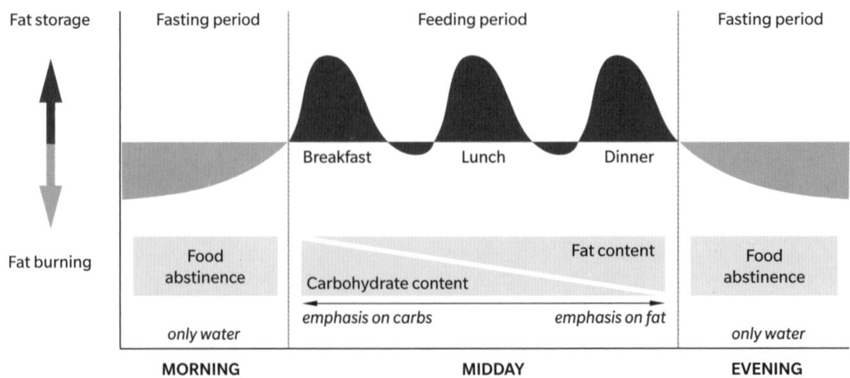

Fig. 29: Intermittent fasting following a 10/14 model[477, 478, 479]

would eat two to four meals, whereas during a shorter feeding window, like the 8/16 method with an 8-hour feeding window, you would probably only eat two to three meals.

The time window is flexible

The precise start and end time of the feeding window can, to a great extent, be adapted to suit your particular circumstances. Ideally, the feeding window should be arranged so that the largest meal of the day is consumed somewhere between midday and 3pm, with only smaller quantities being eaten during the evening hours.[480] For example, for a 10-hour window, the overall feeding window could span the time from 9am to 7pm, with the most calorie-dense meal being consumed in the middle of the day. For an 8-hour feeding window, the period for consuming food could run from 10am to 6pm. As long as the largest meal is consumed in the middle of the day, the feeding period can be shunted slightly earlier or later depending on your personal preference and to make it work for your everyday routine. Water can and should be drunk in unlimited quantities during the fasting phase. Evidence for the time-restricted consumption of food comes from comparative studies on rodents, showing that mice fed the same quantity of food have different increases in their body fat depending on what time they were fed.[481] Mice that were fed during the period when they would normally have been sleeping acquired more body fat than the control group, despite being fed the same number of calories.[482] Although not all observations made for animals can be applied to humans, and bearing in mind the ethical reservations about animal testing, the observations about eating times from the rodent model do appear to be applicable to people. Studies on humans also show that regular food intake during later evening hours increases the proportion of body fat compared with the same number of calories consumed earlier in the day, irrespective of the total quantity of calories consumed.[483] There seems to be some truth to the saying: eat breakfast like a king and dinner like a pauper.[484] As is so often the case, this does not need to be an all-or-nothing principle. What matters is generally eating more generous quantities during the first half of the day and, most importantly, avoiding eating any food in the hours immediately before bedtime. This recommendation is also backed up by a study on overweight people, who were subdivided into two groups, each following a severely calorie-restricted diet. The only difference was that one group ate their main meal at breakfast, while the other group ate their main meal in the evening. Despite being subject to the same calorie restrictions, the group that ate the largest meal at breakfast lost significantly more weight and had better blood fat values than the group eating their main meal in the evening.[485]

Carbohydrates in the morning, fat in the evening

Mediterranean countries, which are generally regarded as having a very healthy diet, often eat very late in the evening, which seems at first sight to contradict these recommendations. However, a closer examination of how calories are distributed over the course of the day suggests that if you compare lots of Mediterranean countries such as Greece, Italy, and Spain to central and northern European countries like Germany, UK, Denmark, and Sweden, the former do eat their largest meal at midday and only eat comparatively light dishes in the evening.[486] It is true that there are no strict overall nutritional guidelines regarding the exact proportions of carbohydrate, protein, and fat that should be eaten (see Tip 2, p.54); however, scientific data does show that people may respond differently to the same meal served at different times of the day when it comes to their blood sugar and insulin levels.[487] The body's insulin sensitivity is generally higher during morning hours and up to midday than it is in the second half of the day,[488] which suggests you should eat meals that are particularly high in carbohydrate with rapidly digestible sugars (such as fruit, white flour, etc.) for breakfast then reduce the quantity of readily available carbohydrates in favour of more healthy fats towards the evening.[489] The second period during which it is acceptable to eat a carbohydrate-rich meal with a high glycaemic load is after sporting activity, because the body's carbohydrate stores will have been emptied during exercise and some fast-acting carbohydrates will be very welcome.[490] The long-term benefits of the TRF approach are presented in a clear summary at the bottom of this page.

So next time you are travelling and there is no vegan food available, you can console yourself with the knowledge that a period of fasting could be positively beneficial for you. Yet despite all the aforementioned benefits of a temporary abstinence from food, it is important to note that this kind of approach is not designed for people who are underweight and that anyone in this category should be concentrating on reaching their normal weight by consuming sufficient calories without watching the clock. In addition, regardless of what time you eat, it is important to provide an adequate average calorific intake in the long term. If you fail to do this, even consuming food at the ideal times will only be of limited use.

Health benefits of a time-restricted feeding regime

- ▲ Better sleep[491] (▼ reduced risk of e.g. heart disease[492] and metabolic disorders[493])
- ▲ Increased insulin sensitivity (▼ reduced risk of e.g. type 2 diabetes[494])
- ▲ Lower blood pressure (▼ reduced risk of e.g. cardiovascular disease[495])
- ▲ Weight stabilization (▼ reduced risk of e.g. being overweight or obese[496])
- ▲ Improved cognitive function (▼ reduced risk of e.g. dementia[497, 498])
- ▲ Reduced IGF-1 level (▼ reduced risk of e.g. certain types of cancer[499])
- ▲ Increased autophagy (▼ slows down the ageing process[500, 501])

Tip 10: Don't be afraid of food supplements

Food supplements are a hotly debated topic. On one side, you have the proponents of orthomolecular medicine, who regard high doses of nutritional supplements as a promising therapeutic approach for a large number of health complaints.[502] On the other side, there are a large number of critics who reject the use of supplements for the vast majority of people and regard them not just as unnecessary but sometimes even potentially harmful.[503] As is so often the case, the real answer to such a complex question is far more subtle, and sweeping statements should be avoided. The fact is, there is not yet any scientific evidence to support the dispensing of isolated nutrients in quantities above the generally recommended intake. In fact, some nutrients have been shown to be potentially harmful if taken in isolation in excessive quantities.[504, 505] Given the abundance of inadequately regulated food supplements, it is often also very difficult to differentiate between high-quality and substandard products.

Despite this situation, this chapter will advocate the targeted intake of certain nutrients in physiologically strategic doses via fortified foods or nutritional supplements. The justification for this is that reviews of nutrient levels for people in Germany[506] and Switzerland[507] have shown that omnivores, vegetarians, and vegans are not getting adequate supplies of specific nutrients and there is probably a need to optimize intake in these areas.

When it comes to meeting nutritional requirements, different diets each have their own strengths and weaknesses. So it is important to understand the potentially critical nutrients that need to be covered for each dietary approach. Figure 30 (see p.76) illustrates the results of comparative studies of people following vegan, vegetarian, and omnivore diets in England and Switzerland. It shows that there are deficiencies on average for each of these diets and in all three groups there is room for improvement in different

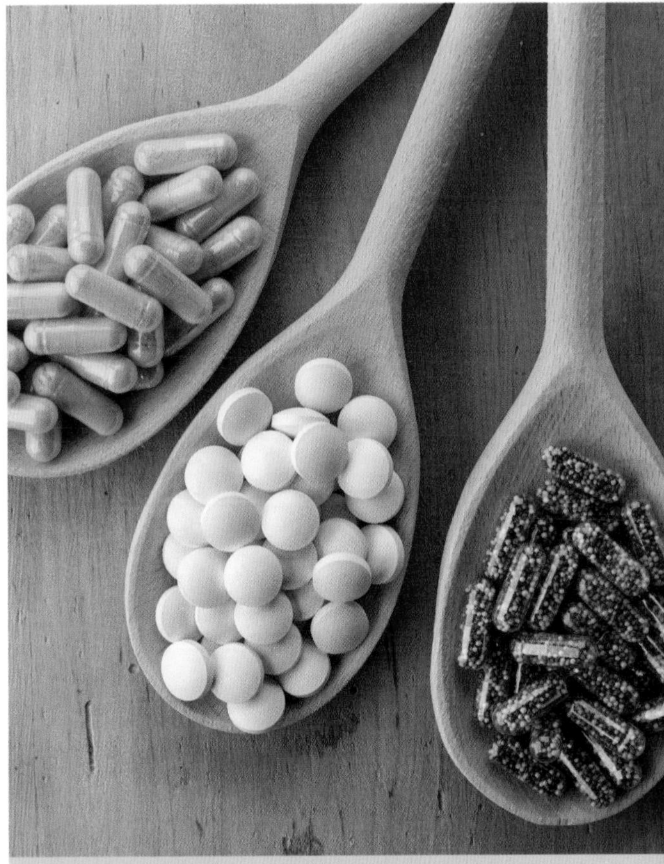

If high-quality food supplements are carefully formulated, these are a good way to provide an additional supply of critical nutrients.

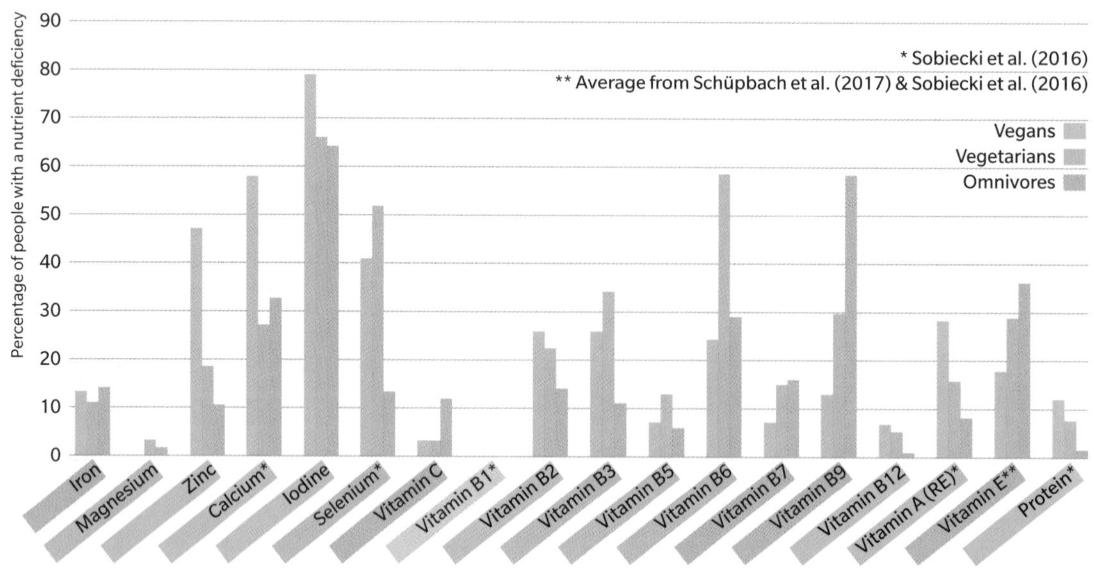

Fig. 30: Prevalence of nutrient deficiencies in vegans, vegetarians, and omnivores in England and Switzerland[509, 510]

areas. It is also important to remember that the strengths of a vegan diet lie primarily in the supply of above-average quantities of bioactive substances (secondary plant substances and fibre), so an exclusive focus on macronutrients and micronutrients does not offer a complete picture of the overall quality of a diet.[508]

As shown in Figure 30, deficiencies in iron, vitamin C, vitamin B7 (biotin), vitamin B9 (folate), and vitamin E were most pronounced in the omnivore group. Among the vegetarians, on the other hand, the most pronounced deficiencies were magnesium, selenium, vitamin B3 (niacin), vitamin B5 (pantothenic acid), and vitamin B6 (pyridoxine). In the vegan group, the most significant deficiencies were in zinc, calcium, vitamin B2 (riboflavin), vitamin B12 (cobalamin), vitamin A, and protein. Iodine was potentially the most critical nutrient, with over 60 per cent of people in all three groups not getting an adequate supply. By contrast, vitamin B1 (thiamine) was not found to be deficient in any of the three groups. This illustrates clearly which nutrients could be deficient in the different dietary groups and highlights where the focus should be in each case.

Food rather than supplements

In the first instance, potentially critical nutrients should be sourced from food rather than dietary supplements. However, depending on your diet, there are certain nutrients that might be lacking for some people, at least in certain countries, perhaps due to local production methods, statutory food regulations, or simply because of a lack of knowledge on the part of the food manufacturers. If specific nutrients cannot easily be obtained in sufficient quantities from the food you eat, taking a nutritional supplement is a well-researched and sensible option to avoid a deficiency. Provided a food supplement is high quality and the dose and type of nutritional compound has been selected appropriately, it does not matter for the human organism what the original source of the nutrient was. In other words, a carefully formulated nutritional supplement can have the appropriate impact.

Take each individual situation into account

The decision as to which nutrients might need supplementing depends greatly on an individual's diet and the rate at which they absorb and convert specific nutrients. A total

NUTRIENT	DOSE	FORM	LABORATORY PARAMETER	REFERENCE RANGE
Long-chain omega-3 fatty acids	250–1000mg	DHA EPA / DHA	HS-omega-3 index	> 8%
Vitamin B12	4–6µg/≥100µg	MHA	Holotranscobalamin (holoTC)	> 50pmol/l
Vitamin D	40–60IU/kg BW (1–1.5µg/kg BW)	Cholecalciferol (vitamin D3)	25-hydroxy vitamin D (25(OH)D)	100–125nmol/l (40–50ng/ml)
Vitamin A	500–1000µg	Retinol	Ratio of vitamin A serum level to retinol binding protein (RBP)	> 0.7
Iodine	100–200µg	Potassium iodide Potassium iodate	Urinary iodine (urine test)	100–200µg/l
Selenium	1–2µg/kg BW	Selenomethionine or sodium selenite/ selenate	Selenium in whole blood	121–168µg /l (1.5–2.1µmol/l)
Zinc	5–10mg	Zinc histidine, gluconate or orotate	Zinc in whole blood	4.0–7.5mg/l (61.2–114.8µmol/l)

Tab. 5: Type, dose, and form of recommended nutritional supplements for a vegan diet[511, 512, 513, 514]

of ten nutrients are specified by the German Nutrition Society as being potentially critical if a vegan diet is not well-balanced. These include vitamins B12, B2, and D, iron, zinc, calcium, iodine, selenium, long-chain omega-3 fatty acids (EPA/DHA), plus protein or the amino acid lysine. However, it is certainly not necessary to provide each of these ten nutrients in the form of supplements. Depending on the composition of an individual's vegan diet, one or more of these substances may need to be supplemented as a simple way of ensuring an adequate supply, at least for people living in Germany, Austria, and Switzerland. Table 5 gives an overview of each nutrient where the recommended intake may be difficult to cover and indicates the daily dose that would normally be sensible in a food supplement. The table also shows in what form the relevant nutrient should be provided and gives details of the laboratory parameters that could be consulted to investigate any potential deficiency, including the optimal range for these reference values.

Not everyone produces enough EPA and DHA

The body is not necessarily dependent on an external supply of the long-chain omega-3 fatty acids EPA (eicosapentaenoic acid) and DHA (docosahexaenoic acid), from food. This is because it can theoretically form both of these fatty acids itself from the alpha-linolenic acid (ALA) that is contained in plant-based foods.[515] However, you will need to provide sufficient basic raw materials by eating linseed, chia seeds, hemp seeds, walnuts, or their oils.

It is also the case that the body's ability to synthesize these fatty acids can fluctuate. The influence of dietary, genetic, and health factors can mean that individuals eating the same amount of ALA can end up with a very different supply of EPA and DHA. An HS-omega-3 test can indicate whether you will be able to produce sufficient EPA and DHA simply by consuming foods containing ALA. An HS-omega-3 index of 4–8 per cent is an acceptable score and a value of > 8 per cent is regarded as optimal.[516] If this value cannot be achieved simply through your food intake, it is worth supplementing with a microalgae oil of 250mg[517] to 500mg[518] with EPA and DHA in a ratio of 1:2. In some situations, higher doses of around 1,000mg or more may be appropriate.[519]

Vitamin B12 is essential

Although it is possible to incorporate larger quantities of bioavailable vitamin B12 in fermented plant-based foods by using the appropriate fermentation technique with special bacterial cultures,[520, 521] and although a number of algae constitute promising sources of B12,[522, 523] neither of the two most comprehensive studies conducted so far have been able to prove that these foods are a good source of vitamin B12 for humans. In addition, these foods are still not readily available. For this reason, all vegans are advised to take the recommended daily dose of vitamin B12 regularly via a fortified food product or nutritional supplement.

Quantity of B12 and intake intervals

Due to the body's very limited ability to absorb vitamin B12, the intervals at which you take this vitamin have a very big impact on the dose of B12. If you eat two to three meals or snacks each day containing foods that are fortified with vitamin B12, such as soya milk or soya yogurt, leaving a gap of at least three hours between meals,[524] a B12 intake of just 4 to 8µg per day will be sufficient.[525] However, if you only take one vitamin B12 supplement per day, the very limited active absorption of B12 per unit time means that the minimum dose including an adequate safety buffer will be 250µg, because only this amount can guarantee that enough B12 will get into the body's cells.[526]

B12: form and test values

For most people, any kind of B12 will work (cyanocobalamin, methylcobalamin, adenosylcobalamin, or hydroxocobalamin).[527] However, smokers[528] and people with a renal impairment[529] should avoid cyanocobalamin and choose another form instead. To err on the side of caution, you could opt for a supplement containing multiple forms of vitamin B12. A so-called MHA supplement offers a combination of the last three types of cobalamin listed above. To check how good your supplies are, you can get a holotranscobalamin (holoTC) test, which is much more informative than the classic serum B12 test.[530] The result should be 50pmol/l or higher.[531]

Vitamin D from sunshine

In principle, the body can produce enough vitamin D by itself if we get sufficient exposure to the sun. However, since many people spend the sunniest hours of the day in summer in enclosed spaces, and in many months of the year the sun is not strong enough even at midday, research suggests that 1 in 5 of the UK population has low vitamin D levels.[532] An adequate supply of vitamin D is by no means just an issue for vegans. If you want to find out how good your vitamin D levels are, you can get your doctor to check your blood count for 25-hydroxy vitamin D (25(OH)D). Based on the latest data, a reference range between 100 and 125 nmol/l seems to be ideal.[533, 534] In the event of inadequate sun exposure, the daily vitamin D supplement dose varies widely from person to person. But a value of 40 to 60IU vitamin D3 per kg body weight is generally established as a good guideline for individuals with a normal weight.[535]

Calculating vitamin D intake

To remedy an existing deficiency, the following formula can be used:

40 × (target value in nmol/l – initial value in nmol/l) × body weight in kg = initial dose in IU.[536]

This initial dose is then divided by 10,000 to determine the number of days you should take 10,000 IU vitamin D3 to make up for the deficiency. Finally, a maintenance dose of 40–60 IU per kg body weight is advised.

Well-supplied with vitamin A

The NHS does not list vitamin A as a critical nutrient in the vegan diet[537] because a daily serving of certain vegetables, for example just 60g (2oz) of carrots or 80g (3oz) of sweet potatoes, already contains sufficient quantities of various carotenoids for the body to synthesize its own vitamin A.[538, 539] Squash, kale, spinach, and red peppers are other good plant-based sources of carotenoids. However, there are big differences between people when it comes to their ability to convert carotenoids from plants into vitamin A in the body.[540, 541] Research into this individual capacity for converting carotenoids into vitamin A has produced mixed results, which may in part be due to the fact that the body's ability to form vitamin A from carotenoids is lower where there is more vitamin A in the diet.[542]

Converting carotenoids into vitamin A

As with the absorption rate and conversion capacity for other nutrients from plants, it is not expedient to test the ability to convert carotenoids into vitamin A in short-term experiments on omnivores. What is needed is an examination of the medium-term adaptations in longer-term studies on people following a vegan diet. Only in this way can we get a true picture of the capacity to convert carotenoids into vitamin A in the vegan diet. If you are one of the poorer converters, you should double the intake of retinol equivalent via food to be on the safe side and eat more products containing carotenoids with sufficient fat to optimize the absorption rate.[543] If you are one of the very rare individuals whose conversion rate is barely perceptible, a vitamin A supplement of 500–1000μg is recommended. It is important not to significantly exceed this dose because the therapeutic range for optimal vitamin A supplementation is narrow.[544] Since the level of vitamin A in serum (retinol level) on its own is not enough to evaluate an individual's supply, the retinol binding protein (RBP) should also be measured. The retinol to RBP ratio should be greater than 0.7.[545]

Supplementing with iodine is essential

Iodine is an important nutrient because it is used by the body to make thyroid hormones, which control how fast your cells work. The recommended amount of iodine per adult is 140μg per day. However, vegans can meet the required iodine intake with just a few grams of dried algae per day, although it is worth noting that iodine levels are highly variable in many algae, which means these are often unpredictable sources of iodine.[546] Of all the different algae, the following dried varieties are best to cover your daily iodine requirements: nori with 35μg/g, wakame with 160μg/g, sea lettuce with 136μg/g, dulse with 173μg/g and lithothamnion with 33μg/g.[547, 548, 549] If you do not regularly eat unpolluted, quality-controlled marine algae, it is sensible to take a supplement containing between 100–200μg iodine (depending on your intake of other foods containing iodine) in the form of potassium iodate or potassium iodide. Unlike other laboratory parameters, your iodine levels are measured in urine rather than in blood, and they should be in the range between 100 and 200μg/l.[550] Individuals suffering from thyroid disorders should consult their doctor about their iodine intake.

Countries with a selenium deficiency

Selenium is similarly a critical nutrient because German soil is very low in selenium compared to other countries, such as Canada,[551] and Germany has not yet opted to implement the kind of soil enrichment programme successfully conducted for selenium in Finland.[552] Instead, animal feed in Germany is enriched with up to 500μg selenium per kg[553] to increase the selenium content of animal food products. This means that meat-eaters get selenium via dietary supplements, albeit circuitously via the animals they consume. Brazil nuts are in principle a good source of selenium for vegans, however, there are significant variations which make precise estimates very difficult.[554, 555] Without Brazil nuts, someone on a vegan diet in Germany should take a food supplement with selenium levels of

1.5 to 2μg/kg body weight in the form of sodium selenite/sodium selenate or selenomethionine.[556] If you decide to use Brazil nuts as a source of selenium, the efficacy of this approach should be checked regularly by testing your selenium levels in serum, which should be between 101 to 139μg/l.[557]

Zinc is not absolutely critical

If you eat a varied, nutritious vegan diet and consume sufficient substances to promote absorption (see Tip 5, p.62), it is not generally necessary to take a zinc supplement. However, if your vegan food is less than optimal, it is possible to boost zinc levels with a daily supplement containing 5–10mg in the form of zinc histidine, zinc gluconate, or zinc orotate.[558] To establish whether this is necessary, you can test your zinc status in a full blood sample (not serum), which should be between 4.0 and 7.5mg/l.[559]

In a nutshell

In summary, the current evidence suggests that at least a vitamin B12 supplement is an essential part of a vegan diet to ensure an adequate supply. In some cases, other nutritional supplements might be beneficial for the sake of convenience.

If you want to make things really simple, you could take a multivitamin compound that is specially designed for the needs of vegans to cover all these essential substances with just a single pill per day. You will find a list of suitable food supplements for people on a vegan diet at the website associated with this book, at www.nikorittenau.com/healthy-vegan.

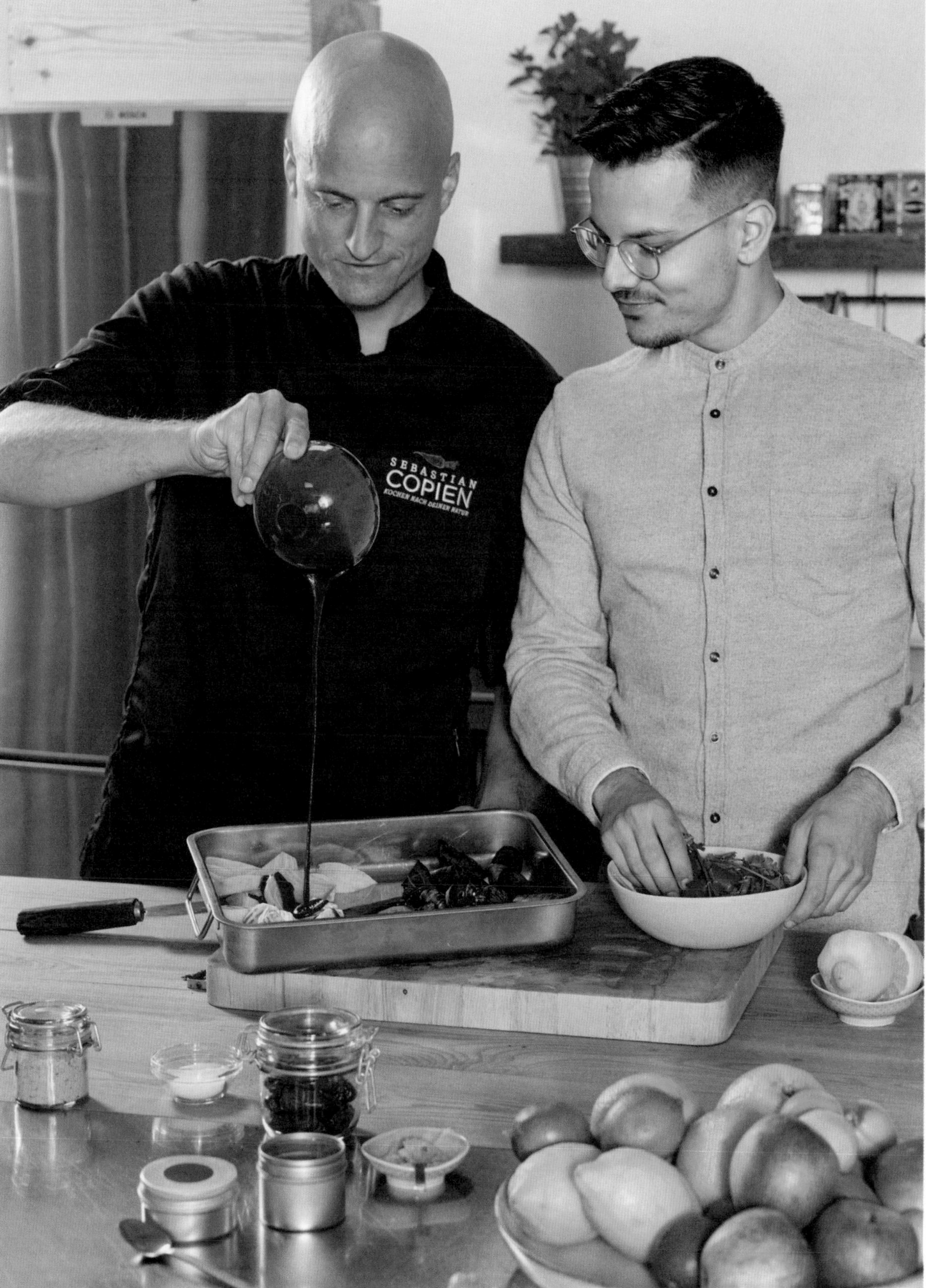
SEBASTIAN
COPIEN

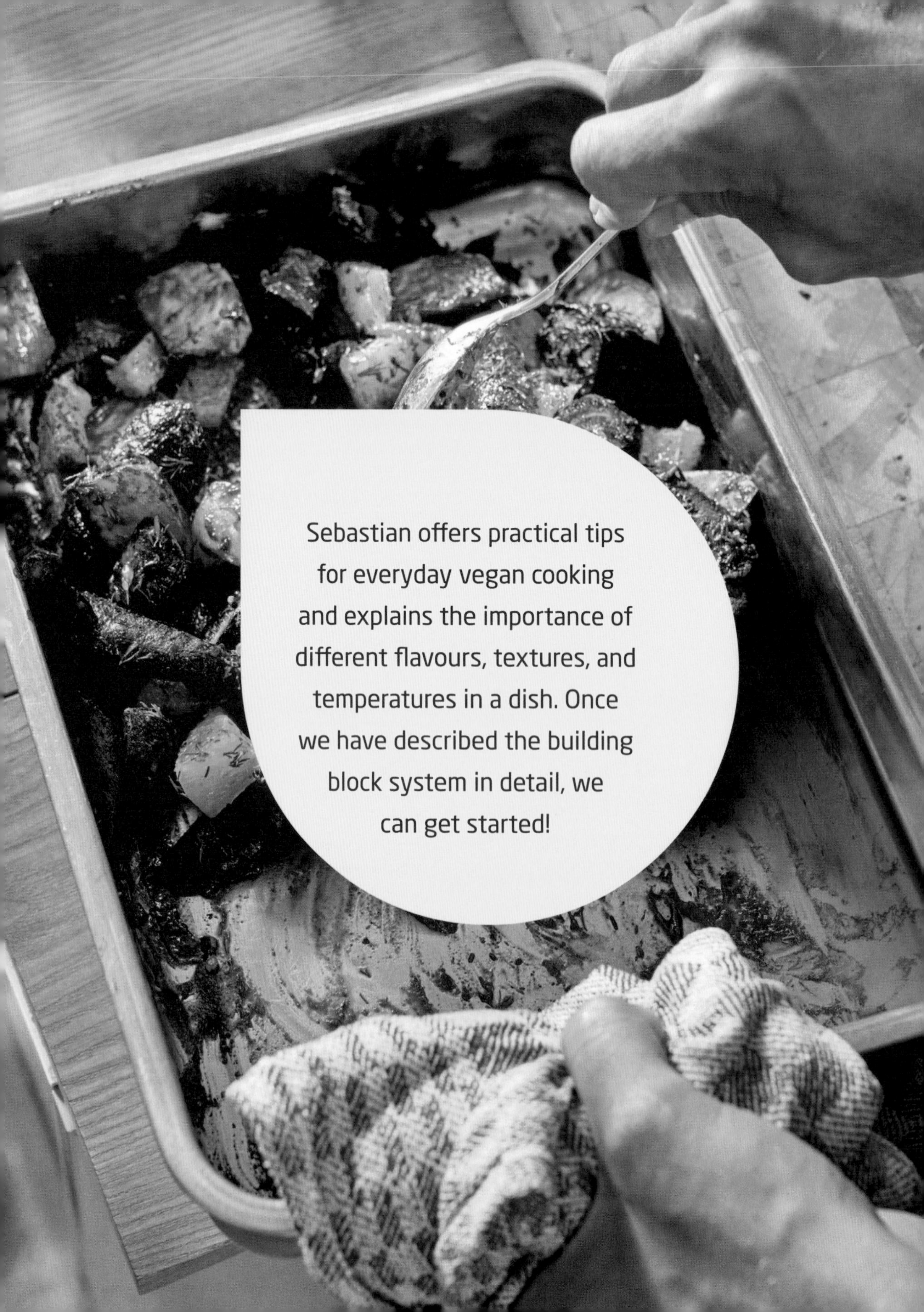

Sebastian offers practical tips for everyday vegan cooking and explains the importance of different flavours, textures, and temperatures in a dish. Once we have described the building block system in detail, we can get started!

Practical tips and recipe building blocks

High-quality gastronomy and healthy eating – a contradiction in terms?

If you are going to serve high-quality food from a gastronomic perspective, you need to get to grips with the theory of cooking and taste. Only then can you really understand how our palate works, allowing you to create healthy dishes that are also incredibly delicious and enjoyable to eat.

The fundamentals of good vegan cuisine
Anyone can make tasty food by using lots of sugar, white flour, fat, and salt, because our sense of taste has evolved to appreciate all these flavours.[1] However, there is plenty of evidence that excess salt, sugar, and calories elevate the risk of chronic-degenerative illnesses.[2] On the other hand, healthy food is often accused of tasting bland, making you feel as if you are missing out. The following recipe section will show in detail how – with just a little bit of practice – you can create healthy food with high gastronomic standards.

We will show you how to cook food that is good for you and tastes delicious. To achieve this, it is crucial to understand the fundamental principles behind flavour and mouthfeel. The model behind this theory of taste is illustrated in Figure 31. Once you have assimilated the vital basic knowledge, you can build on it and use your own creativity to produce delicious food from all sorts of plant-based raw ingredients. After all, fabulous food involves far more than just a single taste sensation – there needs to be a balance between different flavours and a perfect interplay amongst a variety of smells, temperatures, and consistencies.

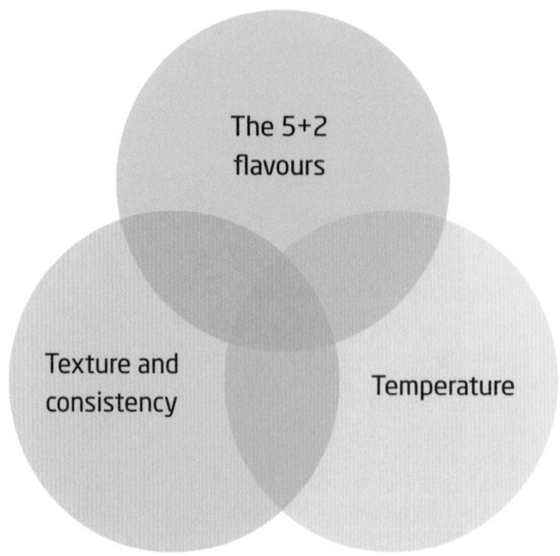

Fig. 31: The fundamentals of good vegan cuisine

The 5 + 2 flavours

Food that harmoniously combines different flavours tastes particularly good. That is the goal in all of Sebastian's recipes. Essentially, there are five main gustatory perceptions that are important in this context, but two others are also worth mentioning. The five fundamental taste perceptions are: **sweet**, **sour**, **salty**, **bitter**, and **umami**.[3]

The two others are **fat** and **spice**. In fact, most recent scientific publications refer to fat as a sixth gustatory perception, for which there are separate receptors in our mouth.[4]

Taste preferences that are essential for survival

A sense of taste and natural preference for fatty, calorific foods were just as important in human evolution as our liking for sweet and salty foods. These preferences allowed our ancestors to reliably identify foods that were safe, and high in calories and nutrients thanks to their rich (fatty), umami (high in protein), and sweet (rich in carbohydrate) flavours.[5] Although there are also lots of very healthy sour and bitter foods in the human diet, in the past our taste buds often used these flavours to detect poisonous plants. Nowadays, however, with a surplus supply of salt, fat, and sugar, these natural human preferences are proving detrimental to our health.[6] That is why it is important to recognize and respond to these preferences without eating too much of the substances that are associated with such negative consequences. While fat is a distinctly promising candidate for classification as an official flavour, the picture for spice is quite different: spicy flavours are only detected thanks to a burning sensation on the tongue and not in the classic manner via our taste buds.[7] Nonetheless, in the right proportions, spicy flavours can make all the difference to the taste of our food.

Balance is vital for good taste

Interesting food relies on the interplay between these 5 + 2 flavours, with one or other flavour being given slightly more prominence in a dish. It is this complexity that ensures you derive pleasure from eating, from the very first spoonful until you have cleared your plate. When the flavours in a dish are perfectly balanced, this can transform your perception from "tastes okay" to "tastes incredible".

A first impression might suggest the need for some more salt, but closer consideration could reveal that additional acidity or sweetness would be a better way to enhance the overall flavour. However, it is not necessary for every individual component on the plate to be in total harmony to make food interesting.

The 5 + 2 recipe building blocks

Using recipe building blocks is a concept that will automatically ensure all the important flavours are present in one dish. It also means that the two cornerstones of great taste are incorporated: consistency and temperature.

The issue of smell is also hugely significant because a large component of what we describe as taste is actually perceived via our sense of smell. Just try tasting a dish while holding your nose and you will notice how much of the flavour is lost. To get a better understanding of the five key flavours, a brief description of each is given on the next page.

Bitter

Foods with bitter components help promote digestion.[8] Lots of the bitter substances they contain also have other health benefits. These substances can be found in foods such as brassicas, citrus fruits, cocoa, herbal teas, and many other plant-based sources.[9] However, bitter flavours should never dominate and are best when subtly perceptible, rounding off the overall profile of the dish.

Sweet

Sweetness is one of the two flavours most often lacking in savoury dishes. In traditional cuisine, it is often introduced through the subtle addition of some sugar or a syrup, but it can also be produced by using alternative sweeteners, such as date sugar or sugar alcohols like erythritol. From a nutritional health perspective, we recommend adding a sweet note by using nutritious fresh or dried fruit or sweeter vegetables, such as sweet potatoes or carrots. In this book, in addition to wholesome fruit, we primarily use our home-made date paste (see p.97).

Salty

Very few cooked dishes lack salt, yet most people instinctively reach for the salt when seasoning their food. However, too much salt is bad for our health (see p.66).[10] That is why salt is only added in small quantities to the recipes in this book; instead we work with home-made stock paste (see p.99), miso, and soy sauce. Some foods, like celery, also introduce a salty flavour to recipes.[11]

Sour

Sourness is another component that is often lacking in food. But a subtle sour note is an excellent way to introduce a fresh flavour to a recipe. Citrus fruits are a great way to incorporate this flavour, but a couple of drops of vinegar or other fruits (such as some varieties of apples) can also add a pleasant sour element. In the recipes from p.102, we focus primarily on lemon juice, lime juice, cider vinegar, and sour fruits.

Umami

The term "umami" was coined in Japan in 1910 and essentially means flavourful, savoury, hearty, and meaty.[12] This rich flavour is found in particular in foods containing glutamates, which are found in protein-rich animal products but also in a range of plant-based foods. These should not be confused with the flavour enhancer monosodium glutamate (MSG).[13] Preparation techniques, such as baking and roasting, can also introduce plenty of umami to a recipe by creating toasted notes. This can even be achieved at low temperatures between 160 and 180 °C (320 and 350°F). This book uses lots of different sources of umami to ensure our plant-based cuisine incorporates this popular savoury flavour. This includes the following ingredients.

High-quality soy sauce: There are huge differences in the quality of soy sauce, which are usually also reflected in the price. Try to choose the highest-quality organic product. Shoyu is a variety of soy sauce that contains gluten, while tamari is gluten-free. The recipes in this book deliberately avoid the use of low-salt soy sauces; instead, they simply use smaller quantities of the tastier, high-salt varieties.

Dried mushrooms: When they are dried, mushrooms develop an incredibly intense umami flavour. Shiitake mushrooms are particularly rich in glutamates, as are maitake mushrooms and porcini. For example, you can grind dried shiitake mushrooms in a food processor and add a level teaspoon to any dish to produce a heartier flavour.

Miso paste: Originally from Japan, this is a spice paste usually produced from fermented soya beans, with lots of different varieties and qualities available. Nowadays you can even get miso made from lupins, lentils, and peas. Varieties like hatcho miso, which are matured for a long time, are dark, firm, and have an intense flavour, while paler varieties like shiro miso are matured for a shorter period and have a more subtle flavour. In our recipes, we mainly use shiro miso as it has a pleasantly mild, slightly sweet taste that is suitable for lots of different dishes. If you are allergic to soya, you should use a pale lupin miso instead.

Nutritional yeast/yeast flakes: These involve yeast that has been deactivated by heat. In addition to containing a high density of B vitamins, this product has very high levels of glutamates. Yeast flakes are a healthy seasoning ingredient; however, people with autoimmune conditions like Crohn's disease should avoid all kinds of yeast (yeast flakes, baking yeast, and brewer's yeast) because it can exacerbate their symptoms.[14] There are lots of different brands which vary in quality and flavour. Good-quality yeast flakes have a pleasantly savoury flavour and should not taste bitter.

A list of specific product recommendations for miso paste, soy sauce, yeast flakes, and other products can be found at www.nikorittenau.com/healthy-vegan.

Fat

Fat is an important flavour carrier, which makes it an essential component in all cuisines. Certain fats also play an important role from a health perspective. The addition of fatty ingredients greatly improves the subjective taste of a dish – whether the fat is from nutritious foods such as nuts, seeds, or avocados, or from virgin vegetable oils. However, oils and margarines, etc. should be used in moderation. Good vegan food can be created with a moderate quantity of fat and, in order to maintain your ideal weight in the long

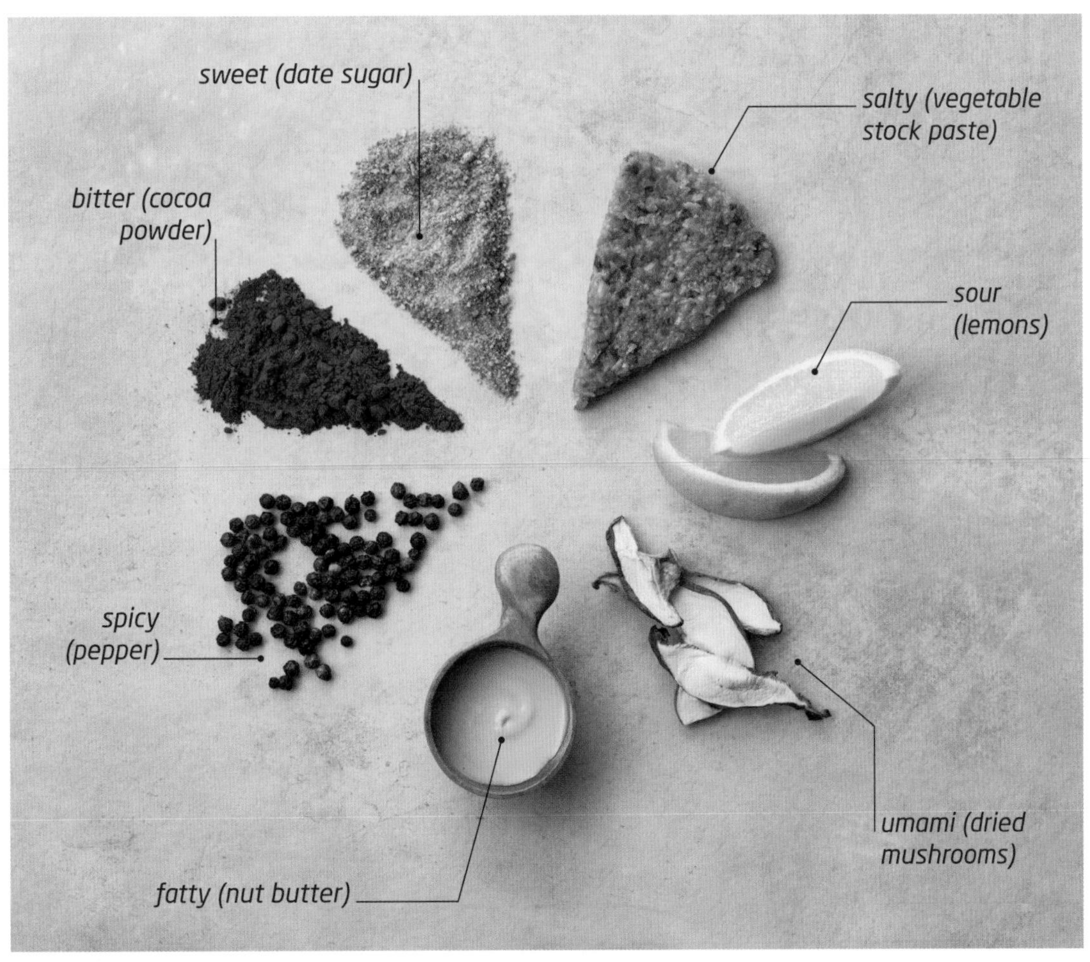

term, it is important to learn how to make things taste good without adding large quantities of fat. Our recipes predominantly use nutritious sources of fat like nuts, seeds, nut butters, and moderate amounts of high-quality oils, e.g. virgin olive oil.

Spice

Spice is not a flavour in the proper sense, being perceived instead as a physical burning sensation. Nonetheless, the right level of spice can create interesting recipes. Caution is needed here, because too much spice can quickly make a dish inedible. Our recipes mainly use pepper, ginger, and hot ground paprika to add a pleasant spicy note to the food.

Temperature, texture, and consistency

In addition to balancing different flavours, the use of different temperatures is another important technique for creating food that tastes and feels more interesting. By incorporating something hot in a dish with cool components, the resulting contrast creates a real wow factor that would be absent if everything was the same temperature. Whether it is a chilled vegetable component as part of a warm dish, a salad as part of a bowl, or a cool "nice cream" (see p.235) served with a slice of freshly baked cake – these temperature differences can greatly enhance the overall impact of a dish.

The third cornerstone for creating delicious healthy food involves texture and consistency. A good example to illustrate the importance of different textures within a dish is a creamy soup. Even if the soup is beautifully seasoned, it can soon seem rather dull thanks to its homogeneous, smooth consistency: every spoonful tastes identical and has the same mouthfeel. The addition of different texture elements helps introduce some variety to the dish. So, you can elevate your pumpkin soup to a whole different level by adding a couple of cubes of umami tofu (see p.201), plus some of the crunchy apple and coriander topping (see p.216) and a blob of the cold yogurt and garlic sauce (see p.211).

The recipe building blocks

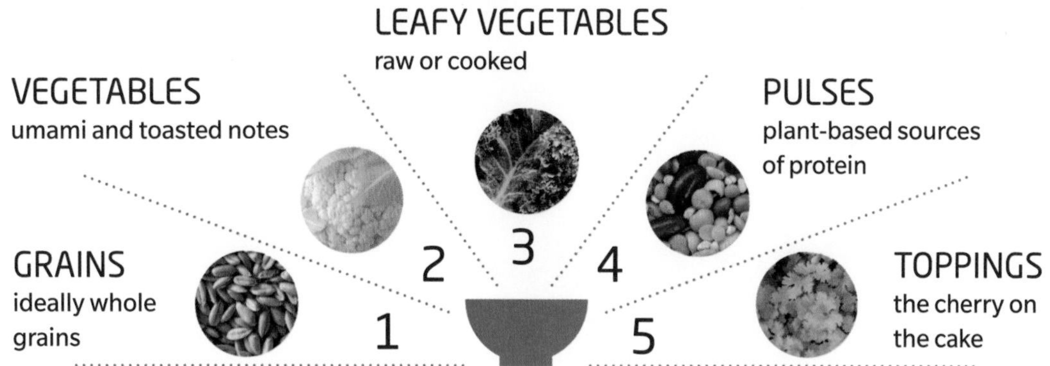

The recipe building blocks in this book are a simple way of creating unbeatable food both in terms of flavour and from a nutritional health perspective. We have both been working with this system for a long time and it has been used as the basis for compiling all the main recipes in this book. That is why the main courses section consists of lots of separate recipes, which can be freely combined depending on what you fancy eating. By combining individual components within this building block system, you can create tasty, nutritious food that is easy to prepare, making it extremely practical for everyday life. The recipe building blocks in this book are limited to main courses. The sections on breakfast and dessert include a whole range of variations and extra ideas to allow for more variety, but these recipes are not building block dishes.

How the recipe building blocks work

Every main dish that is prepared using the building block system should always consist of the following five components:

(whole) grains, vegetables, leafy vegetables, pulses, topping

The recipe sections incorporate the main food groups in a vegan diet, which were discussed in the theory section of this book. An optimal supply of nutrients can be ensured by combining these recipes. While the three main food groups – (whole) grains, (leafy) vegetables, and pulses – turn up in the building block system under the same names that are used in the preceding theory section, the other two categories – fruit and nuts/seeds – are incorporated in the building block system as part of the toppings and also, to some extent, within the other building block components. The combination of recipes ensures the synergistic effect of the individual components from a nutritional perspective, while also creatively incorporating all the previously discussed elements that are vital for gastronomic enjoyment, such as different flavours, textures, and temperatures. The result is healthy food that tastes absolutely delicious. As a bonus, these practical recipes are also perfect for implementing in your everyday life.

Each recipe within the building block system comes from one of the categories for the five components that are described in more detail below. These recipes can be freely combined because they all go beautifully together. For even greater variety, many of the recipes include extra suggested alternatives. This offers an incredible number of combination options, for greater variety and more flexibility in the kitchen.

Version 1: The 5-component system

In the 5-component system you combine at least three gourmet components with two basic components to create a nutritious meal. Of course, other combinations are also possible, such as four gourmet components + one basic dish, or even five gourmet components.

Gourmet component 1: leafy vegetables green salad with date vinaigrette (see p.177)

Gourmet component 2: topping golden yogurt sauce (see p.220)

Basic component 1: vegetables; steamed carrots (see p.154)

Gourmet component 3: pulses; umami bean stew (see p.202)

Basic component 2: grains; millet (see p.135)

Version 2: The 3-component system

If you are short of time, reduce the combination to three components, keeping the grains, pulses, and vegetables. At least two gourmet components should be included to make the meal as interesting as possible.

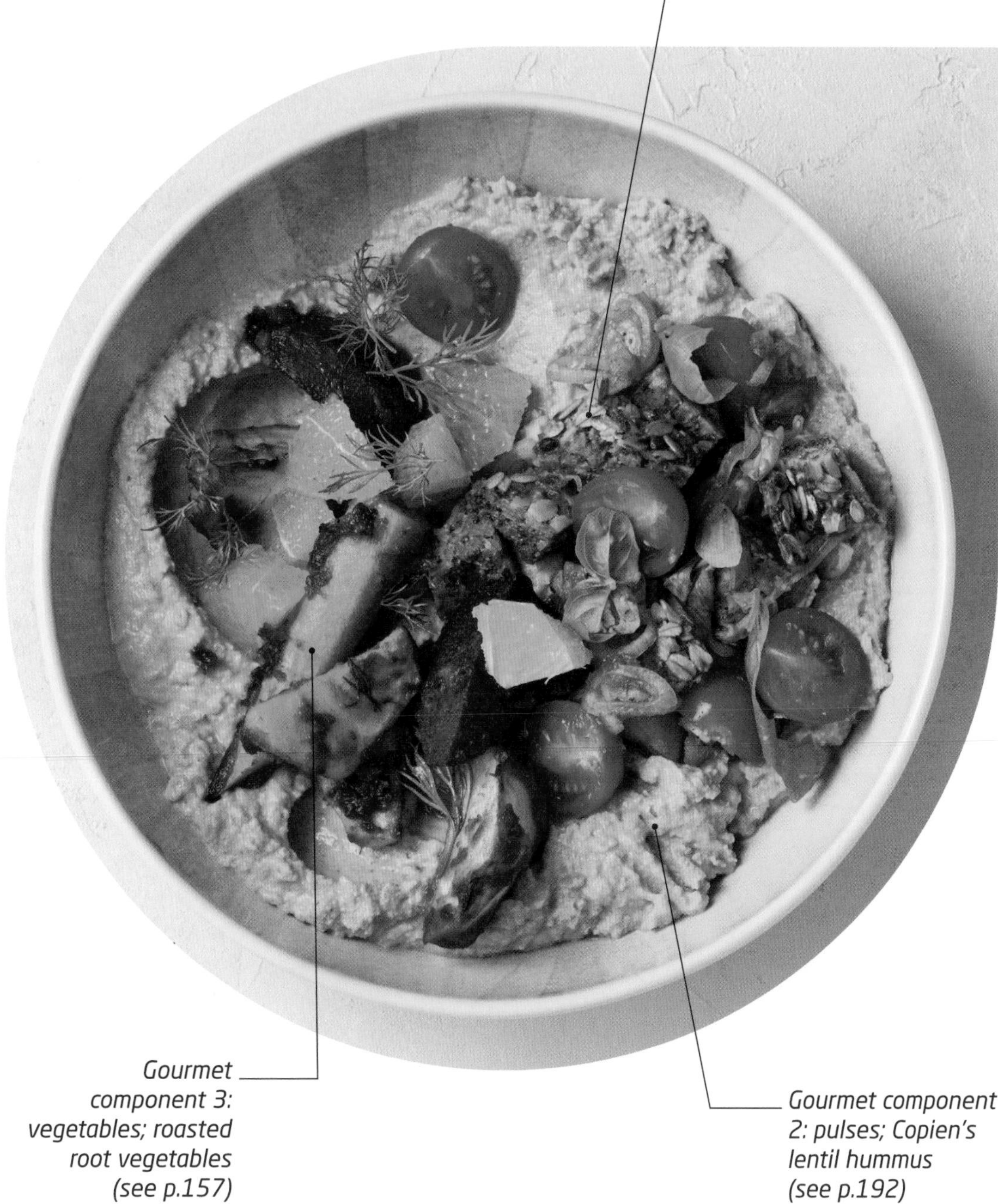

Gourmet component 1: grains; wholegrain panzanella (see p.146)

Gourmet component 3: vegetables; roasted root vegetables (see p.157)

Gourmet component 2: pulses; Copien's lentil hummus (see p.192)

The 5 components

1. Grains

Serve them up in risotto, salads, rissoles, bread, pasta, polenta, or sushi – grains are incredibly versatile and have formed part of the human diet for tens of thousands of years.[15, 16] On pp.135–139, you will find the basic components. These are followed by recipes for transforming the basic ingredients into gourmet components for the building block system (see p.140 onwards). The recipes involve simple yet sophisticated techniques that can be used with all sorts of grains to create meals packed with flavour. There is always the option of preparing a basic component and serving it just as it is. Adding a suitable topping is another way to create a delicious meal.

2. Vegetables

Root vegetables, onions, inflorescence vegetables, and fruiting vegetables – there is such diversity on offer within the vegetable category. With the right preparation, there is something for everyone. We start quite simply with some steamed basic components on p.154, which you can jazz up with an appropriate topping. The gourmet components in the vegetable category (see p.157 onwards) include plenty of tips and are all packed with umami flavours, so vegetables can take a starring role on your plate. If vegetables do not taste great, this is usually down to how they have been prepared rather than the vegetables themselves.

3. Leafy green vegetables

Rocket, kale, spinach, and a wide variety of (wild) herbs make up the group of dark leafy green vegetables. All these plants are very rich in nutrients and should be included in the human diet every day. That is why these foods have been given their own category alongside the other vegetables. You can prepare leafy green vegetables very simply as a basic component – either served raw with a dash of lemon, or steamed. From p.174, you will find recipe ideas for gourmet components using leafy green vegetables, some of which are served raw while others are cooked to create exceptionally delicious dishes.

4. Pulses

Whether used as a topping on bread, or as a veggie burger, in salads, or processed to create tofu and tempeh – pulses represent a high-quality, cheap, and delicious source of nutritious protein. You can easily get started with the straightforward basic components on pp.189–191. After this, you will find the gourmet pulse components (see p.192 onwards) with hearty recipes that are packed with flavour while also being really filling and providing the perfect, protein-rich focus for your meal. From the umami bean stew (see p.202), to the Mediterranean bean salad (see p.196), the tempeh rissoles (see p.200), and the umami tofu (see p.201), there is something here to suit every taste.

5. Toppings

Last but not least, we have the cherry on the cake: the topping. All the topping recipes from p.211 in this book are quick and easy to prepare. The toppings are an important part of the building block system that can enhance even the simplest basic components, so a gourmet topping should always be part of your building block dish. The toppings are particularly interesting because they incorporate ingredients from the food groups containing fruits, nuts, and seeds, enhancing the overall dish both in terms of flavour and from a health perspective. You do not need to prepare toppings from scratch every single day. We always recommend tripling or quadrupling the quantities because all the toppings keep for at least three days if stored in an airtight container in the fridge.

If you are short of time, you can use three components instead of five. There is more information about this on p.95.

Preparing components

When using the recipe building block system to create healthy, nutritious meals, you soon come up against two components that can be tricky to fit into your everyday routine due to the time and flexibility they require. These are the nutritious grains on the one hand, and the pulses and beans on the other. Both these food groups involve long preparation times; they often need to be soaked overnight and are cooked for a very long time. This can be something of a hindrance in our hectic everyday lives. From a nutritional perspective, there is nothing against using beans and lentils from a tin or jar because these have similar nutritional values to the freshly prepared varieties.[17] From a culinary perspective, however, there is a huge difference in quality between the convenience varieties and the ones you cook yourself, which taste far better. So to make the recipe building blocks work in everyday life, you will need to cook larger quantities of both these components in advance and keep a constant supply in your fridge or freezer.

Soaking and cooking do not take time

All you need to do is soak some pulses overnight once or twice a week, then cook them the following day alongside some grains. How difficult is that? Not at all. You just need to make it a habit. Soaking takes less than a minute: put the pulses or beans in a bowl with some water and transfer it to the fridge.

The next day, the soaked pulses can be rinsed and cooked (see p. 189 onwards). The cooking process does not require any intervention on your part and afterwards you will have supplies for almost the whole week. While the pulses are cooking, you can use the time to do other things. You do not need to be constantly standing over the hob as they boil. If you cook the soaked pulses in a pressure cooker, the cooking time will be even shorter. By having these basics in your fridge, it only takes 15–30 minutes to conjure up a dish that is delicious to eat and incredibly good for you, too.

If the pre-cooked grains and pulses are stored as recommended in the recipes, they can be used for a good four to five days without going off. Once you have used up all your supplies, you can always use the quick pulse and grain recipes with shorter cooking times. For grains, these include wholewheat couscous or pearl barley, and for pulses you can use tofu, tempeh, or lentils. Alternatively, of course, you could simply start a new cycle of soaking and cooking to make fresh supplies of pulses and grains for the recipes with longer cooking times.

We recommend choosing one or two days in the week specifically as soaking days, so you can cook the grains and pulses the following day. Friday is a good soaking day for lots of people. Just soak your pulses the evening before the weekend starts, then while you are tidying the house or having a relaxed breakfast the next day, get the grains and pulses cooking at the same time.

The healthy and delicious challenge

The challenge here is to change your old habits. People need to repeat things a few times to make them part of their normal routine. That is why we challenge our readers to implement this system for at least ten weeks. Research shows that people need this long (66 days to be precise) to incorporate new habits permanently in their everyday lives.[18] After a while, you will notice that soaking and cooking the grains and pulses no longer seems like an arduous chore, it just happens seamlessly as a routine part of your everyday life.

Once you are familiar with the recipe building blocks, you will find it greatly enhances the way you feel about everyday food and you won't want to eat any other way.

The implementation

Once your fridge is fully stocked with precooked whole grains and pulses, you have all the basics you need to make nutritious meals in just a few steps. Now there are lots of options for using the recipe building blocks to suit your individual preferences. Whether you need a quick and easy meal, or you have time for more laborious preparation for a real culinary treat, this system opens all sorts of possibilities.

If you are short of time, you should always get at least three components from the building block system on your plate (see opposite). For the full nutritional and culinary scope, however, we recommend using a total of five building block components.

If you choose version 1, so you prepare a recipe from each of the five categories (grains, vegetables, leafy vegetables, pulses, toppings), this may take slightly longer depending on your choice of components and recipes and how skilled a cook you are. If you choose the simplified version 2 of the recipe building blocks, with three components, the preparation time will be much shorter but the result nonetheless delicious. So, you can create satisfying, healthy meals in a short time even on days when life is stressful.

Version 1

Meal with 5 components

min. 3 gourmet components
max. 2 basic components

Version 2

Meal with 3 components

min. 2 gourmet components
max. 1 basic component

You should also watch the video at www.nikorittenau.com/healthy-vegan

Version 1: The 5-component system

There are the following four basic components:

1. **Precooked grains** (already in the fridge – see recipes pp.135–139). Briefly reheat in a pan with no additional fat (e.g. brown rice, millet, couscous, etc.).
2. **Precooked pulses** (already in the fridge – see recipes pp.189 and 191). Briefly reheat in a pan with no fat (e.g. chickpeas, white beans, beluga lentils, etc.).
3. **Steamed vegetables** (see recipe p.154). These should be served with your choice of topping to round off the flavour.
4. **Steamed leafy green vegetables** or dressed leaves. Here you can simply season a handful of leaves with a dash of lemon juice and add them to the meal.

In the 5-component system, your menu plan should include no more than two of these basic components to avoid the final meal being too monotonous. You can then add in your chosen gourmet components. Opposite you will find a couple of examples of possible combinations.

5-component combinations

	GRAINS	PULSES	VEGETABLES	LEAFY VEGETABLES	TOPPINGS
1	Spelt risotto (see p.145)	Umami tofu (see p.201)	Steamed broccoli (see p.154)	Green salad with yogurt dressing (see p.177)	Pear, basil, and walnut topping (see p.220)
2	Cooked millet (see p.135)	Umami bean stew (see p.202)	Steamed carrots (see p.154)	Green salad with date vinaigrette (see p.177)	Golden yogurt sauce (see p.220)
3	Cooked brown rice (see p.136)	Mediterranean bean salad (see p.196)	Risotto-style carrots (see p.158)	Steamed swiss chard (see p.154)	Yogurt and garlic sauce (see p.211)
4	Beetroot pearl barley (see p.146)	Copien's lentil hummus (see p.192)	Steamed beetroot (see p.154)	Steamed pak choi (see p.154)	Yogurt and garlic sauce (see p.211)
5	Cooked pearl barley (see p.138)	Tempeh rissoles (see p.200)	Roasted sweet potato purée (see p.170)	Steamed spinach (see p.154).	Berry and ginger chutney (see p.213)
6	Cooked brown rice (see p.136)	Paneer (see p.207)	Cauliflower steak (see p.160)	Palak (see p.184)	Sesame and coriander pesto (see p.216)
7	Citrus quinoa (see p.141)	Green peppercorn and tempeh in a creamy sauce (see p.204)	Vegetables pickled in vinegar and spice (see p.162)	Steamed savoy cabbage (see p154).	Cheesy pumpkin seed pesto (see p.218)

Version 2: The 3-component system

Of course, we all have days when we are lacking the energy or motivation to cook. That is why we always recommend preparing a bit more of all the components in a larger batch, because you can happily eat the same dish at least twice in a row. By using our meal prep techniques, you can even prepare meals in advance for several days and store them in the fridge, so there will always be something ready to eat on the more stressful days in your week.

As well as using the advance meal prep strategy, you can use a slimmed-down version of the recipe building blocks and make meals using just three components. Below we show a few 3-component combinations that work particularly well in our experience. But all sorts of combinations are perfectly possible. If meals are being prepared following the reduced version of the system, we recommend always including one grain component, one pulse component, and one vegetable component (see table below). The three components should include no more than one basic recipe to avoid the meal being too dull.

3-component combinations

	GRAINS	PULSES	VEGETABLES/LEAFY VEGETABLES
1	Wholemeal panzanella (see p.146)	Copien's lentil hummus (see p.192)	Roasted root vegetables (see p.157)
2	Cooked pearl barley (see p.138)	Tempeh rissoles (see p.200)	Roasted sweet potato purée (see p.170)
3	Smoky millet polenta (see p.150)	Curried legume salad (see p.197)	Cauliflower steak (see p.160)
4	Curried rice rissoles (see p.148)	Green peppercorn and tempeh in creamy sauce (see p.204)	Vegetable gratin with Asian peanut sauce (see p.158)
5	Spelt risotto (see p.145)	Mediterranean bean salad (see p.196)	Steamed beetroot (see p.154)
6	Golden milk couscous (see p.141)	Umami tofu (see p.201)	Greens with peas (see p.180)
7	Cooked brown rice (see p.136)	Umami bean stew (see p.202)	Tahini spinach (see p.174)

Quantities and preparation

This book uses quantities such as tbsp – tablespoon, tsp – teaspoon, g – grams, and oz – ounces. Digital scales are always the most accurate way to measure ingredients.

The terms tbsp and tsp refer to average spoon sizes and these are always slightly heaped. This means a slight curve in your serving of ground paprika, not a mountain! For liquids, tbsp and tsp indicate full level quantities. In some cases, a level tsp is required even when not measuring a liquid. This is always explicitly noted in the relevant recipe.

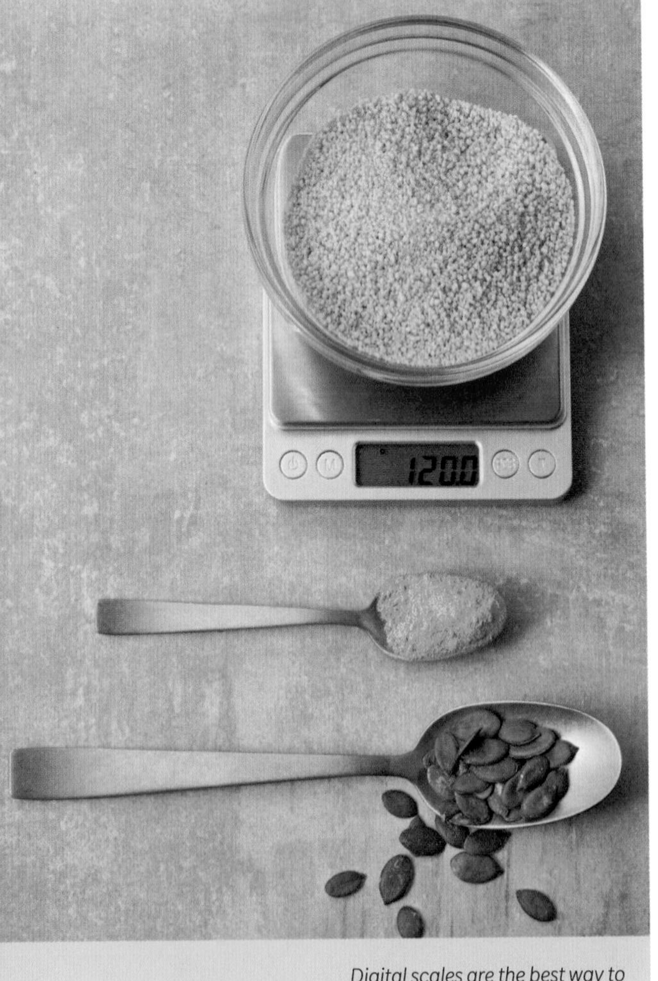

Digital scales are the best way to measure precise quantities.

When you follow a recipe for the first time, it is best to keep strictly to the specified quantities and preparation method. The quantities and process have always been chosen for good reason. Of course, once you have tested the results, we certainly recommend creativity and experimentation. It's a fun way to cook and you will learn a huge amount, too.

To make sure you can follow the instructions easily, we recommend first having a large, clean area to work in, and secondly, good "mise en place" – the preparation of the ingredients in the work area. First, prepare the ingredients. Clean, chop, and put them in little bowls ready for when you start the actual cooking process. Tasks like preheating the oven or boiling water can naturally also be done in advance to save time. But this is always described in detail in each recipe.

If you want to make one of the main meals from the recipe building blocks, we recommend that you read through all the instructions first and check which tasks will take most time. For example, if you are making the umami bean stew (see p.202), which should ideally simmer for at least 15 minutes, you should put this on to cook at the beginning and then perhaps focus on preparing the Mediterranean grain salad (see p.142). The vegetable side dishes can be steamed in the meantime, and it takes no time to add a dash of lemon juice to a handful of rocket for the leafy greens component. As a simple topping, you could scatter over some smoky umami gomasio, and you have a quick, delicious, and exceptionally healthy meal.

Basics: Date paste and vegetable stock paste

Instead of seasoning with salt or adding sugar, in our recipes we use Sebastian's date paste and the reduced-salt vegetable stock.

This has lots of nutritional benefits as well as being very tasty. Both these recipes are ideal for making in advance because they will keep for a while in the fridge.

The perfect sweetener – Copien's date paste

Makes about 500g (1lb 2oz) paste

200g (7oz) soft Deglet Noor dates, stones removed | 300ml (10fl oz) water | 1 slice of organic lemon (about 2cm/¾in thick) | 1 tbsp lemon juice | 1 pinch of salt

Put the dates in a pan with 300ml (10fl oz) of water, cover, and heat. Simmer for about 10 minutes to destroy any possible spores on the fruit. This will prevent the paste going mouldy later.

Now put all the ingredients in a food processor with cooking water and purée until smooth. Transfer the paste to a clean container, screw on the lid, and store in the fridge for up to 2 weeks.

BASTI'S TIP

If the dates are very hard or you do not have a powerful food processor, just soak them in water overnight before blending.

VARIATION

Instead of the lemon, you could use 1 slice of organic orange and add 2 dried rose petals. This gives a wonderfully fruity, floral aroma.
To create an Asian umami sauce, blend 100g (3½oz) of date paste, 1 piece of ginger (3cm/1in), 100ml (3fl oz) of soy sauce, 1 garlic clove, 1 tbsp of shiro miso and 1 tbsp of peanut butter. The sauce will keep for 1–2 weeks in the fridge and can be used to round off various recipes, either cooked with the ingredients or just added at the end.

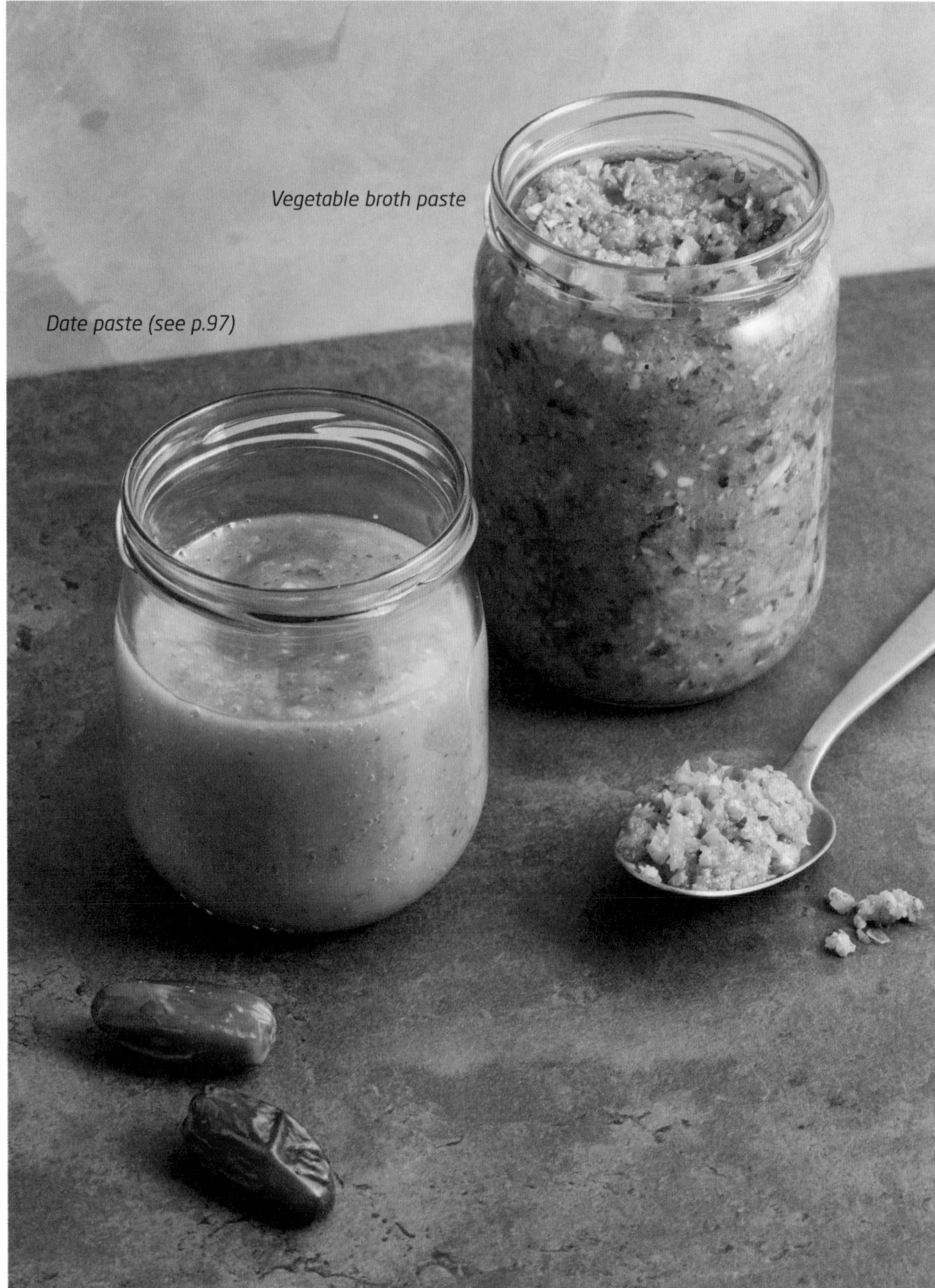
Vegetable broth paste
Date paste (see p.97)

Reduced-salt vegetable stock paste – never be without good-quality stock again

Makes about 1kg (2¼lb)

100g (3½oz) onions, peeled and diced (about 3 small onions) | 100g (3½oz) leek, sliced in rings | 200g (7oz) celeriac, cubed | 100g (3½oz) celery with greens, diced | 200g (7oz) carrots, peeled and finely chopped | 3 garlic cloves, peeled | 30g (1oz) parsley, finely chopped | 100g (3½oz) tomatoes, diced | 2 tbsp dried lovage | 10 black peppercorns | 6 juniper berries | 5g (⅛oz) dried porcini (or dried shiitake mushrooms) | 7 bay leaves | 6 Deglet Noor dates, stones removed | 4 tbsp shiro miso | 5 tbsp olive oil | 110g (4oz) sea salt (or rock salt)

Put all the ingredients except the salt into a food processor and purée until you have a thick but slightly coarse-grained paste. Stir in the salt. Transfer the vegetable purée to a pan and simmer gently for 15 minutes. Decant the hot paste into clean screw-top jars, seal and turn upside down before leaving to cool. Keeps for a couple of months in the fridge.

Important: The consistency should be very slightly coarse and not like a smoothie, otherwise the stock paste will froth up too much. The salt is essential as a preservative. Normally my stock pastes have a ratio of six parts vegetable to one part salt. In which case you can also preserve them raw. In this recipe, we use a ratio of eight parts vegetable to one part salt and we boil the paste, so it keeps for longer. This paste can also be made with a standard blender. In which case, add no more than two handfuls of roughly chopped vegetables to the container and use the pulse function to process to a rough consistency. Then empty it out and continue until everything has been processed. Otherwise there is a danger that the mixture can end up being too fine or runny.

Use: Add as much paste as required to a pan with water – roughly 2 tbsp–1 litre (1¾ pints) of water – and simmer gently for 15 minutes. This will produce a wonderful stock.

Sometimes in this book, we recommend replacing salt with your stock paste to further reduce the quantity of salt. It makes a perfect salt substitute to add flavour to your food.

BASTI'S TIP

The quantity is designed for a large clip-top jar with a capacity of 1.5 litres (2¾ pints), which will accommodate about 1kg (2¼lb) of vegetable stock paste. If that is too much for you, simply halve the quantities for all the ingredients.

For more flavour, just fry the paste in a pan with no oil until brown. Add a splash of water, loosen the bits that have stuck to the pan, let the water simmer off and fry the paste once more. This process is known as deglazing and it helps produce a more intense flavour. Repeat this process two to three times, then cover the paste with water and simmer for at least 15 minutes.

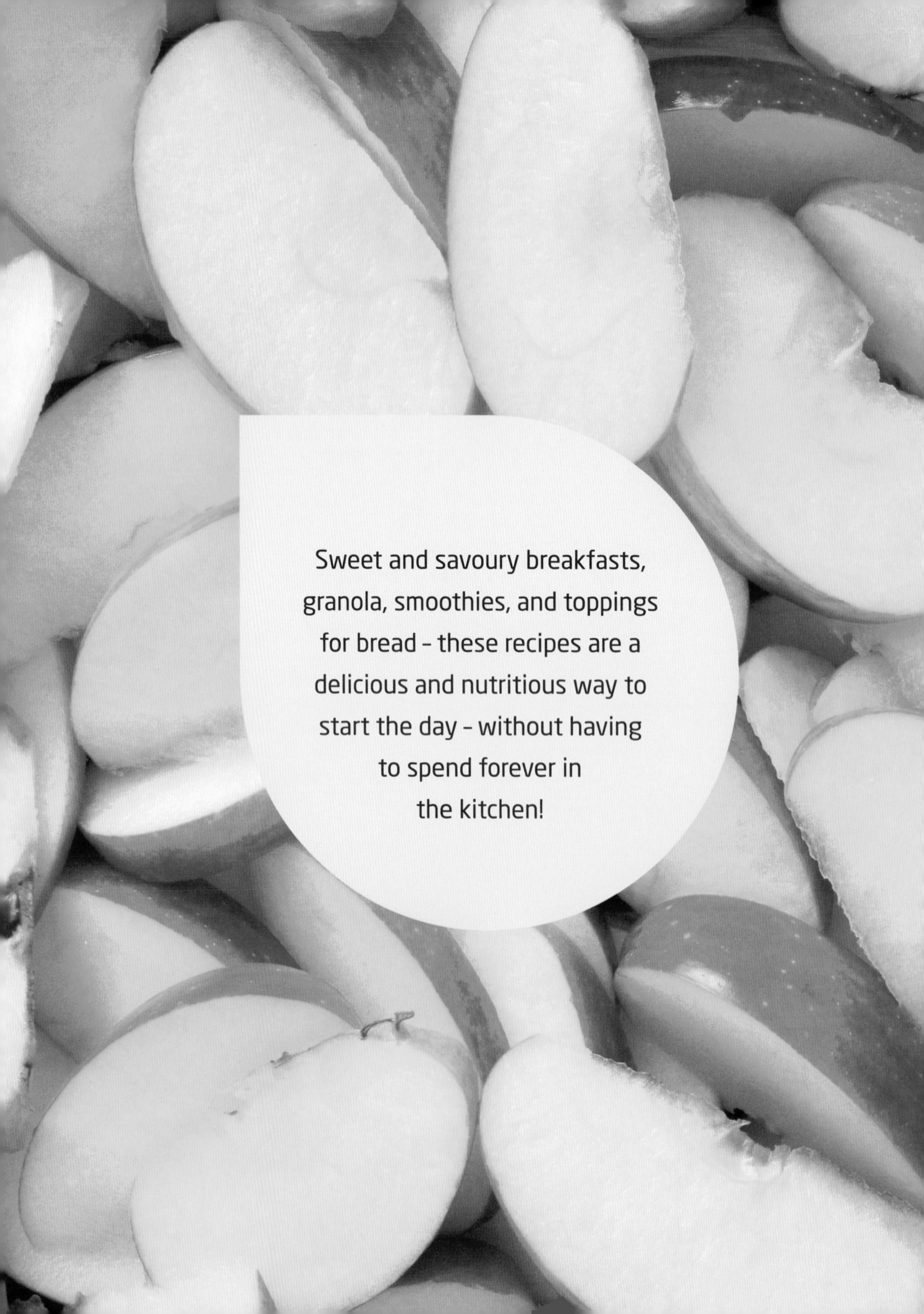

Sweet and savoury breakfasts, granola, smoothies, and toppings for bread – these recipes are a delicious and nutritious way to start the day – without having to spend forever in the kitchen!

Breakfast

Zen oats with poached pears and almond cream

Serves 3

Zen oats: 4 Deglet Noor dates, stones removed | 100g (3½oz) oat flakes (if desired, gluten-free or sprouted) | 50g (1¾oz) buckwheat grains | 1 tsp organic lemon zest | pinch of salt
Poached pears: piece of fresh root ginger (2cm/¾in), peeled | 1 slice of organic lemon (2cm/¾in) | 1 cinnamon stick (or 2 star anise) | 2 small, slightly firm pears (e.g. Williams)
Almond cream: 50g (1¾oz) white almond nut butter | 75ml (2½fl oz) hot cooking liquid from the pears | 1 tbsp frozen blueberries | pinch of salt
Topping: 2 tbsp pumpkin seeds, toasted | 4–6 tbsp frozen blueberries

Nutritional values per portion: 418 kcal | 52.9g carbohydrate | 17.2g fat | 12.6g protein | 8.2g fibre | 0.1g ALA | 584mg lysine | 70mg calcium | 2.8mg zinc | 3.6mg iron | 0.1mg B2 | < 0.1mg RE | 2µg iodine | 0.7g salt

To make the porridge, finely chop the dates and add them to a small pan with the oats, buckwheat, 600ml (1 pint) of water, lemon zest, and salt. Bring to the boil briefly, then cover, turn off the heat and leave to stand for 10 minutes.

For the poached pears, first put the ginger, slice of lemon, and cinnamon into a small pan with 300ml (10fl oz) of water and bring to the boil. Meanwhile, wash, quarter, and core the pears and add them to the spiced cooking liquid. Return to the boil and leave the pears to steep for 10 minutes.

To make the almond cream, stir all the ingredients together with a balloon whisk until well combined. Divide the zen oats between three bowls. Top with almond cream, poached pears, and pumpkin seeds, then garnish with frozen blueberries to serve.

BASTI'S TIP

If you don't want to make the components separately, slice the pears into 1cm (½in) cubes and finely chop the ginger, then cook everything in water together with the cinnamon stick, slice of lemon, and grains. Scatter over the seeds and berries and stir in a spoonful of almond butter. And it's ready!

A dash of beetroot juice in the cooking water will give the pears a wonderful colour.

Drink the leftover poaching water from the pears as tea with your breakfast.

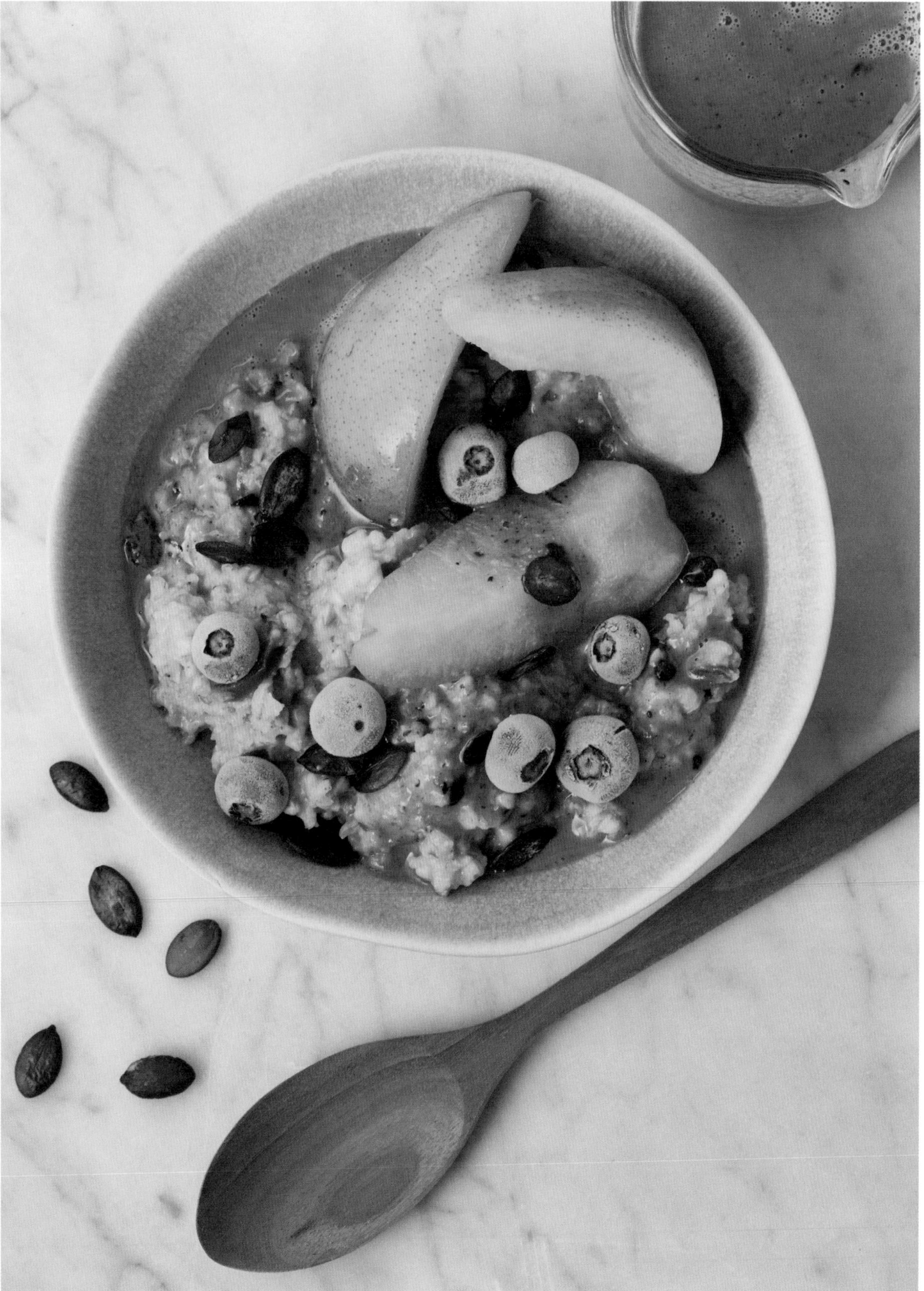

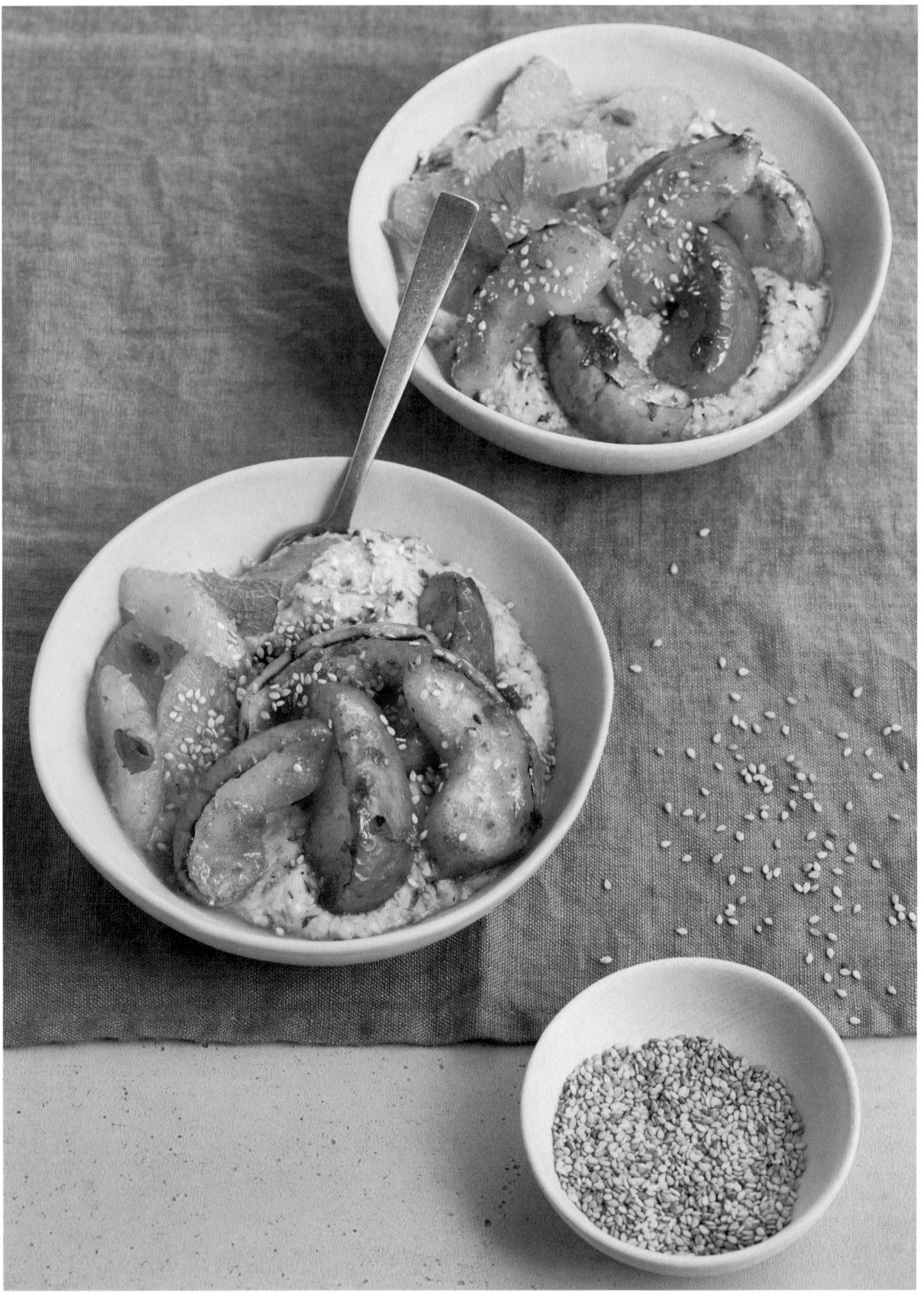

Pumpkin seeds and oats with citrus salad, baked apples

Serves 3

Oats: 60g (2oz) pumpkin seeds | pinch of salt | 120g (4oz) oat flakes | 4 Deglet Noor dates, stones removed
Baked apples: 2 small, slightly tart apples (e.g. Braeburn) |1 tsp olive oil | 2 tbsp date paste (see p.97) | pinch of vanilla powder (or ground cinnamon)
Citrus salad: 1 juicy orange | 1 lemon | 4 mint leaves | 1 tbsp date paste (see p.97)
Topping: 3 tbsp sesame seeds, toasted

Nutritional values per portion: 505 kcal | 62.3g carbohydrate | 19.3g fat | 16.5g protein | 13g fibre | 0.1g ALA | 120mg lysine | 139mg calcium | 3.7mg zinc | 4.8mg iron | < 0.1mg B2 | < 0.1mg RE | 5µg iodine | 0.3g salt

Preheat the oven to 200°C (180°C fan/400°F/Gas 6).

Put the pumpkin seeds in a pan with 600ml (1 pint) of water and the salt, bring to the boil briefly then blend in a food processor to make a smooth pumpkin seed milk. Pour the oats into a bowl and cover with the pumpkin seed milk. Finely chop the dates, add to the mix, and leave everything to stand for about 10 minutes.

Wash, quarter, and core the apples ready for baking. Mix the apples, olive oil, date paste, and vanilla in a bowl and rub in the marinade well. Place the apples on a baking tray lined with baking paper, slide into the oven roughly 10cm (4in) below the grill element and grill for 6–8 minutes until the apples are turning brown.

Segment the citrus fruit for the salad by removing the flesh from the membrane. Shred the mint leaves. Gently mix the citrus fruit segments, mint, and date paste in a bowl. Once the oats have steeped sufficiently but still have a bit of bite, divide them between three bowls and garnish with the baked apples, citrus salad, and sesame seeds.

VARIATION

You can add other dried fruits to the oats rather than dates. Instead of the pumpkin seeds, try sunflower seeds or cashews, or leave out the seeds and replace half the water for the oats with coconut milk, oat cream, or soya cream.

BASTI'S TIP

Instead of cooking the oats until slimy, they are simply immersed in hot liquid and left to stand. This produces a lovely creamy consistency with a slight bite.

Wholemeal pancakes with creamy mushrooms and apple salsa

Serves 3

Pancakes: 150g (5½oz) wholemeal spelt flour | 25g (scant 1oz) cornflour | 1 tsp bicarbonate of soda | 1 tsp cider vinegar | 1 tbsp date paste (see p.97) | ½ tsp salt | 150g (5½oz) smoked tofu | olive oil for cooking
Creamy mushrooms: 50g (1¾oz) onion, peeled | 1 tbsp shiitake mushroom powder (about 4g/scant 1 tsp; see tip p.144) | 450ml (15fl oz) light vegetable stock | 2 tsp cider vinegar | 50g (1¾oz) white almond nut butter (or cashew nut butter) | 50g (1¾oz) button mushrooms, cleaned and quartered | freshly ground pepper | salt
Apple salsa: 1 small, slightly tart apple, thinly sliced |1 tbsp lemon juice (or lime juice) | 4 tbsp finely chopped herbs (e.g. dill, parsley, rocket)

Nutritional values per portion: 596 kcal | 79.9g carbohydrate | 20.4g fat | 19.1g protein | 14.9g fibre | 2.5g ALA | 739mg lysine | 101mg calcium | 4.7mg zinc | 5.8mg iron | 0.2mg B2 | < 0.1mg RE | 5µg iodine | 1.6g salt

Combine the spelt flour, cornflour, and bicarbonate of soda in a bowl. In a second bowl, mix 250ml (9fl oz) of water, vinegar, date paste, and salt, then add this to the bowl with the flour mix and stir everything together to create a smooth batter. Slice the tofu into roughly 5mm (¼in) cubes and stir these into the mix. Heat a large non-stick pan over a moderate heat. Add 1 teaspoon of olive oil to the pan and spread it out using a heat-resistant brush or cloth.

Use a ladle to scoop three to four blobs of batter into the pan, each measuring 5cm (2in), and cook for 2–3 minutes until the edges are turning slightly brown. Carefully flip the pancakes and cook for 2–3 more minutes on the other side. Stack the cooked pancakes on a plate and cover with a clean kitchen towel. Cook the rest of the batter in the same way.

To make the creamy mushrooms, heat a large pan, finely chop the onion and add to the pan with 1 tablespoon of water, then brown the onion slightly for 2–3 minutes. Sprinkle over the mushroom powder and fry for 30 seconds. Deglaze the contents of the pan with the stock and simmer gently for 5 minutes. Add the vinegar and stir in the nut butter. Cook the sauce down until it is thick and creamy. Add the mushrooms, toss in the sauce, leave to stand for 5 minutes, then season with pepper, salt, and vinegar.

For the salsa, gently mix all the ingredients in a bowl. Stack three to four pancakes on a plate. Drizzle with mushroom cream, garnish with salsa, and eat immediately.

BASTI'S TIP

Since there is no protein in vegan pancakes, it is important to stack the pancakes and leave them to stand for 5–10 minutes after cooking. This allows the starches in the mixture to relax slightly, making the pancakes less doughy and giving them a more uniform texture.

VARIATION

Paprika sauce: when browning the onions, use 50g (1¾oz) of finely diced red pepper instead of the mushrooms, and paprika instead of mushroom powder. But take care: fry the paprika very briefly and deglaze immediately, otherwise it will go bitter. Season the finished sauce with 1 tbsp of soy sauce.

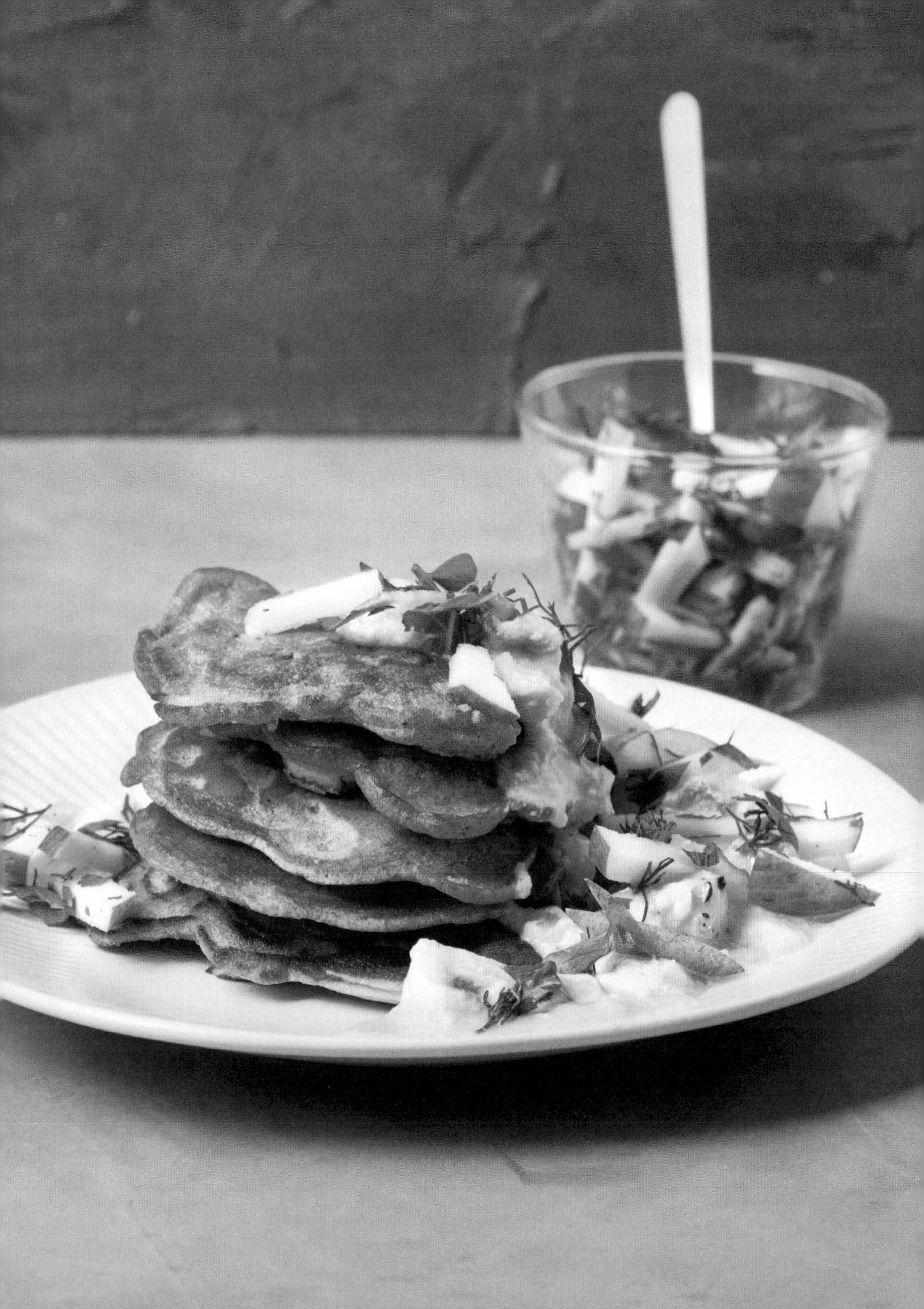

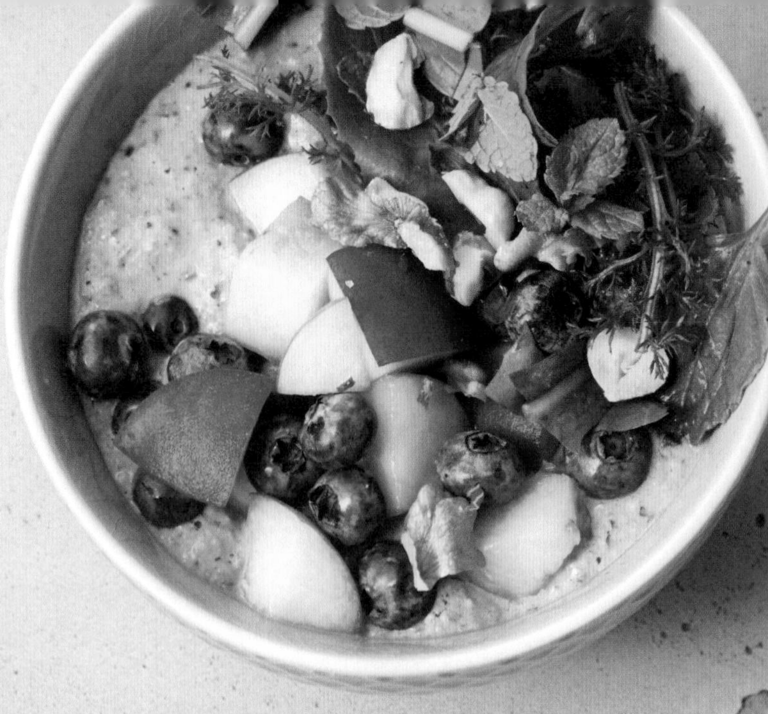

Surfer's protein bowl

Serves 2

Bowl: ½ organic lemon | 1 apple | 100g (3½oz) pumpkin seeds | 20g (¾oz) sesame seeds | 4 Deglet Noor dates, stones removed | 75g (2½oz) cooked chickpeas (or white beans; see p.191) | 125g (4½oz) mixed frozen berries | 75g (2½oz) oat flakes (or sprouted oats) | pinch of salt | good pinch of ground cloves | good pinch of ground turmeric | pinch of freshly ground pepper | 750ml (1¼ pints) soya milk with calcium (or almond milk)

Topping: 6 tbsp blueberries | 2 flat peaches | 2 small handfuls of wild herbs (e.g. ground elder, mint, thyme, ribwort) | 4 tbsp nuts (or seeds), toasted

Nutritional values per portion: 871 kcal | 82.4g carbohydrate | 38.3g fat | 33.5g protein | 19.6g fibre | 0.6g ALA | 2427mg lysine | 576mg calcium | 7.4mg zinc | 10.2mg iron | 0.2mg B2 | < 0.1mg RE | 50µg iodine | 1.1g salt

Wash the lemon in hot water, dry it, then chop into small cubes, including the skin. Wash the apple, then dice it finely, including the core. Put both in a powerful food processor with all the other ingredients for the bowl and blend to a creamy consistency.

Wash the blueberries and peaches for the topping. Dab dry the blueberries, halve the peaches, remove the stones, and chop into cubes. Finely chop the herbs. Divide the cream between two bowls and garnish with the fresh fruit, herbs, and nuts.

BASTI'S TIP

Due to the lemon zest, this mixture soon becomes bitter. It is always best freshly prepared and eaten immediately.

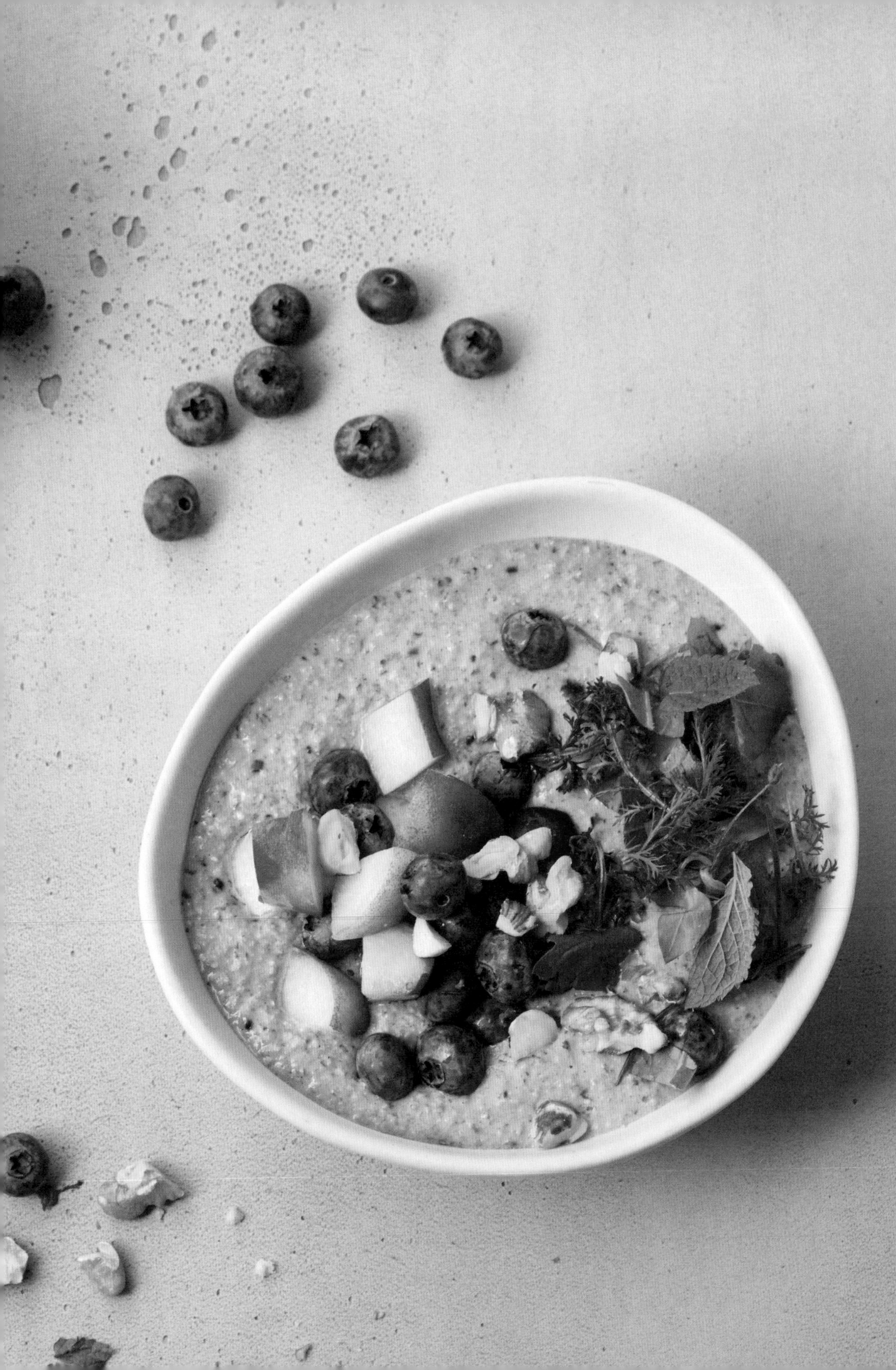

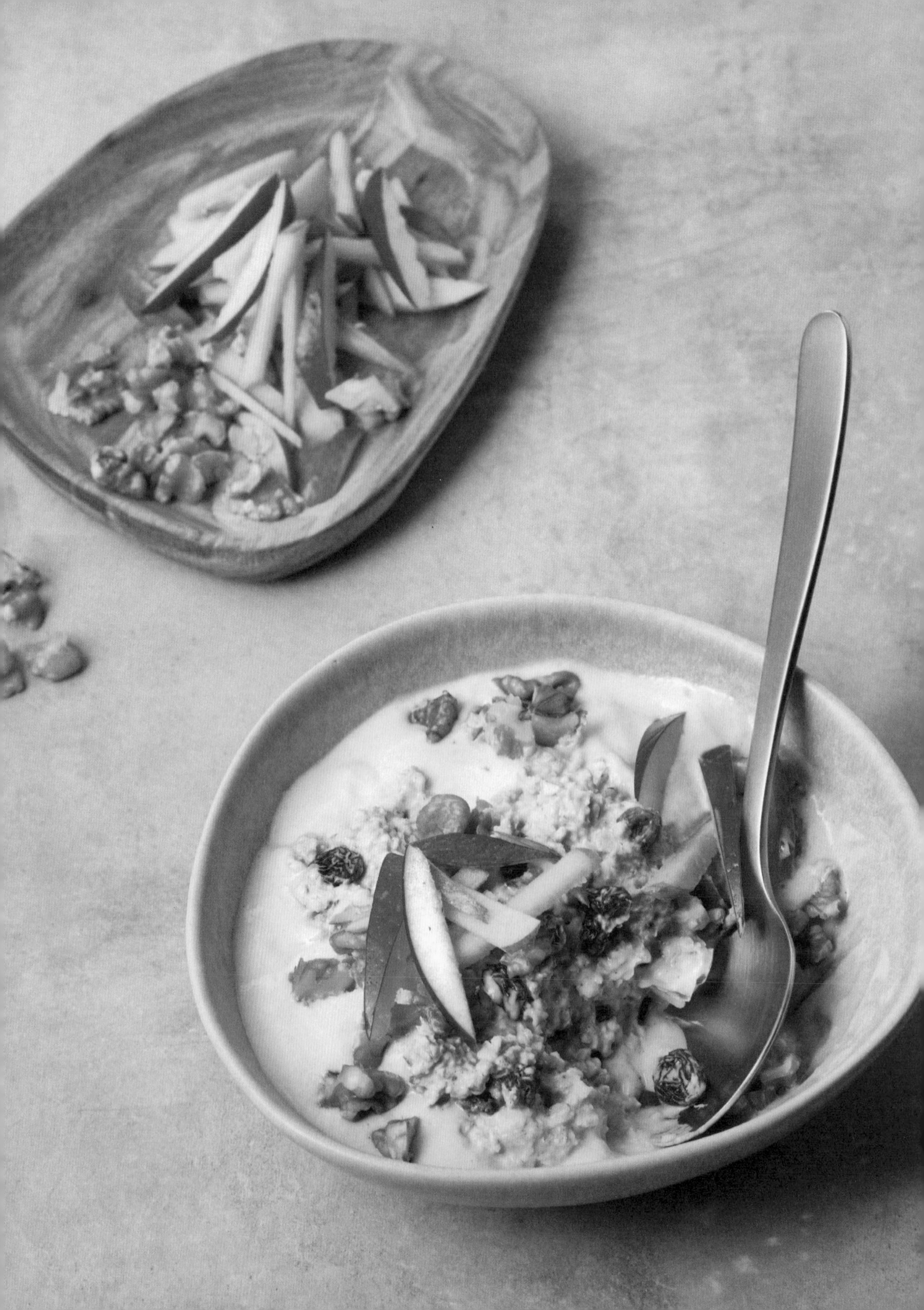

Bircher-style overnight oats with peach cream

Serves 3

Overnight oats: 200g (7oz) oat flakes | 400ml (14fl oz) soya milk with calcium (or other plant-based milk) | 4 tbsp raisins (or other dried fruit) | 1 tsp organic lemon zest | 2 tbsp lemon juice | pinch of salt | pinch of ground cinnamon
Peach cream: 200g (7oz) soya yogurt (or other plant-based yogurt) | 1 tbsp white almond nut butter | 100g (3½oz) ripe peach flesh (2 peaches) | 1 tbsp lemon juice
Topping: 50g (1¾oz) walnuts | 1 apple

Nutritional values per portion: 638 kcal | 77.8g carbohydrate | 25g fat | 20.8g protein | 11.8g fibre | 1.9g ALA | 895mg lysine | 242mg calcium | 3.7mg zinc | 5.9mg iron | 0.1mg B2 | < 0.1mg RE | 19µg iodine | 0.5g salt

Prepare the overnight oats the evening before you want to eat them by combining the oats with the soya milk, raisins, lemon zest, lemon juice, salt, and cinnamon in a bowl, which you put in the fridge.

For the peach cream, put the yogurt, almond nut butter, peaches, and lemon juice into a food processor, process until smooth then chill. For the topping, cover the walnuts with water in a bowl and soak.

The next morning, wash, quarter, core, and thinly slice the apple. Tip the walnuts into a sieve, rinse under running water, and chop finely. Stir the oat mixture well and divide it between three bowls. Mix the peach cream and add to the oat mixture as a garnish. Finally, scatter over the walnuts and sliced apple.

VARIATION

Instead of peach, you could also use apricots or 50g (1¾oz) of berries.

BASTI'S TIP

You can also slice the apple the previous evening – just drizzle with 2 tbsp of lemon juice to stop it going brown.

If you prefer your oats less runny, just reduce the quantity of plant-based milk.

Although it is not necessary to soak the walnuts from a nutritional perspective, it helps reduce their bitter edge and improves their flavour.

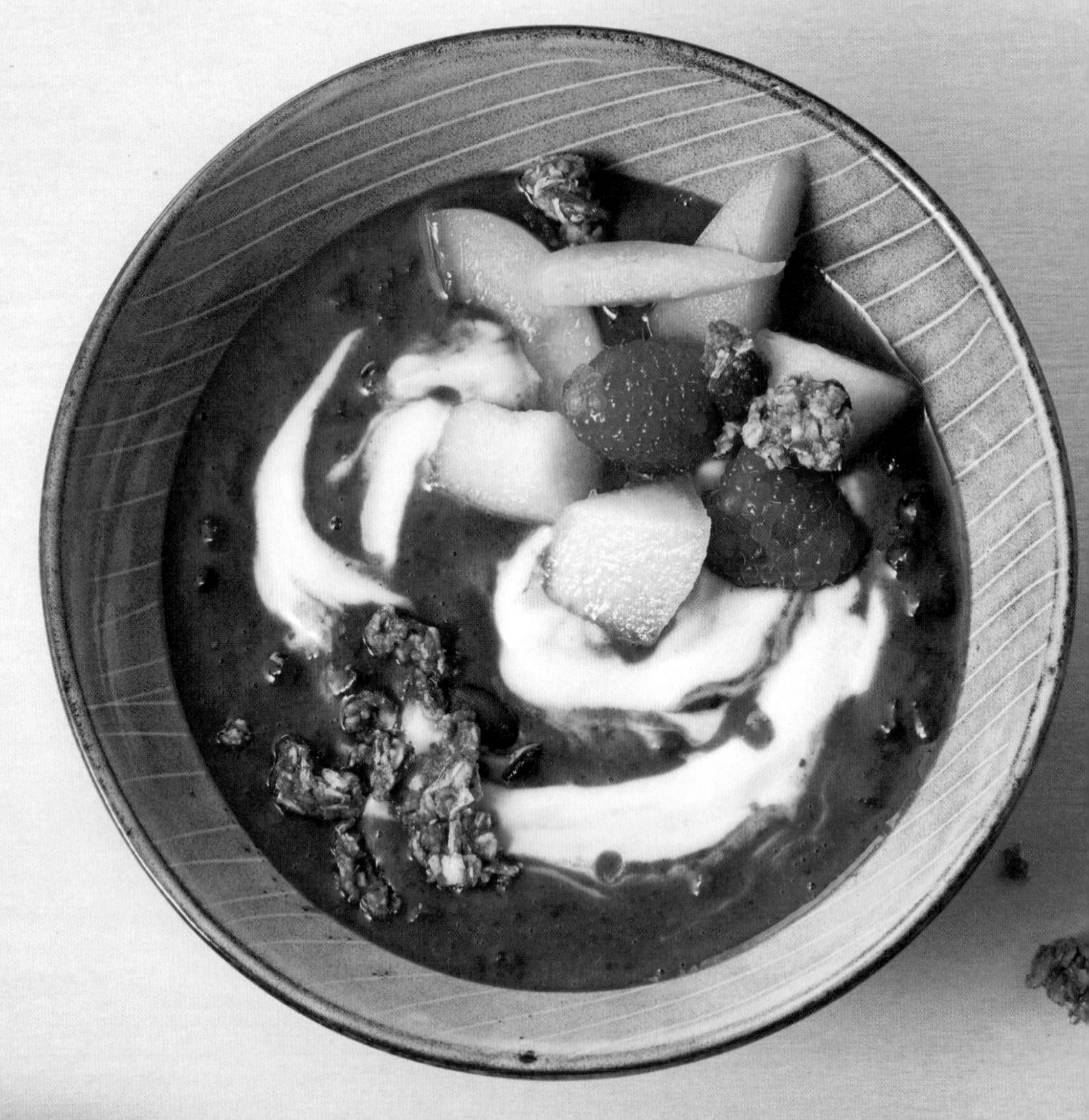

BASTI'S TIP

Ideally, make this granola in quadruple quantities on a regular basis once every couple of weeks so you always have some in your store cupboard. It keeps very well and provides an instant delicious breakfast.

Blueberry cream yogurt with super miso granola

Serves 3

Super miso granola: 30g (1oz) light tahini (sesame seed paste; see tip p.192) | 150g (5½oz) date paste (see p.97) | 2 tbsp shiro miso | 100g (3½oz) oat flakes | 50g (1¾oz) pumpkin seeds | 20g (¾oz) desiccated coconut | 1 tsp ground cinnamon
Blueberry cream yogurt: 100g (3½oz) frozen blueberries | 2 tbsp date paste (see p.97) | 100g (3½oz) white almond nut butter (or other nut butter) | 400g (14oz) soya yogurt (or coconut yogurt)
Topping: 15 tbsp washed, finely chopped seasonal fruit

Nutritional values per portion: 746 kcal | 65g carbohydrate | 40.7g fat | 21.4g protein | 14.9g fibre | 0.3g ALA | 1223mg lysine | 194mg calcium | 3.9mg zinc | 6mg iron | 0.3mg B2 | < 0.1mg RE | 6µg iodine | 0.9g salt

Preheat the oven to 120°C (100°C fan/250°F/lowest gas) to cook the granola. Add the tahini, date paste, and miso to a bowl and mix. Then stir in the oats, pumpkin seeds, desiccated coconut, and cinnamon. Lay the granola mix out on a baking tray lined with baking paper and bake for 20 minutes in the centre of the oven. Break up the granola again and continue baking for another 20 minutes, then mix it once more and bake for a final 20 minutes. Let the granola cool down then transfer into a suitably large screwtop jar.

To make the blueberry cream yogurt, mix the berries with 100ml (3½fl oz) of water, date paste, and nut butter in a small pan. Bring to the boil briefly and mix everything together well using a balloon whisk. Divide the yogurt between three bowls, scatter over the berries and stir just enough to create a lovely marbled effect. Serve with granola and fruit.

VARIATION

Instead of using nut butter, you could finely mash 1 small avocado and mix this with the date paste and blueberries. In which case, do not add any water or heat the cream. Sweet mango or other berries also taste great instead of blueberries in the cream.

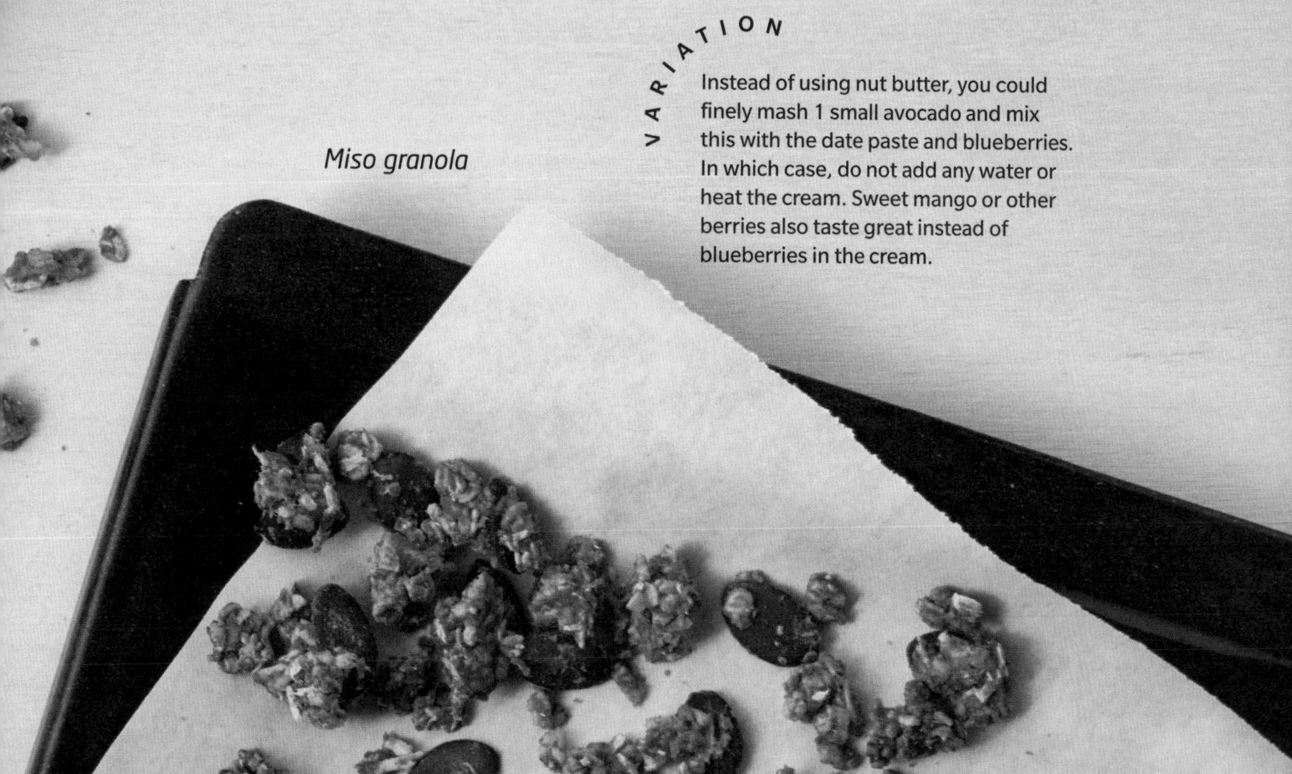

Miso granola

Hearty quinoa porridge with beans and miso

Serves 3

200g (7oz) quinoa | 500ml (16fl oz) mild vegetable stock | 200g (7oz) sweet potato, peeled and cut into cubes | 2 tbsp white almond nut butter | 100g (3½oz) cooked beans (see p.191) | pinch of salt | 1 tbsp lemon juice | ½ tsp freshly ground pepper | 2 tbsp shiro miso | 3 tbsp pumpkin seeds, toasted | 1 tsp sesame seeds, toasted | 2 tbsp finely chopped parsley | 1 apple, cored and diced

Nutritional values per portion: 630 kcal | 82.2g carbohydrate | 22.3g fat | 20.4g protein | 14.6g fibre | 0.3g ALA | 1273mg lysine | 119mg calcium | 3.4mg zinc | 5mg iron | 0.2mg B2 | 0.9mg RE | 8µg iodine | 1.7g salt

Put the quinoa in a sieve and rinse thoroughly under hot running water, then add to a pan with the vegetable stock and cubes of sweet potato. Boil for 15 minutes until the quinoa is cooked and has a slightly creamy consistency.

Stir in the almond butter and beans, season everything with salt, lemon juice, and pepper, mixing well, then stir in the miso. Gradually add some more salt and pepper to taste, divide between three bowls, garnish with pumpkin seeds, sesame seeds, parsley, and diced apple – and enjoy!

VARIATION

Instead of quinoa, you could use 400g (14oz) of cooked brown rice or cooked millet. In this case, use half the quantity of stock and reduce the cooking time to 10 minutes. The porridge works well with other vegetables instead of sweet potato, too.

Green power bowl

Serves 2

Bowl: 75g (2½oz) spinach | 2 oranges | 5 sprigs of parsley | 10 mint leaves | 75g (2½oz) cooked chickpeas (see p.191) | 1 banana, peeled | ½ organic lemon | 3 Deglet Noor dates, stoned | 1 piece of fresh root ginger (2cm/¾in), peeled and finely diced | 1 tbsp linseed (or sesame seeds) | pinch of salt | pinch of ground turmeric

Topping: 4 tbsp plant-based yogurt | 1 banana, peeled and cubed | 4 tbsp super miso granola (see p.113) | 8 Cape gooseberries, halved

Nutritional values per portion: 293 kcal | 50.5g carbohydrate | 3.7g fat | 9.9g protein | 14.6g fibre | 1.5g ALA | 523mg lysine | 209mg calcium | 1.4mg zinc | 3.8mg iron | 0.2mg B2 | 0.3mg RE | 11µg iodine | 0.5g salt

Sort and wash the spinach. Peel and dice the oranges. Finely chop the parsley and mint. Add the spinach, oranges, herbs, and all the other ingredients for the bowl to a powerful food processor along with 300ml (10fl oz) of water and process until you have a smooth, creamy, thick mixture. Divide between two bowls, garnish each with 2 tablespoons of yogurt, a couple of cubes of banana, some granola, and Cape gooseberries.

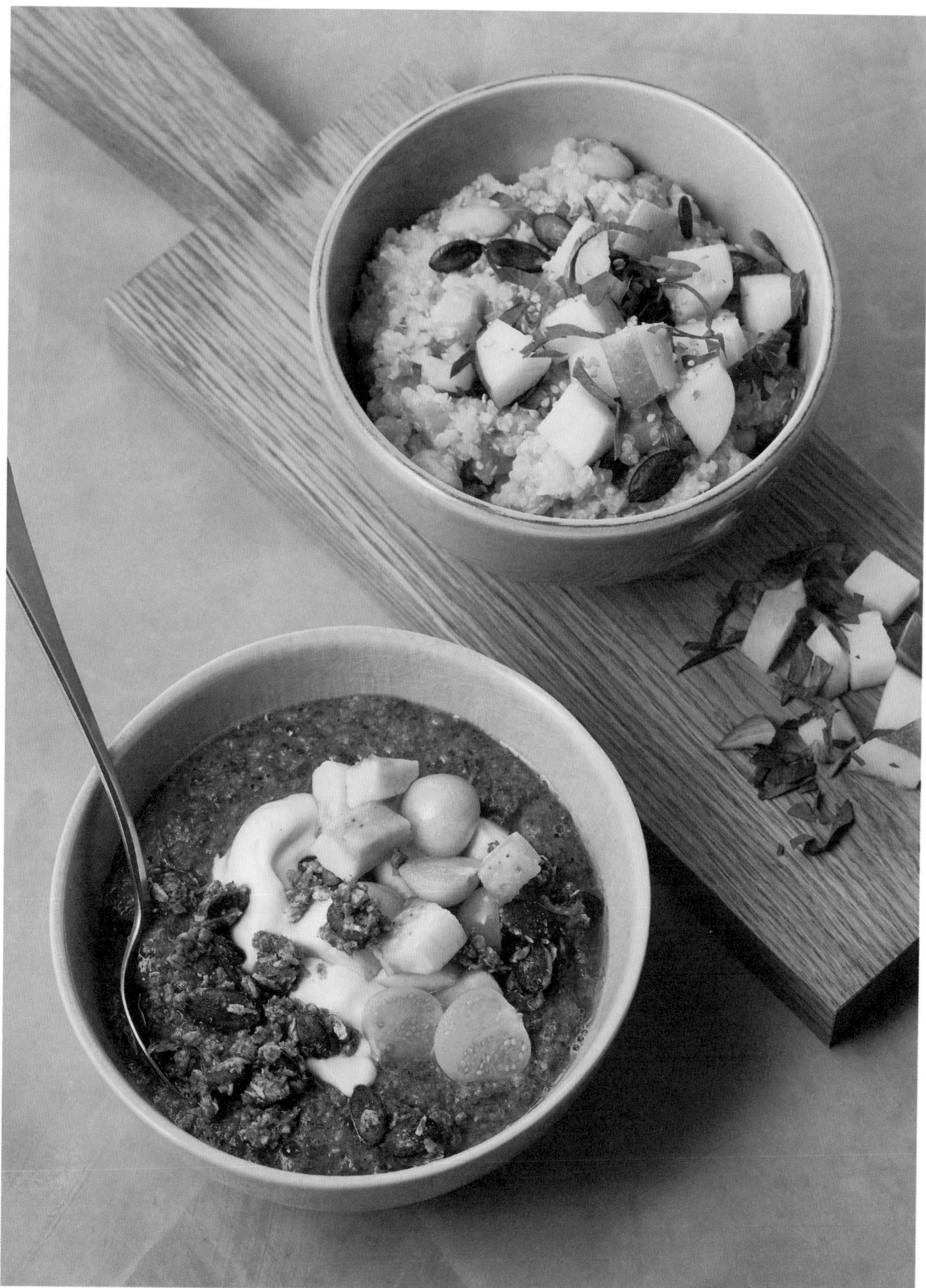

Asian baked beans with crunchy tempeh and chive bread

Serves 3

Baked beans: 2 tbsp date paste (see p.97; about 30g/1oz) | 2 tbsp yeast flakes | 150g (5½oz) passata | 2 garlic cloves (optional), peeled | 2 tsp dried oregano | ¼ tsp ground cinnamon | ¼ tsp ground turmeric |1 tbsp olive oil | 1 tbsp organic soy sauce | 600g (1lb 5oz) cooked white beans (see p.191)
Herby yogurt: 4 sprigs of parsley | 4 sprigs of dill | 200g (7oz) soya yogurt (or other plant-based yogurt) | 1 tbsp almond nut butter (or cashew nut butter) | salt
Tempeh: 200g (7oz) tempeh | 1 tsp olive oil | salt | freshly ground pepper
Chive bread: 3 slices wholemeal bread | 6 tbsp vegan spread (e.g. pepper and sunflower seed spread, see p.127) | 1 bunch of chives, finely chopped
Also: baking dish (about 20 × 20 × 4cm/8 × 8 × 2in)

Nutritional values per portion: 726 kcal | 69.8g carbohydrate | 26.2g fat | 50.8g protein | 20g fibre | 1.5g ALA | 3253mg lysine | 344mg calcium | 7.5mg zinc | 13.1mg iron | 0.8mg B2 | 0.1mg RE | 8µg iodine | 1.8g salt

Preheat the oven to 180°C (160°C fan/350°F/Gas 4) ready to cook the baked beans. Purée the date paste, yeast flakes, passata, 150ml (5fl oz) of water, garlic, oregano, cinnamon, turmeric, olive oil, and soy sauce in a food processor until smooth. Mix the purée with the cooked beans and transfer to the baking dish. The bean mixture should be roughly 2cm (¾in) deep. Bake the beans in the oven (middle shelf) for 30–40 minutes until the sauce has thickened nicely.

Finely chop the parsley and dill, then mix with the yogurt and nut butter in a bowl. Lightly season the herb yogurt with salt.

Cut the tempeh into wafer-thin strips using a peeler and transfer these to a bowl. Drizzle the strips with olive oil, then toss gently to ensure everything is coated in oil. Heat a non-stick pan and fry the tempeh strips for about 4 minutes until crisp. Season with salt and pepper and keep warm.

Toast the bread, top with the vegan spread and sprinkle generously with chopped chives. Divide the baked beans between deep plates, garnish with the tempeh and herby yogurt and eat with the chive bread.

BASTI'S TIP

These baked beans are best prepared the previous evening, then reheat for 10 minutes in an oven preheated to 80°C (60°C fan/175°F/lowest gas). Breakfast will be ready in no time.

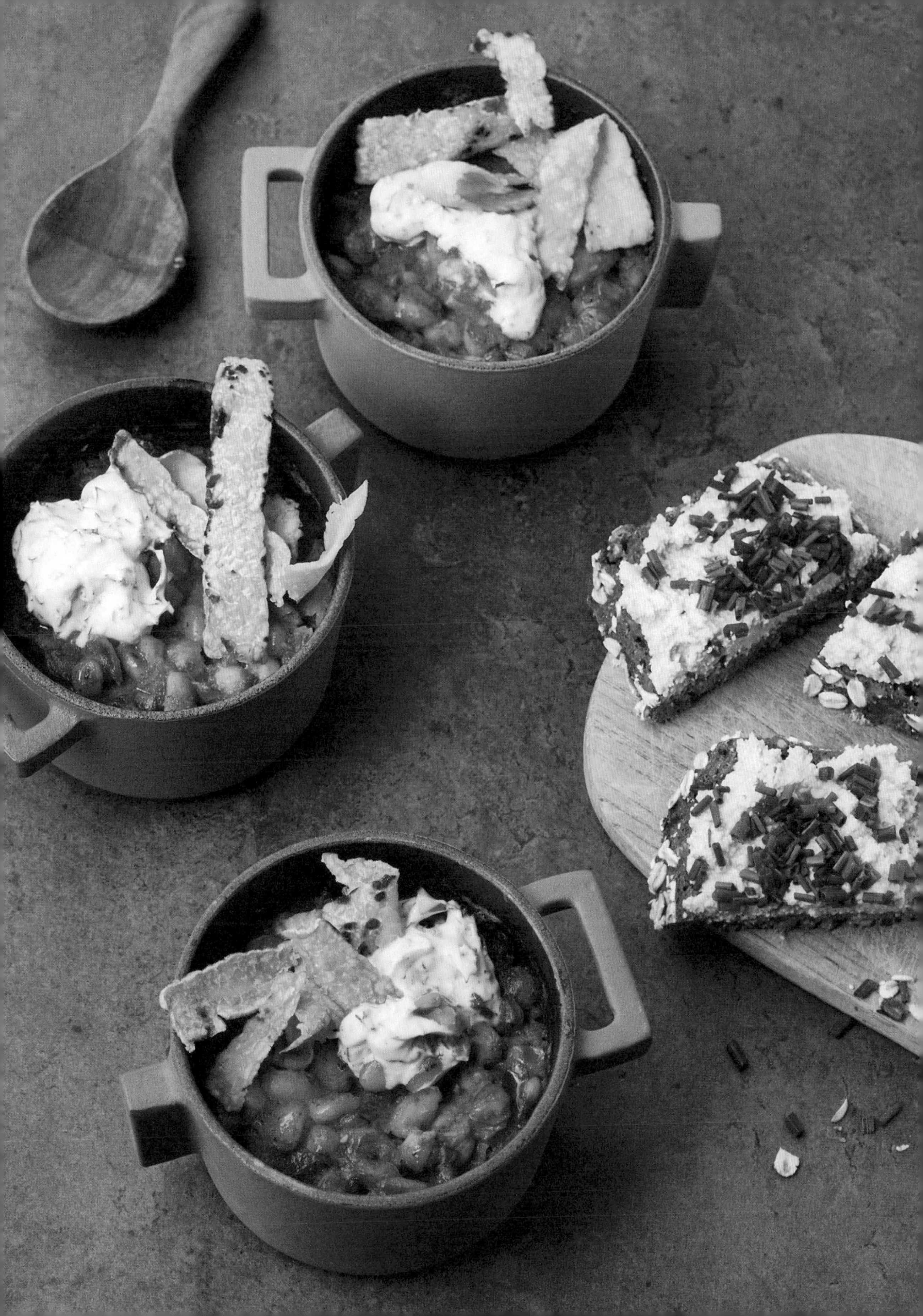

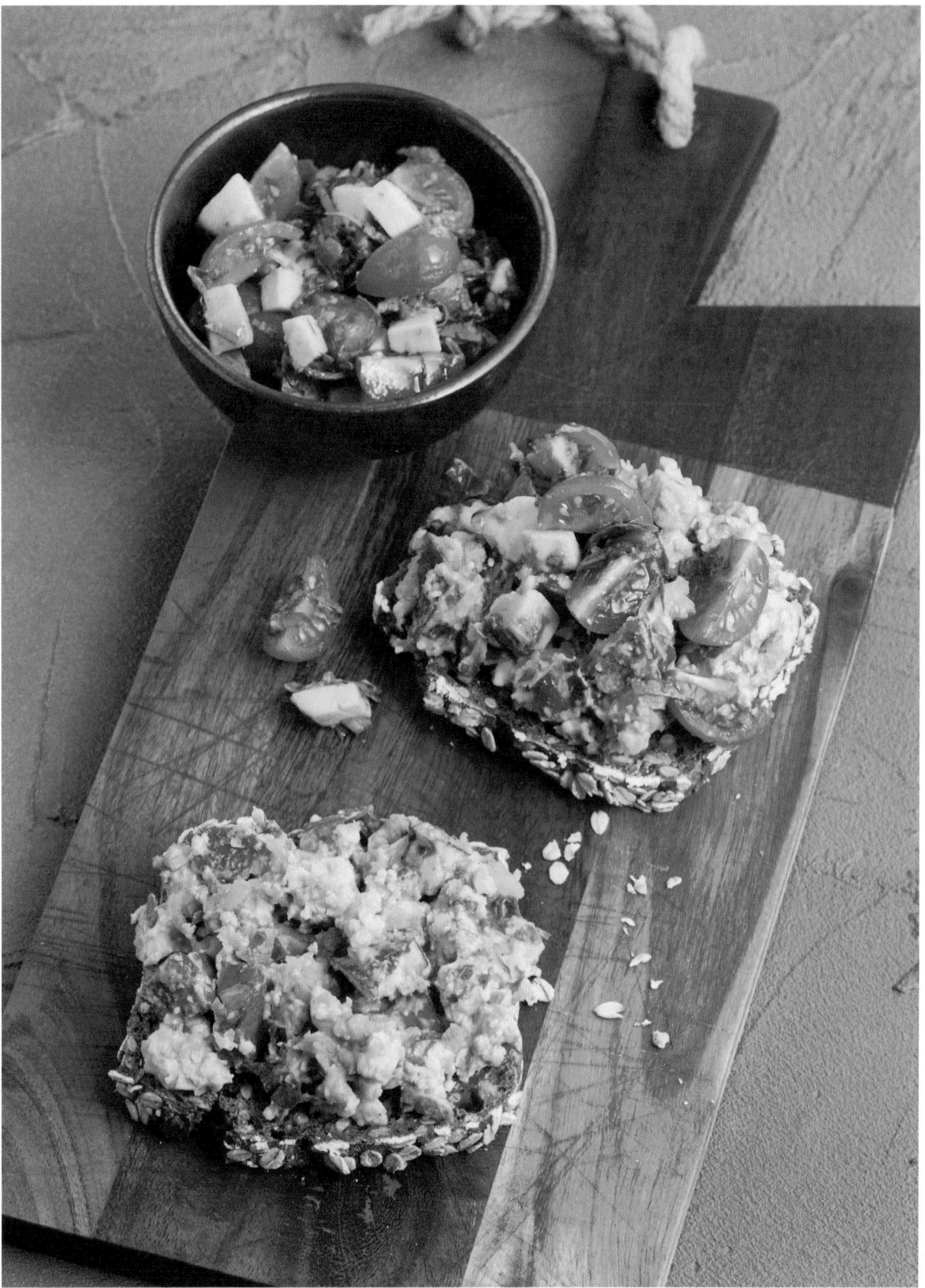

Scrambled tofu on toast with tomato and rocket salsa

Serves 3

Scrambled tofu on toast: 1 onion, peeled | 200g (7oz) tofu | 200g (7oz) smoked tofu | 2 small pieces of celery | 1 tbsp olive oil | 5 sprigs of parsley | salt | freshly ground pepper | 2 slices of wholemeal bread per portion, toasted
Kala namak cream: 2 tsp kala namak (see tip) | ¼ tsp ground turmeric | 160g (5½oz) cooked chickpeas (see p.191) | 160ml (5fl oz) light vegetable stock | 1 tbsp olive oil | 2 tbsp yeast flakes
Salsa: 10 cherry tomatoes | 20g (¾oz) rocket | 1 tbsp date paste (see p.97) | 1 small ripe avocado, cut into cubes | 2 tbsp lemon juice

Nutritional values per portion: 658 kcal | 60.5g carbohydrate | 28.6g fat | 39.3g protein | 19.6g fibre | 1.1g ALA | 2508mg lysine | 405mg calcium | 5.6mg zinc | 9.7mg iron | 0.5mg B2 | 0.1mg RE | 20µg iodine | 1.9g salt

Finely chop the onion. Crumble both varieties of tofu into fine crumbs with your hands. Wash and finely dice the celery. Heat a large non-stick pan until nice and hot. Add the tofu crumbs, celery, and chopped onion to the pan and drizzle with olive oil. Mix everything well and sauté over a high heat for 3 minutes, stirring occasionally. Lower the temperature and continue cooking over a moderate heat for another 8 minutes. Meanwhile, finely chop the parsley.

Put all the ingredients for the kala namak cream into the food processor and blend until you have a smooth purée. Wash and quarter the cherry tomatoes for the salsa. Finely chop the rocket and combine it with the cherry tomatoes, date paste, avocado, and lemon juice in a bowl.

Add the kala namak cream and parsley to the tofu and cook down the liquid over a high heat until the mixture no longer looks runny. Season the tofu mixture with salt and pepper. Place the toasted wholemeal bread on plates and top with the tofu mixture. Garnish with the salsa and enjoy.

BASTI'S TIP

There are so many different brands of tofu and they vary greatly in quality. You just have to try them out until you find the right brand for you.

Kala namak is an ayurvedic, sulphurous salt which has a very eggy smell and taste.

VARIATION

Be adventurous and try out different spices, vegetables, and herbs in the scrambled tofu. It tastes great with mushrooms and courgette, or even with pickled capers, olives, and a generous handful of basil.

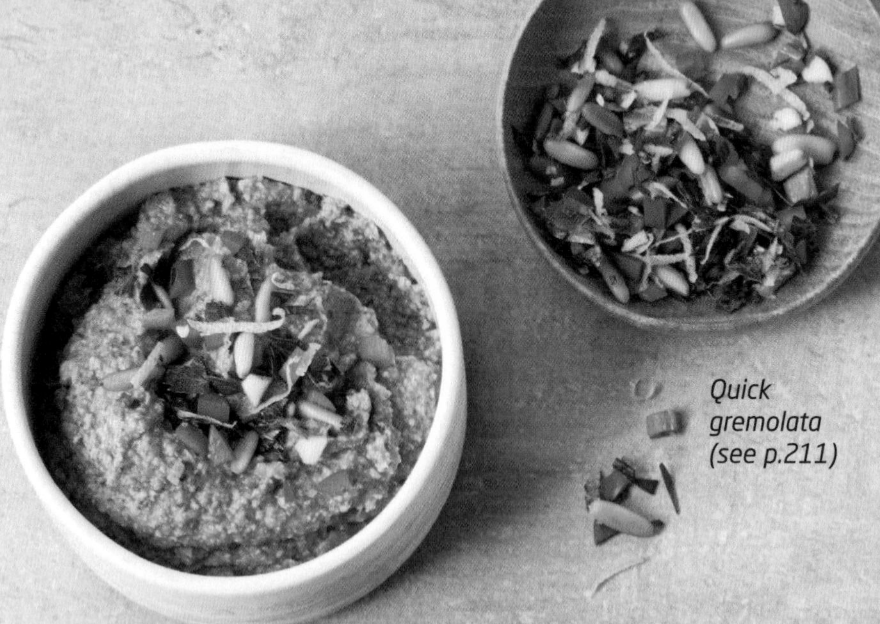

Quick gremolata (see p.211)

Kidney bean and tempeh spread

Makes about 550g (1¼lb) or 12 portions

1 onion, peeled | 1 garlic clove, peeled | 200g (7oz) tempeh (soya or lupin) | 2 tbsp olive oil | 200g (7oz) cooked kidney beans (or other beans; see p.191) | 50ml (1¾fl oz) bean cooking water (see p.191) | 1 tsp cider vinegar | 20g (¾oz) tomato purée | 1 tbsp date paste (see p.97) | ½ tsp freshly grated nutmeg | 1 tsp dried marjoram | 15g (½oz) shiro miso | 2 tbsp organic soy sauce | pinch of hot paprika | salt | freshly ground pepper

Nutritional values per portion: 72 kcal | 4.1g carbohydrate | 4g fat | 5g protein | 3g fibre | 0.2g ALA | 321mg lysine | 33mg calcium | 0.9mg zinc | 1.3mg iron | 0.1mg B2 | < 0.1mg RE | 1μg iodine | 0.3g salt

Finely chop the onion and garlic. Slice the tempeh into roughly 2cm (¾in) cubes. Heat a pan. Add the onion, garlic, and tempeh, drizzle with 1 tablespoon of olive oil and sauté until the diced onion is browning slightly. Meanwhile, put the remaining ingredients with the rest of the oil (1 tablespoon) into a food processor. Add the onion and tempeh mixture and process everything until you have a smooth, creamy consistency. Season with salt and pepper, let the flavours infuse in the fridge for at least 2 hours then adjust the seasoning again.

VARIATION

If you just mash the tempeh with a fork and add 100g (3½oz) of cooked quinoa you can shape the mixture into rissoles. Fry until crisp for a delicious treat.

BASTI'S TIP

Some types of tempeh can have a slightly bitter aftertaste. You can either steam these beforehand for about 10 minutes, or buy the garlic and coriander variety from an organic tempeh manufacturer. The cooking water from the beans is packed with umami flavours, so you must include it. This spread tastes great topped with the quick gremolata (see p.211).

Pepper and walnut spread

Makes about 550g (1¼lb) or 12 portions

2 large red peppers | 200g (7oz) walnuts | 1 tbsp sweet paprika | 2 tsp hot paprika | 1 tsp ground cumin | 1 tsp ground cinnamon | 1 tbsp date paste (see p.97) | 1 small garlic clove, peeled | 1½ tbsp shiro miso | 2 tbsp olive oil | 100g (3½oz) cooked pulses (see from p.189, e.g. white beans) | 2 tbsp organic soy sauce | 1 tbsp lemon juice, plus extra to taste | 1 tsp grated organic lemon zest | salt | freshly ground pepper

Nutritional values per portion: 172 kcal | 6g carbohydrate | 14.9g fat | 4.2g protein | 2.7g fibre | 1.8g ALA | 184 mg lysine | 25mg calcium | 0.6mg zinc | 0.9mg iron | 0.1mg B2 | 0.1mg RE | 1µg iodine | 0.4g salt

Preheat the grill to a high heat. Wash, halve, and remove the seeds from the peppers. Place the pepper halves on a baking tray skin side up and grill for 10–15 minutes until the skins are black all over.

Meanwhile, put the walnuts in a pan with 1 litre (1¾ pints) of water, bring to the boil and simmer gently for 10 minutes. Tip the walnuts into a sieve and rinse under running water. Remove the peppers from the oven, cover with a damp kitchen towel and leave to cool for 10 minutes. Pull off the charred skin with a knife. Finely chop the peppers and put three-quarters into the food processor. Add all the remaining ingredients except the walnuts to the food processor and purée to a smooth, creamy consistency. Add the nuts and process everything again until you have a fine, crumbly mixture. Fold in the remaining pepper pieces and season the spread to taste with salt, pepper, and lemon juice.

BASTI'S TIP

The walnuts should taste delicious before you boil them – it is important they do not smell old or musty, otherwise this will impair the overall flavour of the dish. This spread goes beautifully with a topping of fresh pomegranate seeds, finely chopped parsley, and a few toasted walnuts.

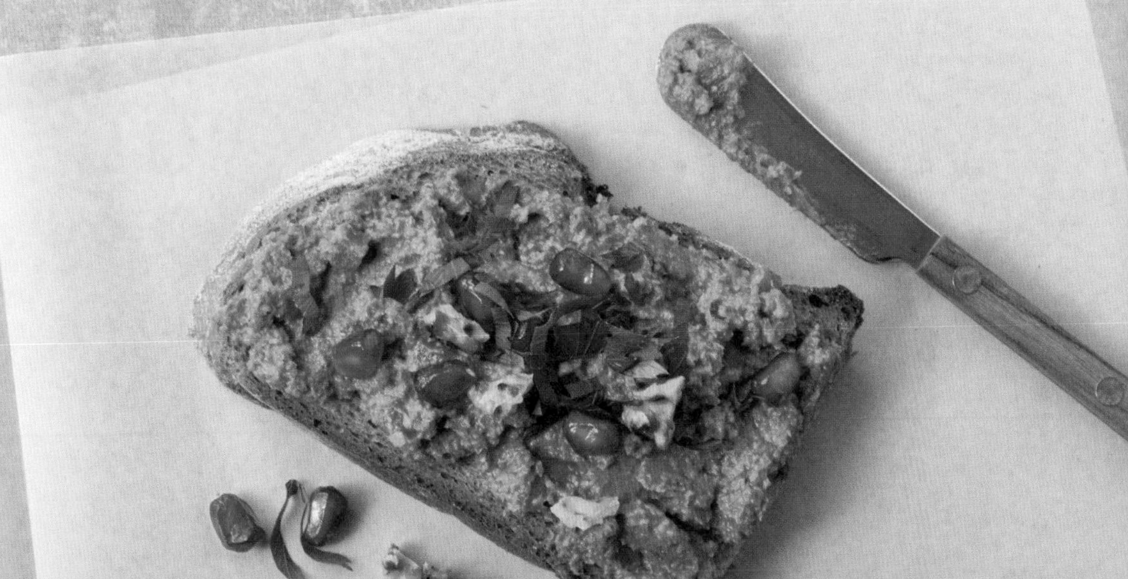

Spicy quark spread

Makes about 600g (1lb 5oz) or 12 portions

400g (14oz) tofu | 1 onion, peeled | 2 tbsp curry powder (see tip) | 2 level tsp salt | 2 tbsp date paste (see p.97) | 2 tbsp olive oil | 1 juicy orange, peeled | pinch of vanilla powder | 1 tbsp shiro miso | lime juice | freshly ground pepper
Topping: 1 yellow banana | ½ bunch of fresh coriander (or basil) | 1 tbsp black sesame seeds (or white sesame seeds), toasted | juice of 1 lime

Nutritional values per portion: 102 kcal | 7g carbohydrate | 5.2g fat | 6.1g protein | 1.9g fibre | 0.24g ALA | 373mg lysine | 88mg calcium | 0.7mg zinc | 1.4mg iron | < 0.1mg B2 | < 0.1mg RE | 3µg iodine | 1g salt

Preheat the oven to 200°C (180°C fan/400°F/Gas 6). Slice the tofu and onion into 2cm (¾in) cubes. Place on a baking tray lined with baking paper, toss with the curry powder, 1 level teaspoon of salt, date paste, and 1 tablespoon of olive oil and bake for 13 minutes in the oven (middle shelf).

Remove the seeds from the orange, dice it and add to the food processor with the remaining salt (1 level teaspoon), vanilla, the remaining oil (1 tablespoon), and miso paste. Purée until smooth. Take the cooked tofu mixture out of the oven, add it to the food processor and process again to a smooth cream. Depending how sour the orange is, adjust the flavour of the cream with lime juice, salt, and pepper. Chill in the fridge for at least 2 hours. Finally, adjust the flavour of the spread with extra salt, pepper, and lime juice.

To make the topping, peel and dice the banana. Finely chop the coriander. Mix the banana, coriander, and sesame seeds and add lime juice to taste. Spread a generous layer of the tofu cream on bread and garnish with the topping.

BASTI'S TIP

Curry powders are spice mixes consisting of at least seven spices. They vary hugely in terms of flavour and quality. It can take some hunting around to find one you really like. Organic curry powder is usually very good quality. Different fruits vary greatly in terms of taste and how sweet or sour they are. You will need to allow for this when you tweak the flavour of the spread.

The topping is essential for a rounded flavour, but other options are also available. This spread works beautifully with steamed potatoes or sweet potatoes. Serve with a nice salad and the pear, basil, and walnut topping (see p.220) for an exquisite combination.

VARIATION

Instead of the orange or banana, you could easily use a sweet, juicy mango.

Anyone who is allergic to soya can use 300g (10oz) of cooked white beans instead of the tofu. In which case, just roast the diced onion on its own.

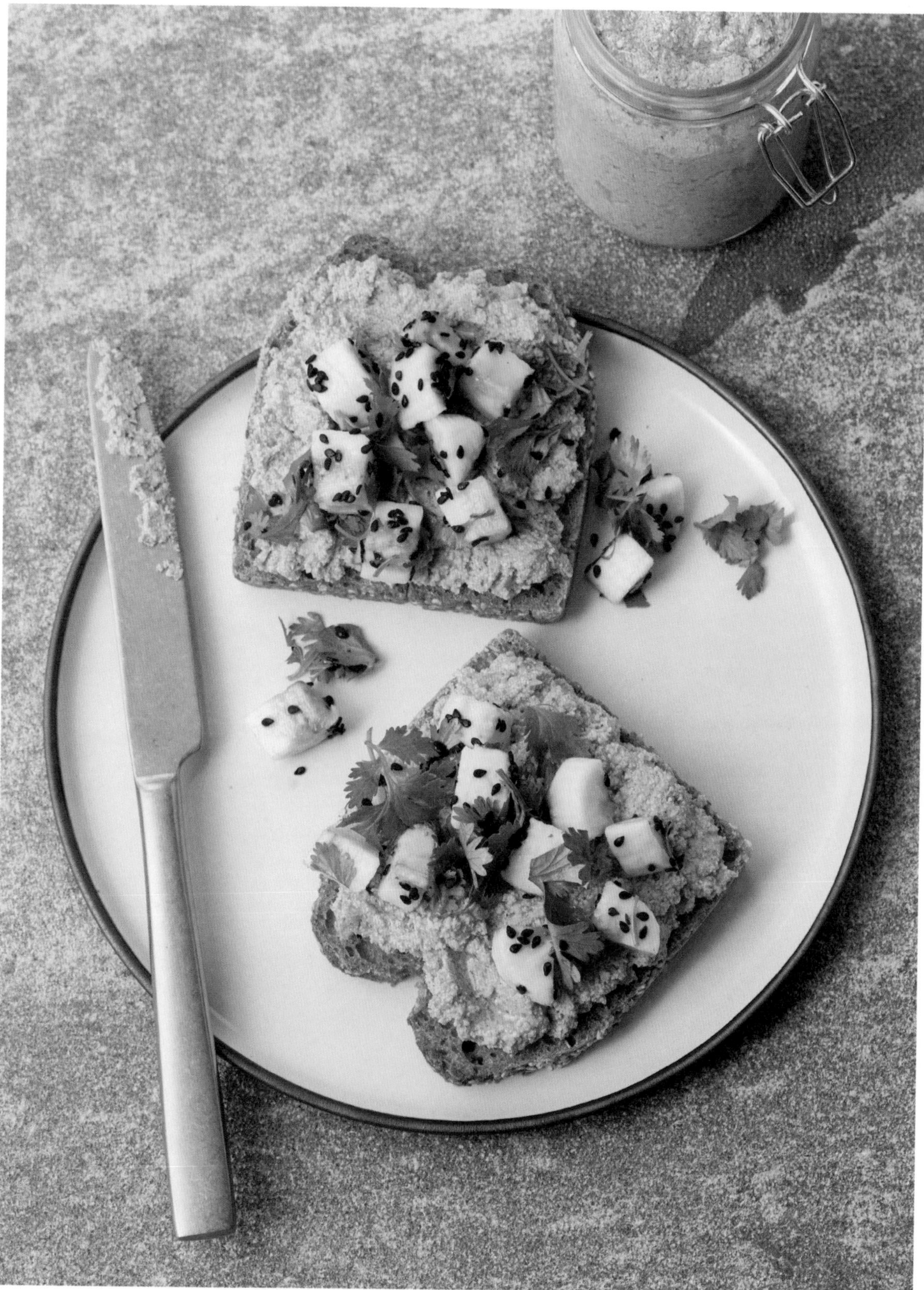

Creamy spinach spread

Makes about 600g (1lb 5oz) or 12 portions

200g (7oz) frozen spinach | 8 sprigs of parsley | 300g (10oz) cooked pale pulses (e.g. chickpeas or beans; see p.191) | 40g (1¼oz) shiro miso | 40g (1¼oz) light tahini (sesame seed paste; see tip p.192) | pinch of ground cloves | pinch of ground cumin | 1 tsp freshly ground pepper | 2 tsp cider vinegar | salt (to taste)

Nutritional values per portion: 59 kcal | 5.8g carbohydrate | 2.2g fat | 3.6g protein | 3.3g fibre | 0.1g ALA | 227mg lysine | 47mg calcium | 0.6mg zinc | 1.4mg iron | 0.1mg B2 | 0.1mg RE | 4µg iodine | 0.1g salt

Defrost the spinach. Finely chop the parsley. Add the spinach and parsley to the food processor with all the other ingredients and purée to a smooth, creamy consistency. Season the spread to taste with salt and pepper. Roasted cubes of sweet potato make a delicious accompaniment.

VARIATION

Instead of spinach, this spread works beautifully with cooked Swiss chard or broccoli.

Just replace the miso paste with 3 tbsp of yeast flakes to make the spread suitable for anyone with a soya allergy.

Mushroom spread

Makes about 600g (1lb 5oz) or 12 portions

700g (1½lb) button mushrooms, cleaned (or oyster or shiitake mushrooms) | 2 onions, peeled | 1 tsp salt (or vegetable stock paste, see p.99) | 2 tbsp olive oil | 1 tsp smoked paprika | 40g (1¼oz) tomato purée | 1 tsp ground coriander | 2 tbsp organic soy sauce | 2 tbsp orange juice (optional) | 1 tbsp shiro miso | 200g (7oz) cooked pulses (see from p.189) | freshly ground pepper | 1 tbsp lemon juice

Nutritional values per portion: 62 kcal | 4.5g carbohydrate | 2.9g fat | 4.4g protein | 3.2g fibre | 0.1g ALA | 256mg lysine | 19mg calcium | 0.6mg zinc | 1.2mg iron | < 0.1mg B2 | < 0.1mg RE | 11µg iodine | 0.7g salt

Preheat the oven to 200°C (180°C fan/400°F/Gas 6). Halve the mushrooms and roughly dice the onions. Put the chopped onion, mushrooms, salt, 1 tablespoon of olive oil, paprika, tomato purée, and coriander in a bowl, mix well, then transfer to a baking tray and cook in the oven (middle shelf) for 15 minutes until brown.

Remove the tray from the oven. Leave the mushroom mixture to cool slightly, then add it to the food processor with the soy sauce, orange juice (if using), miso, the remaining olive oil (1 tablespoon), and pulses and process to create a smooth spread that still has a slight texture. Season with salt, pepper, and lemon juice and eat lukewarm or leave to chill in the fridge.

BASTI'S TIP

Once the mushroom mixture has cooled down, you should adjust the seasoning as mushrooms are very absorbent.

This mushroom spread tastes fantastic with the pear, basil, and walnut topping (see p.220).

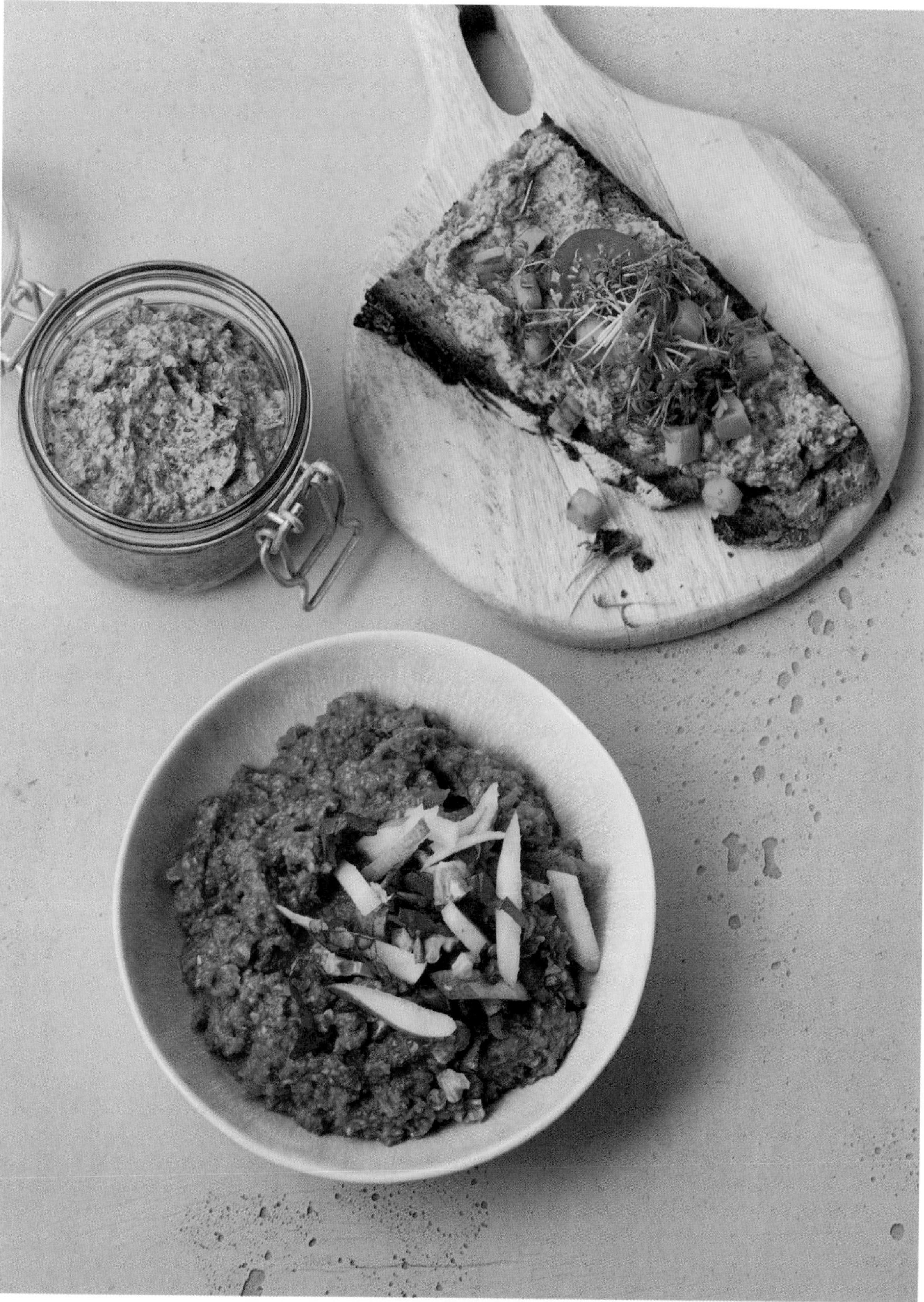

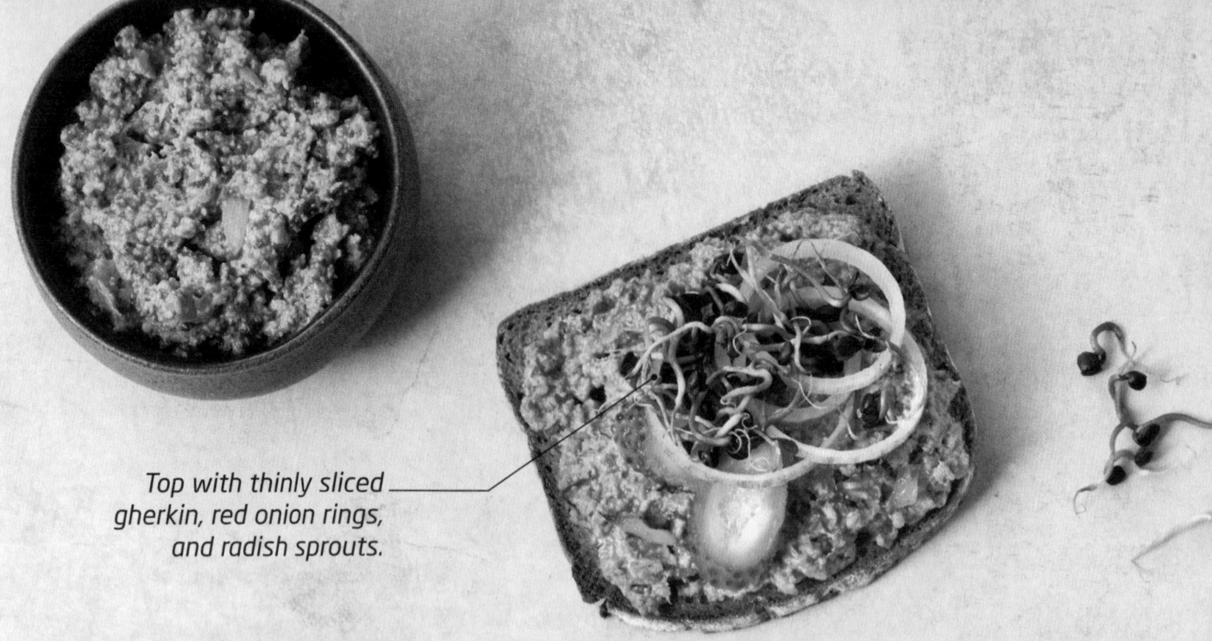

Top with thinly sliced gherkin, red onion rings, and radish sprouts.

Smoky umami spread

Makes about 600g (1lb 5oz) or 12 portions

250g (9oz) smoked tofu | 1 medium onion, peeled | 3 garlic cloves, peeled | 2 tbsp olive oil | 1 tbsp date paste (see p.97) | 1 tbsp sweet paprika | 150g (5½oz) cooked kidney beans (see p.191; or red lentils, see p.189) | 50–100ml (1¾–3½fl oz) light vegetable stock | 30g (1oz) white almond nut butter (or soaked pumpkin seeds) | 2 tbsp cider vinegar | 3 tsp dried oregano | 1 tsp hot paprika | 1 tsp smoked paprika | 3 tbsp organic soy sauce | 2 tbsp yeast flakes | freshly ground pepper

Nutritional values per portion: 97 kcal | 4.4g carbohydrate | 6g fat | 6.3g protein | 1.9g fibre | 0.2g ALA | 455mg lysine | 75mg calcium | 0.8mg zinc | 1.5mg iron | 0.1mg B2 | < 0.1mg RE | 2µg iodine | 0.7g salt

Preheat the oven to 200°C (180°C fan/400°F/ Gas 6). Slice the tofu into 2cm (¾in) cubes.

Cut the onion into 1cm (½in) wide wedges. Put both these ingredients in a bowl with the garlic and toss with 1 tablespoon of olive oil, the date paste, and sweet paprika. Transfer the tofu and onion mixture to a baking tray and roast in the oven (middle shelf) for 15 minutes until the onion is browning and completely cooked.

Meanwhile, put all the other ingredients and the remaining olive oil (1 tablespoon) into the food processor and blitz until smooth. Then add the tofu and onion mixture from the tray, including any cooking liquid, and process everything to a slightly lumpy consistency. Season to taste with pepper and soy sauce. Chill the spread in the fridge for at least 2 hours.

BASTI'S TIP

If you prefer a milder flavour, start by using just half the spices. For a hearty, savoury taste, this makes the perfect spread.

The spread tastes fantastic on toasted rye bread with thinly sliced gherkins, red onion rings, and radish sprouts.

Pepper and sunflower seed spread

Makes 600g (1lb 5oz) or 12 portions

100g (3½oz) sunflower seeds | 1 large red pepper (about 200g/7oz) | 400g (14oz) fermented tofu (Feto from Taifun) | 150ml (5fl oz) light vegetable stock | 2 tsp olive oil | 2 tbsp yeast flakes (or shiro miso) | 1 tsp salt (or vegetable stock paste, see p.99) | 1 tsp cider vinegar | freshly ground pepper

Nutritional values per portion: 101 kcal | 4.7g carbohydrate | 5.6g fat | 8g protein | 1.6g fibre | 0.2g ALA | 456 mg lysine | 73mg calcium | 1.1mg zinc | 1.7mg iron | 0.1mg B2 | 0.1mg RE | 3μg iodine | 1.2g salt

Preheat the grill to a high heat. Put the sunflower seeds in a pan with 500ml (16fl oz) of water, bring to the boil and simmer gently for 10 minutes. Meanwhile, wash, halve, and deseed the pepper then place the pieces skin-side up on a baking tray. Grill the pepper for 10 minutes until the skin has turned completely black. Remove and cover with a damp kitchen towel. Once the pepper is lukewarm, pull off the skin and finely chop the remaining flesh.

Crumble the fermented tofu into the blender beaker. Pour away the sunflower seed cooking water, tip the seeds into a sieve and rinse with fresh water. Add the seeds, stock, olive oil, yeast flakes, salt, vinegar, and half the diced pepper to the blender beaker, then process everything to a creamy consistency. Season the mixture with salt, pepper, and vinegar, then fold in the remaining diced pepper pieces. Leave the spread for at least 2 hours in the fridge to allow the flavours to develop, then adjust the seasoning again.

VARIATION

If you need the spread for a sweet combination, just leave out the pepper or replace it with another type of vegetable or fruit, e.g. mango, cooked beetroot, or strawberries.

This spread also makes a great base for a pasta filling (e.g. for tortellini). Just add a bit more seasoning for the perfect pasta dish.

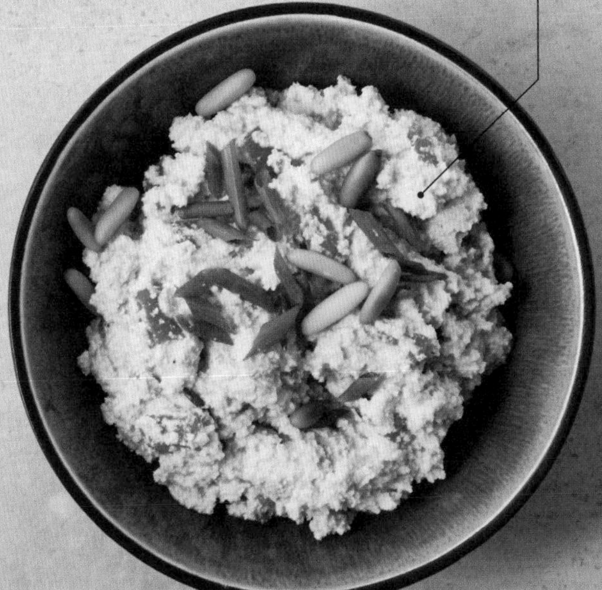

A topping of toasted pine nuts and chives rounds off this spread perfectly.

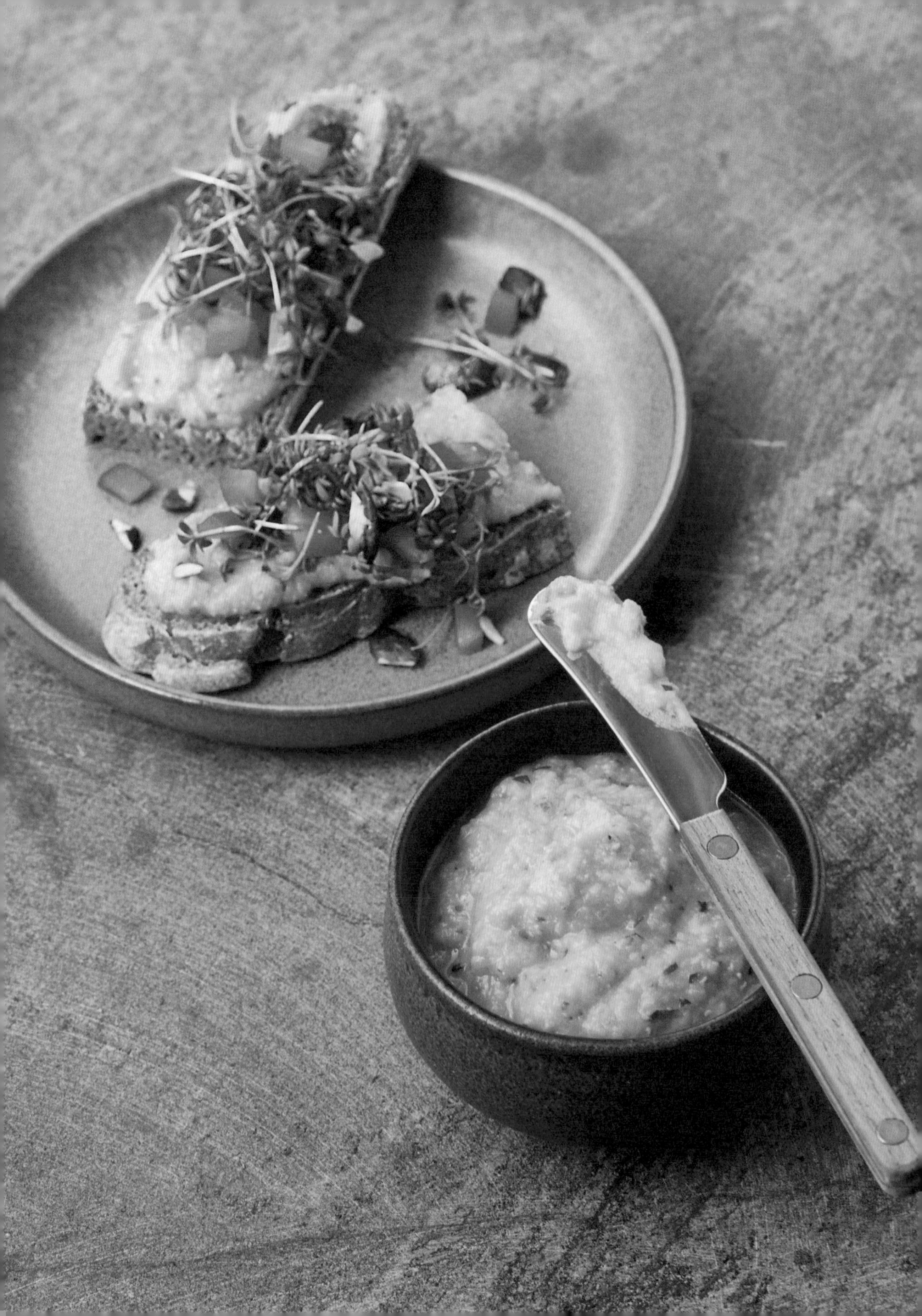

Granny's lentil spread

Makes about 600g (1lb 5oz) or 12 portions

200g (7oz) uncooked red lentils | 1 large carrot, cleaned | 1 onion, peeled | 100g (3½oz) celeriac, peeled | 5 sprigs of parsley | 3 tbsp cider vinegar | 2 tsp salt (or vegetable stock paste, see p.99) | 1 tsp almond nut butter | 2 tbsp olive oil | 1 tsp freshly ground pepper

Nutritional values per portion: 85 kcal | 9.6g carbohydrate | 3.3g fat | 4.2g protein | 2.2g fibre | < 0.1g ALA | 303mg lysine | 18mg calcium | 0.7mg zinc | 1.3mg iron | 0.1mg B2 | 0.2mg RE | 1µg iodine | 0.8g salt

Wash the lentils well in warm water. Slice the carrot and onion, and cut the celeriac into 2cm (¾in) cubes. Put the chopped vegetables and lentils in a pan with 1 litre (1¾ pints) of water, bring to the boil, and simmer for 20 minutes until the vegetables are soft.

Meanwhile, finely chop the parsley. Tip the vegetables and lentils in a sieve and leave to drain for 10 minutes, saving the cooking water (which you can store in the fridge and use as the base for a soup). Add the drained vegetables and all the remaining ingredients to a food processor and blend to a slightly lumpy, creamy consistency. Season to taste, if needed.

VARIATION

This spread tastes great with beluga lentils or green lentils. You can swap in all sorts of other vegetables, too.

Just add an extra 400ml (14fl oz) of flavoursome vegetable stock and you have a delicious soup. Add texture and spice with some toasted wholemeal croutons and a couple of spoonfuls of the quick gremolata (see p.211).

BASTI'S TIP

This spread is incredibly versatile and makes a delicious purée. Try it topped with fresh cress, toasted pumpkin seeds, and some finely diced peppers.

Pea and herb spread

Makes about 650g (1½lb) or 12 portions

1 bunch of basil (about 30g/1oz) | 4 sprigs of dill | 450g (1lb) frozen baby peas, defrosted | 2 tsp olive oil | 75g (2½oz) cashews (see tip) | 1 garlic clove, peeled | 30g (1oz) shiro miso | 1½ tsp salt (or vegetable stock paste, see p.99) | 1½ tsp cider vinegar | 120ml (4fl oz) light vegetable stock | freshly ground pepper

Nutritional values per portion: 83 kcal | 2.8g carbohydrate | 4.1g fat | 4.3g protein | 2.7g fibre | 0.1g ALA | 307mg lysine | 25mg calcium | 0.7mg zinc | 1.3mg iron | 0.1mg B2 | 0.1mg RE | 2μg iodine | 0.8g salt

Finely chop the basil and dill. Put all the ingredients except the dill in the food processor and blend to a smooth, creamy purée. Season the mixture with additional salt, pepper, and cider vinegar as desired. Stir in the dill and chill in the fridge for at least 2 hours to let the flavours develop before adjusting the seasoning again.

VARIATION

Instead of cashews, you could use white almond nut butter or cashew nut butter. You can also use whatever herbs you fancy. The same goes for the spices. This creamy purée is incredibly versatile.

Just add 200g (7oz) of the purée to 200ml (7fl oz) of vegetable stock, bring to the boil briefly and mix again – and you have a delicious soup.

Chocolate hazelnut spread

Makes about 550g (1¼lb) or 12 portions

130g (4½oz) Deglet Noor dates, stones removed | 200g (7oz) hazelnut butter | 25g (scant 1oz) cocoa powder | 100g (3½oz) cooked chickpeas (see p.191) | 1 tsp vanilla powder | 1 tbsp shiro miso (or ¼ tsp salt)

Nutritional values per portion: 163 kcal | 10.5g carbohydrate | 11.5g fat | 4.4g protein | 3.5g fibre | < 0.1g ALA | 180mg lysine | 42mg calcium | 0.6mg zinc | 2mg iron | < 0.1mg B2 | < 0.1mg RE | 1μg iodine | 0.1g salt

Add the dates to a small pan with 150ml (5fl oz) of water, bring to the boil briefly and simmer for 10 minutes until the dates are soft. Put the dates and their cooking water into a food processor with the remaining ingredients and blend until smooth. It keeps in a jar in the fridge for 4–5 days.

VARIATION

Replace the cocoa powder with 3 tsp of vanilla powder and 1 tbsp of grated organic orange zest.

BASTI'S TIP

This wonderful chocolate spread goes beautifully with some sweet banana or juicy peach plus a few chopped, toasted hazelnuts.

It also tastes fantastic on pancakes or bread and makes a great filling for a cake or pralines.

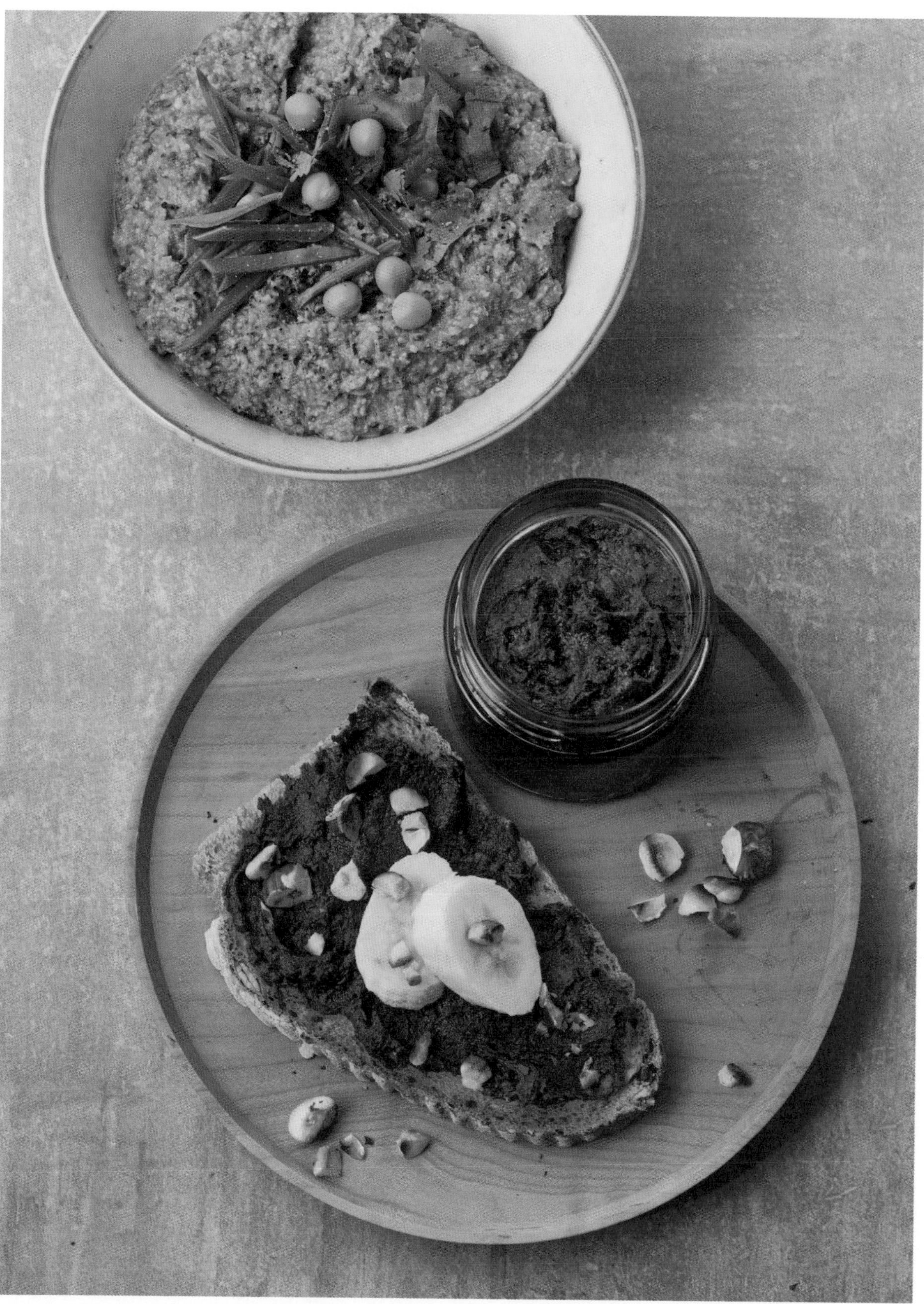

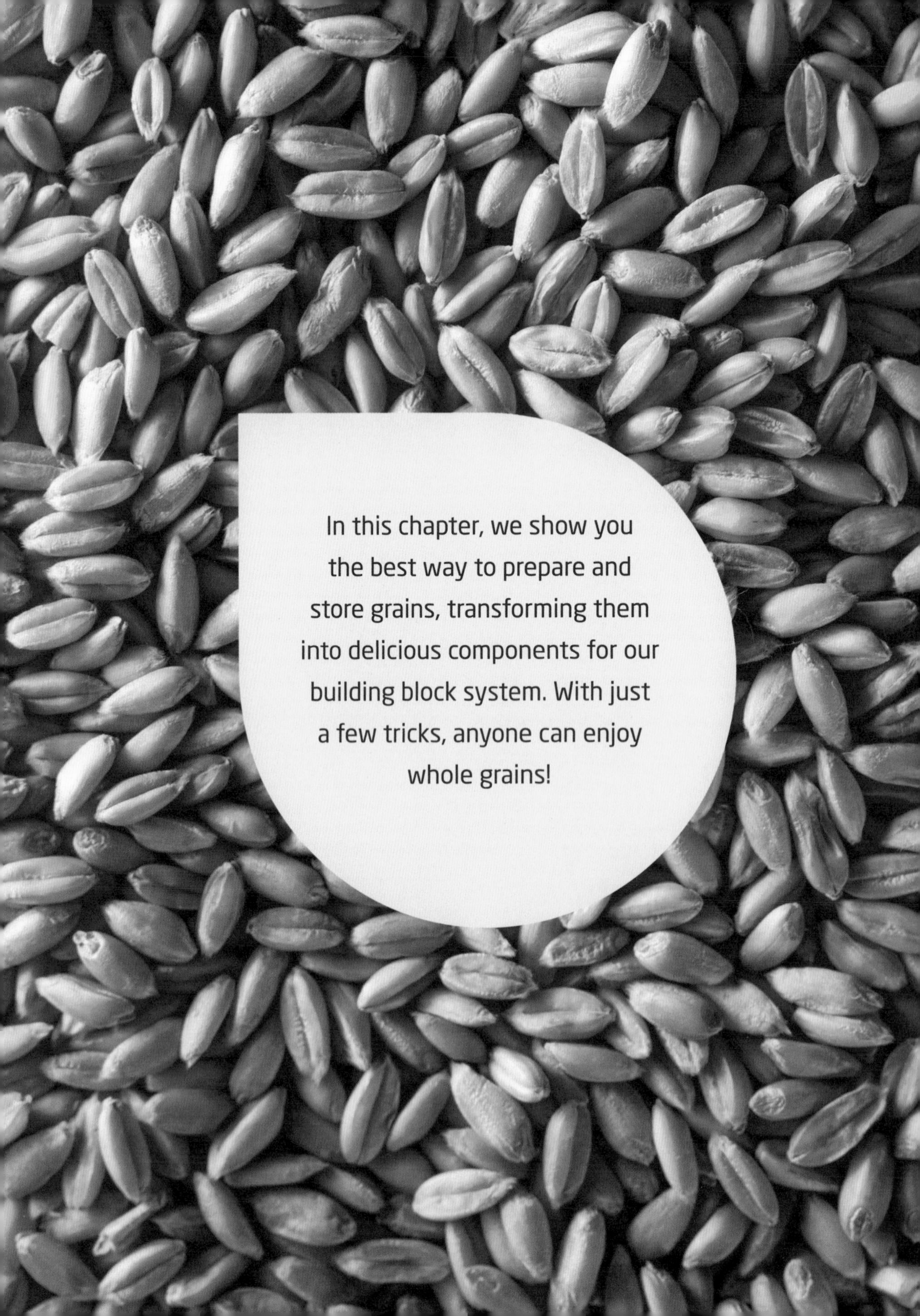

In this chapter, we show you the best way to prepare and store grains, transforming them into delicious components for our building block system. With just a few tricks, anyone can enjoy whole grains!

Grains

Building block basics: grains

By following our tips, your grains will always be cooked perfectly in future: not too hard, and not too mushy. With the right instructions, millet, brown rice, etc. can be a real gourmet treat. The quantities specified here are always for a whole packet, i.e. 500g (1lb 2oz), as this makes it incredibly easy to rustle up all sorts of delicious, wholesome meals over several days.

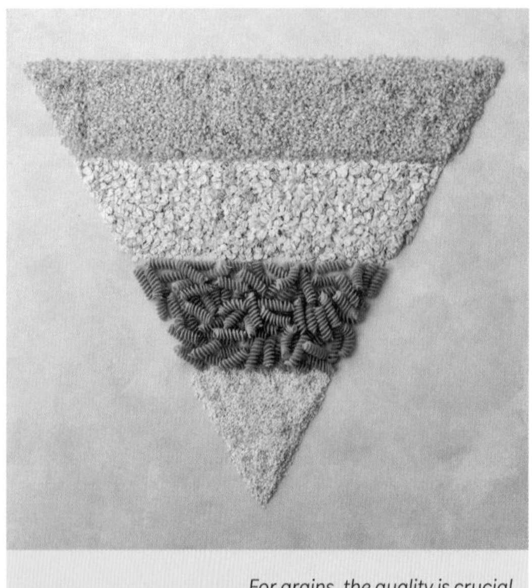

For grains, the quality is crucial (see whole grain hierarchy p.17).

General note

The volume of water required can vary slightly depending on what type of hob you have and how hot it gets. It may take one or two attempts to find the perfect product and technique for you. Once you have decided on a brand or product, just experiment a bit until you are serving up perfect results.

Whatever variety of grain you are using, once it has been cooked to perfection, we always recommend spreading it out on a baking tray to cool. This stops the grains cooking any further and they can be stored for days without clumping together. Transfer the cooled grains into jars with a capacity of 1–1.5 litres (2¾ pints), seal so they are airtight, and keep in the fridge.

Basic variations for all kinds of grains

The quickest and simplest transformation can be achieved simply by adding some spices, herbs, juice, or vegetables to create a wide range of different dishes. Below you will find a few suggestions for a variety of delicious grains.

Add one of the following spice ingredients to the cooking water for 500g (1lb 2oz) of grain:

- 1 tbsp ground turmeric
- 1 tbsp curry powder (see tip p.122) or curry paste
- 1 tbsp harissa
- 1 tbsp tomato purée
- 2cm (¾in) kombu seaweed
- 1 umeboshi plum
- 1 tbsp dried thyme
- 2 tbsp curry leaves
- 5 bay leaves
- 5 kaffir lime leaves
- replace 100ml (3½fl oz) of cooking water with 100ml (3½fl oz) of beetroot or carrot juice
- for any variety of grain that is cooked for at least 10 minutes, add 1 diced onion plus spices

Millet

Makes about 1.2kg (2¾lb) cooked millet

500g (1lb 2oz) fine millet | 1 tsp salt (or 2 tbsp vegetable stock paste, see p.99)

Put the millet in a large bowl and cover with roughly 1 litre (1¾ pints) of lukewarm water. Wash the millet by hand until the water is milky. Carefully pour off the water and replace with fresh lukewarm water. Repeat this process five to seven times until the water remains clear. It might take 5 minutes, but this essential step is well worth it!

Drain the millet in a sieve and transfer to a pan (roughly 3 litres [5¼ pints] capacity). Pour in 1 litre (1¾ pints) of cold water, add the salt, cover, and bring to the boil. You will need to keep an eye on it as the millet easily boils over.

Once the water is boiling, leave the lid on and simmer the millet gently over a low heat for 10 minutes until soft. Turn off the hob and leave the millet to stand for a further 15 minutes. Eat the millet immediately or tip it out onto a baking tray, loosen the grains, and let the steam evaporate. Once it is cool, gently crumble using your fingers, transfer into a large screwtop jar and store in the fridge. It will keep for up to 5 days.

BASTI'S TIP

There are lots of kinds of millet, but most are simply labelled 'millet' or 'golden millet'. The varieties with smaller kernels are generally tastier and easier to prepare.

VARIATION

The final product will contain more iron if you replace 100ml (3½fl oz) of the cooking water with beetroot juice.

Photo see p. 137 top

Brown rice

Makes about 1.2kg (2¾lb) cooked brown rice

500g (1lb 2oz) brown short-grain rice | ½ tsp salt

Put the rice in a large bowl, cover with about 1 litre (1¾ pints) of lukewarm water and gently massage and wash the grains by hand until any loose material comes away and floats to the surface. Carefully pour away the water along with any of this loose material and cover with fresh water. Repeat this process two to three times until the water remains clear. Pour the rice into a sieve, leave to drain briefly, and transfer to a pan (roughly 3 litres/5¼ pints capacity).

Pour in 1.15 litres (2 pints) of lukewarm water, add the salt and leave the rice to swell for 2 hours. Then bring the contents of the pan briefly to the boil with the lid on. You will need to keep an eye on it as the rice easily boils over.

Once the water boils, turn down the heat so it just continues gently simmering. Carefully, place a kitchen towel over the pan with the lid on top so the cloth is clamped between the pan and the lid, press down firmly and ideally add a weight to keep it in place. Cook the rice with the lid on for 40 minutes.

Turn off the hob, remove the lid, and allow the rice to steam openly for 10–15 minutes. You can either eat the rice straight away or spread it out on a baking tray and leave to cool. Loosen the grains of rice with a fork, transfer to a large screwtop jar and store in the fridge. It will keep for up to 4 days.

BASTI'S TIP

There are lots of kinds of brown rice available and the quality varies widely. Organic brown rice from Italy is particularly delicious.

The longer the rice is left to soak, the shorter the subsequent cooking time will be. Overnight soaking produces the best results. The cooking time will then be just 25–30 minutes.

To reheat, mix the grains with stock at a ratio of 100g (3½oz) of rice to 1 tbsp of vegetable stock. Put the rice in an ovenproof dish and heat for 15 minutes at 180°C (160°C fan/350°F/Gas 4) in a preheated oven. You could also add a few nuts, herbs, or dried fruit immediately before reheating.

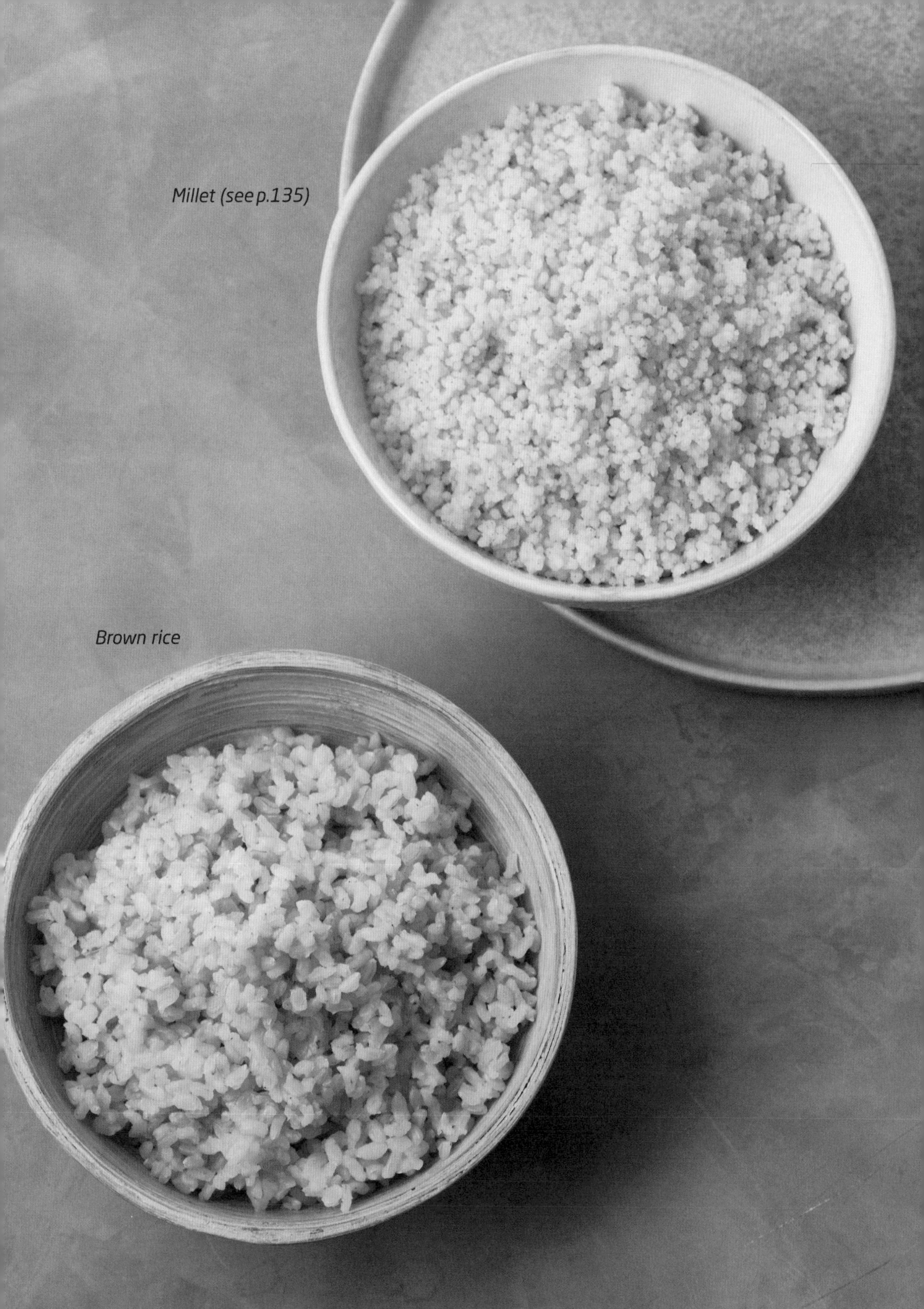

Millet (see p.135)

Brown rice

Quinoa

Makes about 1.2kg (2¾lb) cooked quinoa

500g (1lb 2oz) quinoa | ½ tsp salt

Put the quinoa in a large bowl, cover with roughly 1 litre (1¾ pints) of lukewarm water and gently wash by hand until the water is slightly cloudy. Carefully pour this away and add fresh water. Repeat this process one or two times until the water remains clear.

Tip the quinoa into a sieve, leave to drain briefly then transfer into a pan (roughly 3 litres/5¼ pints capacity). Pour over 1 litre (1¾ pints) of lukewarm water, add the salt and bring briefly to the boil. You will need to keep an eye on it as quinoa easily boils over.

Once the water is boiling, leave the lid on and simmer gently over a low heat for 10 minutes until soft. The quinoa should still have a slight bite. Turn off the hob and allow the quinoa to steam openly for 10 minutes. You can eat it straight away or leave it to cool and transfer to a large screwtop jar to store in the fridge. It will keep for up to 4 days.

Pearl barley

Makes about 1.2kg (2¾lb) cooked pearl barley

500g (1lb 2oz) pearl barley | 2 litres (3½ pints) light vegetable stock

Add the pearl barley to a pan with the vegetable stock, bring to the boil uncovered then put the lid on and simmer gently over a low heat for 25 minutes. There are all kinds of different varieties and sizes of pearl barley, so the first time you cook it, test after 10 minutes' cooking time to see if it is ready, then every 5 minutes after that. The pearl barley is ready when the grains are soft all the way through but still intact.

Drain the cooked pearl barley in a sieve, making sure to keep the broth, which you can use as the base for a soup – it contains lots of nutrients. Leave the pearl barley to steam for 10 minutes and either use immediately or leave to cool completely and store in the fridge in a large screwtop jar. It will keep for up to 4 days.

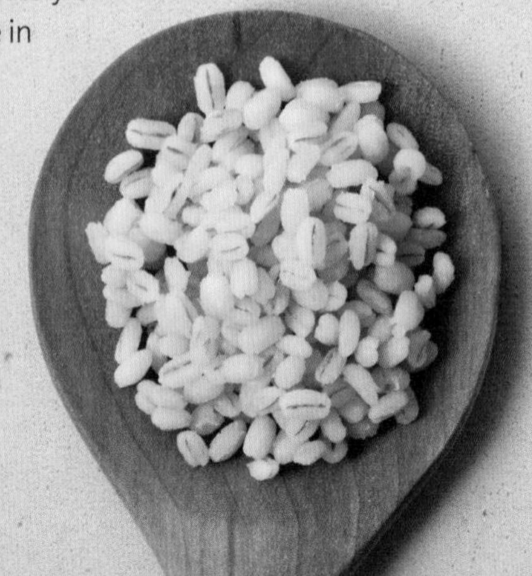

Wholewheat couscous

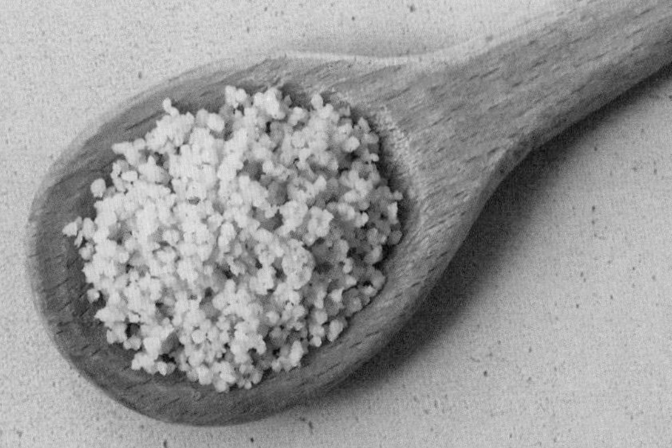

Makes about 1.2kg (2¾lb) cooked couscous

750ml (1¼ pints) light vegetable stock | 500g (1lb 2oz) wholewheat couscous made from spelt (or wheat) | 1 tbsp olive oil | 1 tsp grated organic lemon zest | 2 tbsp lemon juice

Put the stock in a pan and bring to the boil. Add the couscous to a second pan, pour over the boiling stock, and leave the couscous to swell with the lid on for 5 minutes.

Mix the olive oil, and lemon zest and juice. Test the couscous to see if it is done. Different varieties of couscous will need slightly different quantities of liquid. Usually a ratio of 1:1.5 couscous to stock is appropriate. The couscous should have a soft, loose consistency and should not be sticky. If it is still slightly too firm, add a small amount of hot stock, mix this in and leave the couscous to stand again. When the couscous is ready, drizzle over the lemon and oil mixture and fork through until combined. Eat the couscous straight away or spread it out on a baking tray to steam. Store in an airtight container in the fridge for up to 4 days.

Pearled spelt

Makes about 1.2kg (2¾lb) cooked spelt

500g (1lb 2oz) pearled spelt | 2 litres (3½ pints) light vegetable stock

Add the spelt to a pan with the stock and bring to the boil, uncovered, then add the lid and continue simmering gently over a low heat for about 20 minutes. There are all kinds of different varieties of pearled spelt with different cooking times, so the first time you make it, test after 15 minutes to see if it is ready, then every 5 minutes after that. The grains are cooked when they are soft all the way through but still intact.

Drain the cooked spelt in a sieve, making sure to keep the broth, which you can use as the base for a soup – it contains lots of nutrients. Leave the spelt to steam for 10 minutes and either use immediately or leave to cool completely and store in the fridge in a large screwtop jar. It will keep for up to 4 days.

BASTI'S TIP

Pearled spelt has been pre-steamed so the cooking time is much shorter. Make sure you buy the right variety!

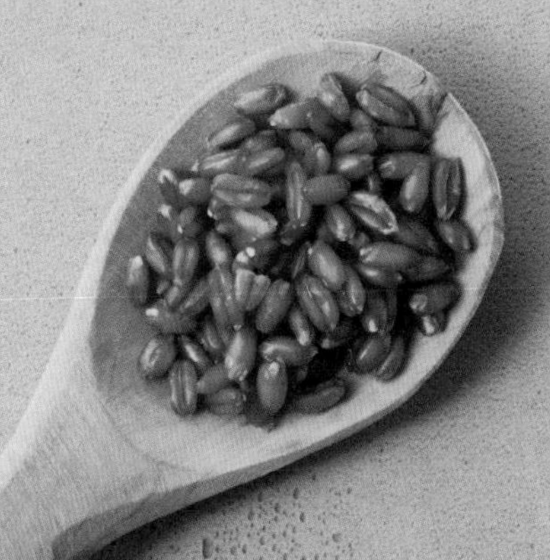

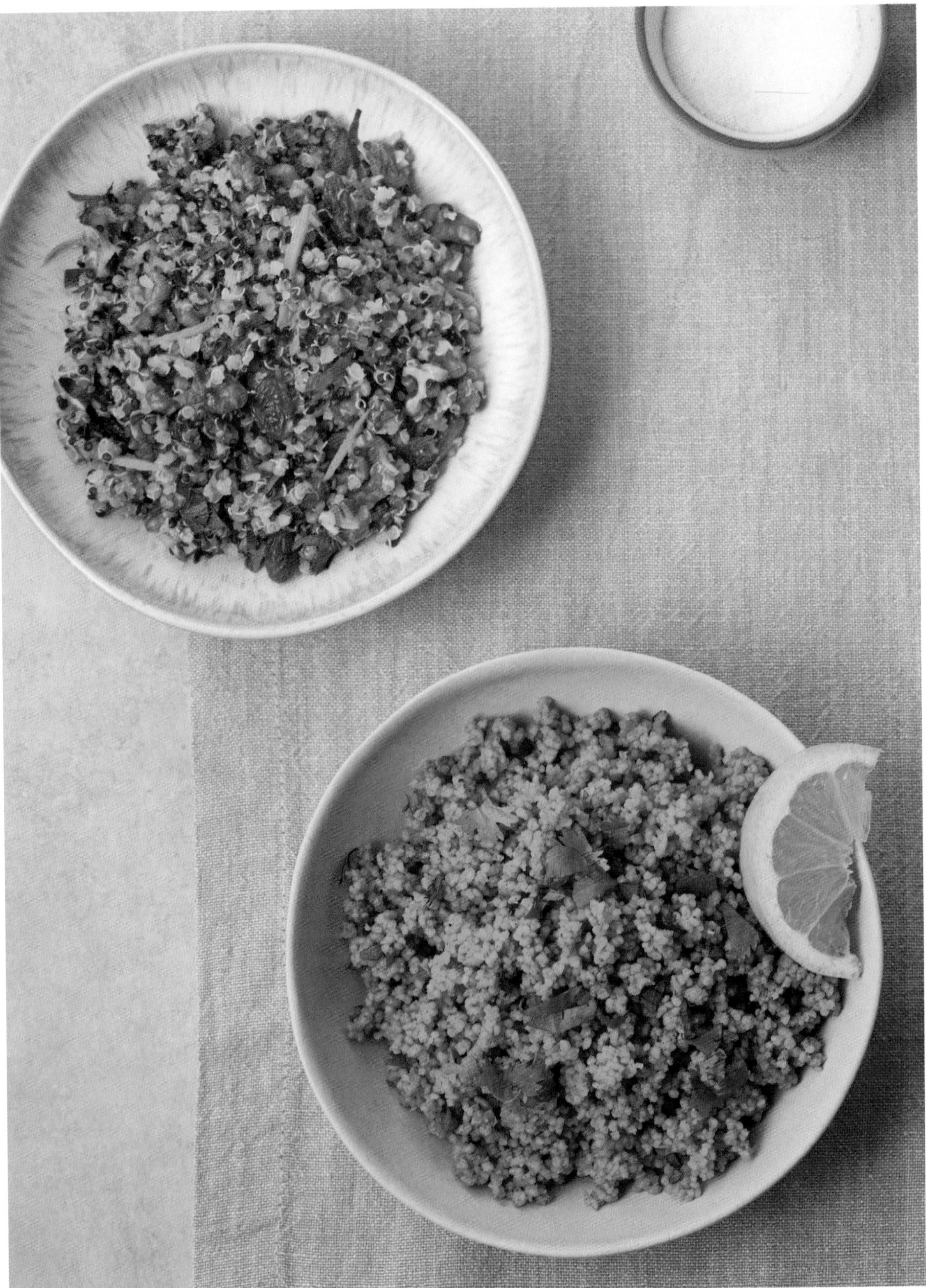

Citrus quinoa

Serves 2

30g (1oz) raisins | 50ml (1¾fl oz) vegetable stock | 1 tbsp lemon juice | 50g (1¾oz) walnuts (or other nuts) | 1 organic orange | 1 tsp olive oil (optional) | 240g (9oz) cooked quinoa (see p. 138, or other grain) | 5 sprigs of parsley (or other herbs)
Also: small ovenproof dish (about 15 × 15 × 4cm/6 × 6 × 2in)

Nutritional values per portion: 428 kcal | 44.1g carbohydrate | 21.8g fat | 10.1g protein | 9g fibre | 2.7g ALA | 470mg lysine | 118mg calcium | 2mg zinc | 2.5mg iron | 0.1mg B2 | < 0.1mg RE | 8µg iodine | 0.4g salt

Put the raisins in a pan with the stock and lemon juice, bring to the boil, and allow the liquid to gently simmer for 4 minutes to a quarter of its original volume until the raisins are saturated.

Preheat the oven to 200°C (180°C fan/400°F/Gas 6). Roughly chop the walnuts. Wash the orange in hot water then dry it. Remove two long strips of orange zest using a peeler and use a knife to slice these into wafer-thin 2cm (¾in) long strips. Squeeze the juice of the orange. Put the orange juice, desired quantity of olive oil, stock, and raisins into the ovenproof dish with the quinoa and mix well.

Scatter the walnuts over the quinoa mixture and bake in the oven (middle shelf) for 15 minutes. Meanwhile, finely chop the parsley. Stir the cooked quinoa mixture to combine, fold in the parsley and serve.

Golden milk couscous

Serves 2

130ml (4fl oz) soya milk with calcium (or other plant-based milk) | 130ml (4fl oz) light vegetable stock | ½ tsp freshly ground pepper | 1 piece of fresh root ginger (1cm/½in), peeled and finely grated | 1½ tsp ground turmeric | ½ tsp ground cinnamon | 2 small garlic cloves, peeled and crushed | 120g (4oz) wholewheat couscous | 1 tbsp lemon juice | ½ bunch of fresh coriander (or chives) | salt

Nutritional values per portion: 239 kcal | 45g carbohydrate | 2.2g fat | 9.3g protein | 4.1g fibre | 0.1g ALA | 322mg lysine | 94mg calcium | 1.5mg zinc | 2.1mg iron | < 0.1mg B2 | < 0.1mg RE | 9µg iodine | 0.7g salt

Put the soya milk, stock, pepper, ginger, turmeric, cinnamon, and garlic in a small pan, bring to the boil and simmer for 2 minutes with the lid on.

Add the couscous and remove the pan from the heat. Mix in the couscous, cover, and leave to stand for 3 minutes. Drizzle over the lemon juice, fluff the couscous with a fork and leave to stand for another 3 minutes. Finely chop the coriander and stir into the couscous. Season the golden milk couscous to taste with salt, serve on two plates and enjoy.

VARIATION

You can stir other herbs or toasted nuts into the couscous. If you are using quinoa, simmer the grains with 120ml (4fl oz) each of vegetable stock and a plant-based milk over a low heat with the lid on for 10 minutes.

North African pepper and millet salad

Serves 2

½ small red pepper | 1 small celery stick | 4 Deglet Noor dates, stones removed | 10 large mint leaves | 5 sprigs of parsley | ½ organic lemon | 1 tsp olive oil | 200g (7oz) cooked millet (see p.135) | salt | freshly ground pepper

Nutritional values per portion: 236 kcal | 41.2g carbohydrate | 4.5g fat | 5.2g protein | 5.4g fibre | 0.1g ALA | 160mg lysine | 26mg calcium | 1.3mg zinc | 3.4mg iron | 0.1mg B2 | 0.2mg RE | 3µg iodine | 0.4g salt

Halve and deseed the pepper, then cut into 3cm (1in) long strips. Wash and finely dice the celery. Finely dice the dates. Finely chop the mint and parsley.

Wash the lemon in hot water and dry it, grate 1 teaspoon of zest and squeeze the juice. Mix the lemon juice, olive oil, and lemon zest in a bowl. Add the prepared vegetables, dates, herbs, and millet, mix roughly and season the salad with salt and pepper.

VARIATION

You can use any other variety of grain here and substitute whatever herbs you fancy.

Mediterranean grain salad

Serves 2

1 shallot, peeled | 4 dried apricots | 10 black olives, pitted | 1 organic lemon | 1 tsp olive oil | 1 small cucumber | 6 cherry tomatoes | 10 large basil leaves | 10 rocket leaves | 200g (7oz) cooked grain (see from p.135, e.g. brown rice) | salt | freshly ground pepper | 2 tbsp pine nuts, toasted

Nutritional values per portion: 344 kcal | 44.8g carbohydrate | 12.1g fat | 8.5g protein | 8.7g fibre | 0.2g ALA | 365mg lysine | 64mg calcium | 1.5mg zinc | 4.3mg iron | 0.1mg B2 | 1.6mg RE | 4µg iodine | 0.4g salt

Dice the shallot and apricots very finely, and halve the olives. Wash the lemon in hot water and dry it, grate 1 teaspoon of zest and squeeze the juice.

Combine the lemon juice, olive oil, diced shallots and apricots, olives, and lemon zest in a bowl. Wash the cucumber, cut into 1cm (½in) cubes. Wash and quarter the cherry tomatoes. Finely chop the basil and rocket.

Add the cucumber, tomatoes, basil, rocket, and grain to the dressing in the bowl and gently toss the salad. Season with salt and pepper, divide between two plates and scatter over the pine nuts to serve.

VARIATION

You can substitute other vegetables and herbs as preferred. This salad always tastes delicious.

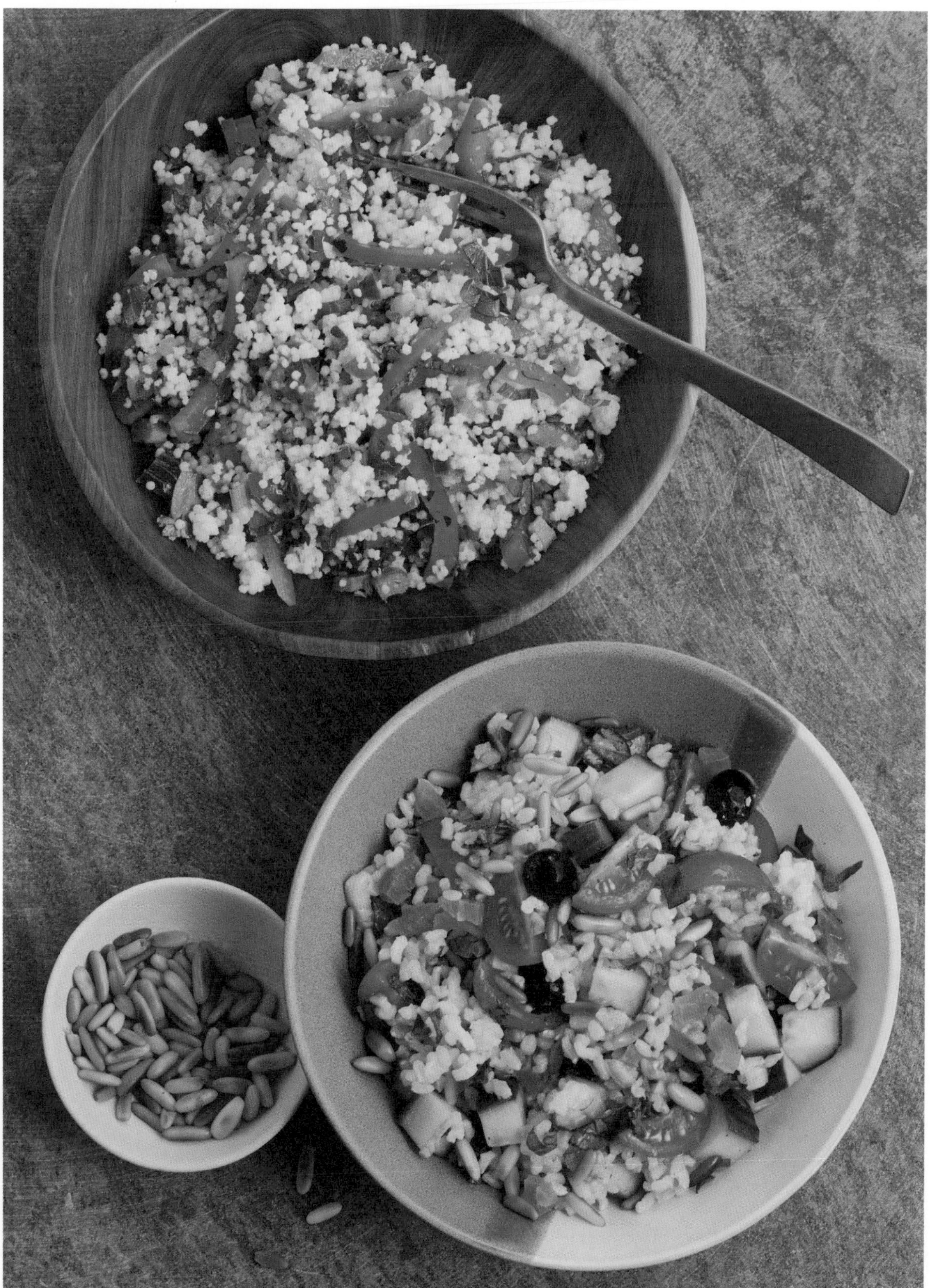

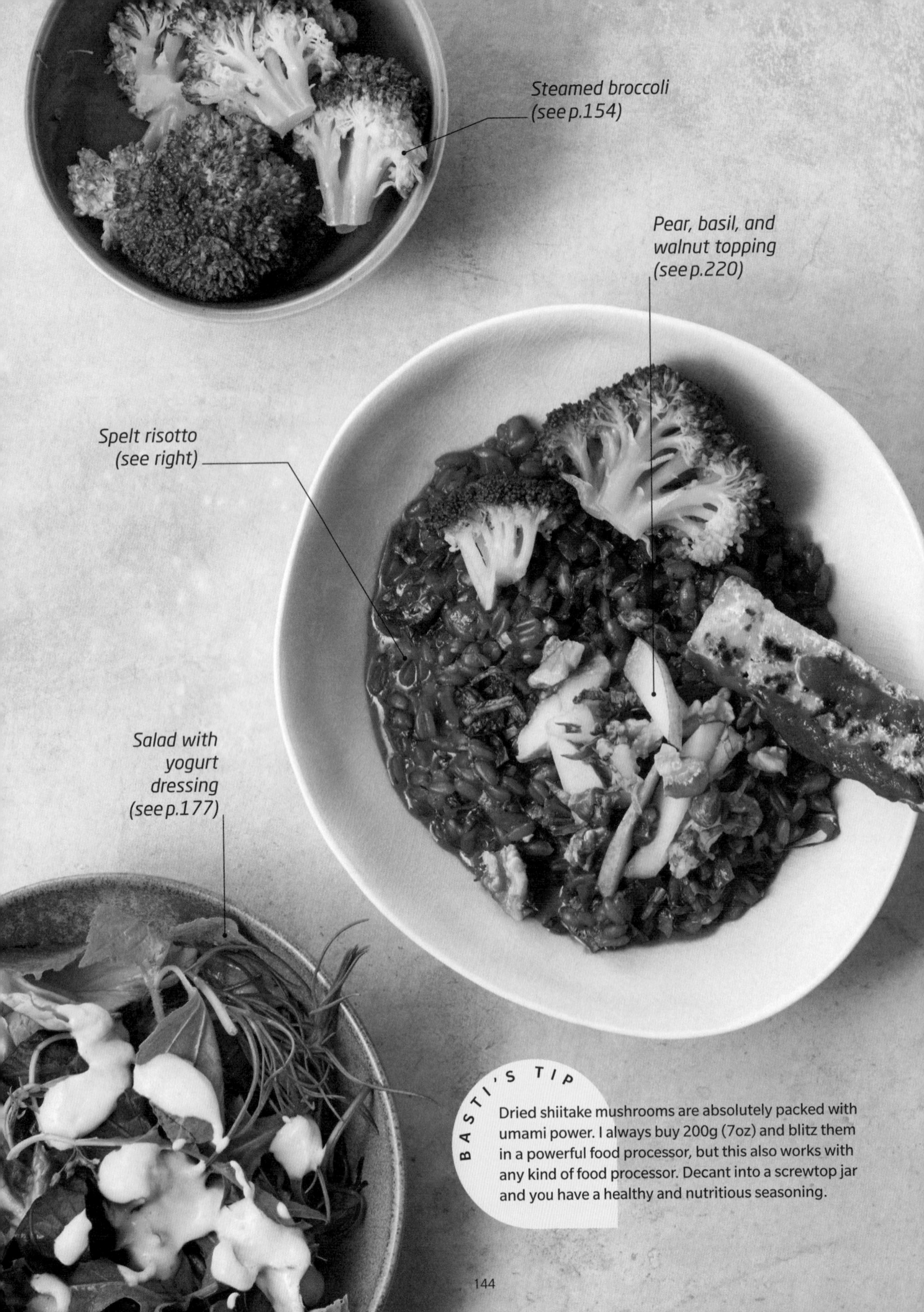

BASTI'S TIP

Dried shiitake mushrooms are absolutely packed with umami power. I always buy 200g (7oz) and blitz them in a powerful food processor, but this also works with any kind of food processor. Decant into a screwtop jar and you have a healthy and nutritious seasoning.

Spelt risotto

Serves 2

1 onion, peeled | 1 tsp dried thyme | 1 tbsp shiitake mushroom powder (see tip) | pinch of ground turmeric | 1 tsp olive oil | 250ml (9fl oz) light vegetable stock | 50ml (1¾fl oz) beetroot juice | 1 tsp white almond nut butter | 200g (7oz) cooked spelt (see p.139) | 1–2 tbsp yeast flakes | 1 tsp organic lemon zest | 1 tbsp lemon juice | 1 handful of finely chopped herbs (e.g. rocket, basil, coriander, or parsley) | salt (or vegetable stock paste, see p.99) | freshly ground pepper

Nutritional values per portion: 241 kcal | 31.1g carbohydrate | 6.6g fat | 11.2g protein | 5.5g fibre | 0.2g ALA | 423mg lysine | 49mg calcium | 2.2mg zinc | 3.1mg iron | 0.3mg B2 | < 0.1mg RE | 1µg iodine | 1.3g salt

Finely chop the onion. Heat a pan and add the onion, thyme, mushroom powder, and ground turmeric. Drizzle with olive oil and sauté for about 1 minute until browning slightly. Then deglaze the pan with stock and beetroot juice and loosen any bits that are stuck to the base.

Add the almond butter and stir in with the balloon whisk. Next, add the spelt and cook over a high heat for 3 minutes, stirring constantly. Lower the heat. Add the yeast flakes, lemon zest and juice, and continue cooking the risotto for another 5 minutes over a moderate heat until it is thick and creamy. Fold in the herbs, season with salt and pepper, and serve.

VARIATION

Of course, you can also incorporate the vegetable component directly into the risotto. Just cut the vegetable of your choice into 5mm (¼in) cubes and sauté briskly with the chopped onion. Then proceed as described in the recipe.

Instead of using spelt, you could substitute pearl barley, brown rice, quinoa, or millet. For grains with smaller kernels, just halve the cooking time.

Umami tofu (see p.201)

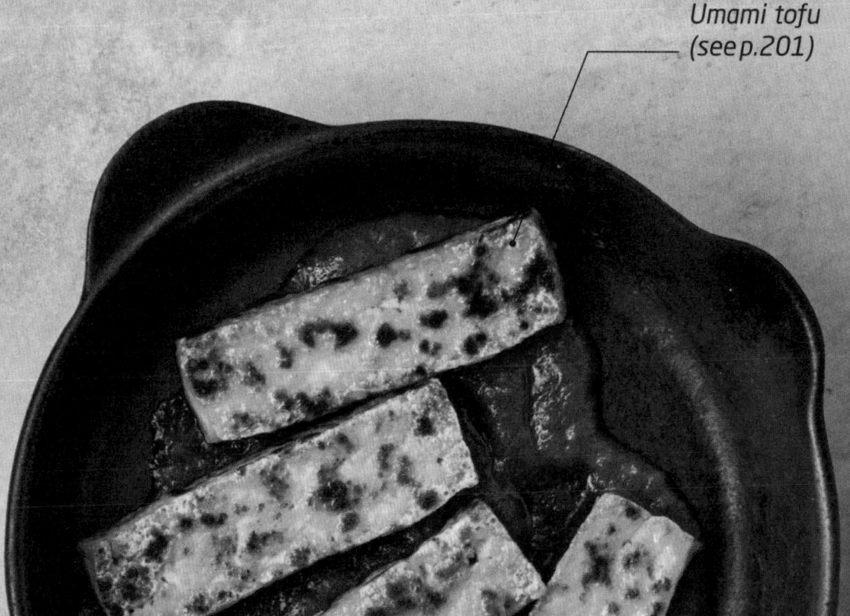

Wholemeal panzanella

Serves 2

2 garlic cloves, peeled | 1 tbsp olive oil | 200g (7oz) wholemeal bread | 1 shallot, peeled | salt | 10 cherry tomatoes | 10 basil leaves | ½ avocado, diced | 100g (3½oz) cooked beans (see p.191) | 1 handful of fresh coriander, finely chopped | 4 tbsp lemon juice | 2 tbsp date paste (see p.97) | 1 tsp organic lemon zest | freshly ground pepper

Nutritional values per portion: 304 kcal | 46.6g carbohydrate | 9g fat | 8.4g protein | 10.1g fibre | 0.1g ALA | 333mg lysine | 51mg calcium | 1.7mg zinc | 2.5mg iron | 0.2mg B2 | 0.1mg RE | 4µg iodine | 0.5g salt

Preheat the oven to 150°C (130°C fan/300°F/Gas 2). Finely grate the garlic and mix with the olive oil in a bowl. Cut the bread into 2cm (¾in) cubes and toss in the garlic oil. Place the cubes of bread on a baking tray and roast in the oven (middle shelf) for 15 minutes until crisp.

Slice the shallot into wafer-thin rings, add a small amount of salt and leave to stand for 2 minutes. Wash and halve the tomatoes. Tear the basil leaves. Add the tomatoes, basil, avocado, beans, and coriander to a bowl with the shallots, lemon juice, date paste, and lemon zest, and combine. Remove the toasted croutons from the oven and mix these into the salad. Season with salt, pepper, and more lemon juice to serve.

Beetroot pearl barley

Serves 2

1 small onion, peeled | 1 tbsp shiitake mushroom powder (see tip p.144) or yeast flakes) | 1 tsp ground cumin (or dried thyme) | 100ml (3½fl oz) light vegetable stock | 50ml (1¾fl oz) beetroot juice (or 50g/1¾oz beetroot, finely grated) | 5 small sprigs of dill | 100g (3½oz) cucumber | 30g (1oz) white almond nut butter | 200g (7oz) cooked pearl barley (see p.138) | 1 tbsp cider vinegar | salt | freshly ground pepper

Nutritional values per portion: 246 kcal | 32.2g carbohydrate | 9.6g fat | 7g protein | 3.2g fibre | 0.1g ALA | 233mg lysine | 69mg calcium | 1.3mg zinc | 1.9mg iron | 0.1mg B2 | 0.1mg RE | 3µg iodine | 1g salt

Finely chop the onion, add to a non-stick pan with 1 tablespoon of water and sauté until brown. Add the mushroom powder and cumin and continue frying for 30 seconds. Pour in the stock and beetroot juice, bring to the boil and simmer gently for 5 minutes.

Finely chop the dill. Wash the cucumber and slice into 5mm (¼in) cubes. Add the almond butter to the sauce and stir in using a balloon whisk. Cook the sauce down over a low heat until thick and creamy. Add the pearl barley, cucumber, dill, and vinegar and continue gently simmering until the mixture has thickened slightly. Season the beetroot pearl barley with the vinegar, salt, and pepper before serving.

VARIATION

Replace the dill with 5 large sprigs of basil and use brown rice, quinoa, pearled spelt, or millet instead of the pearl barley.

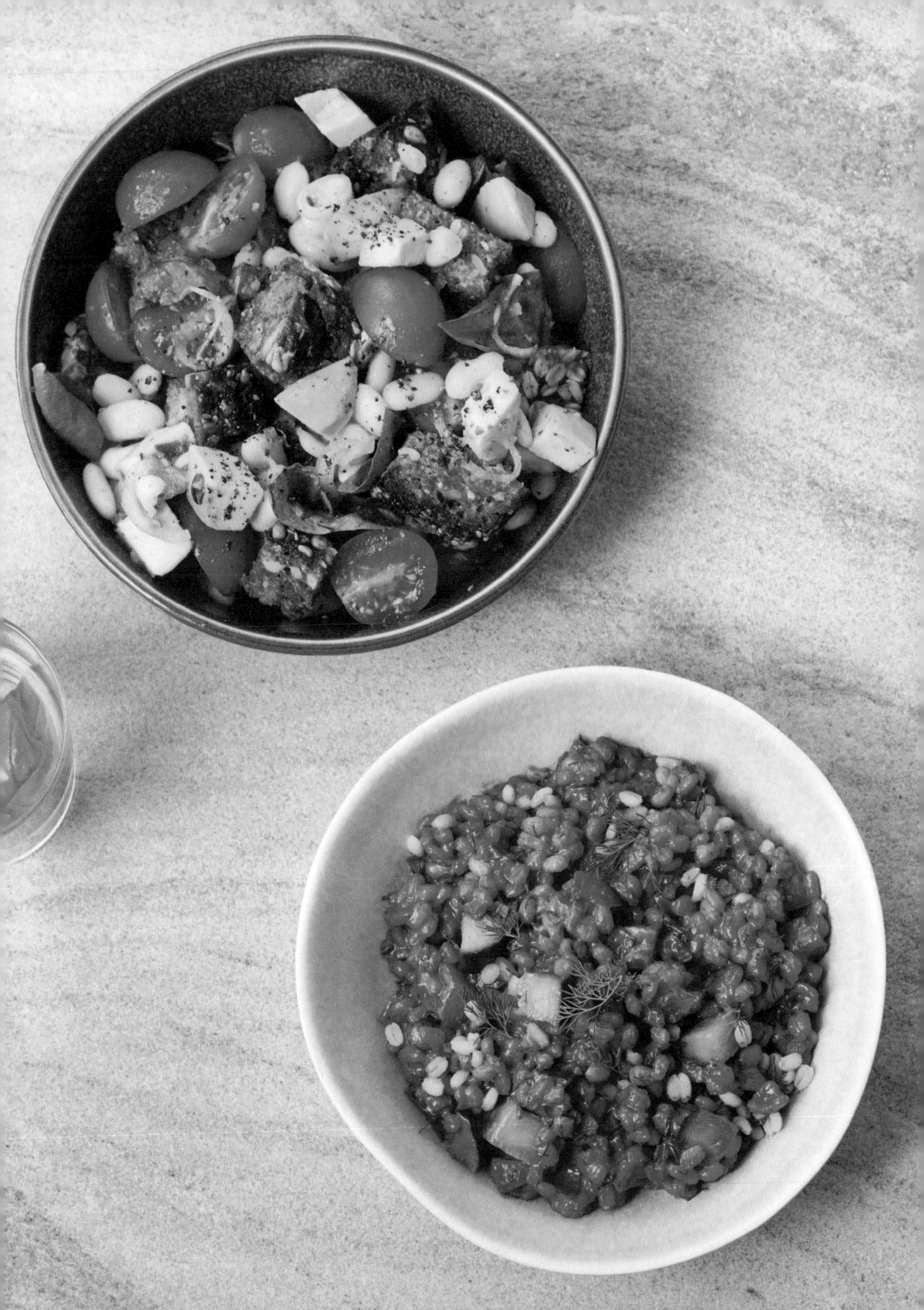

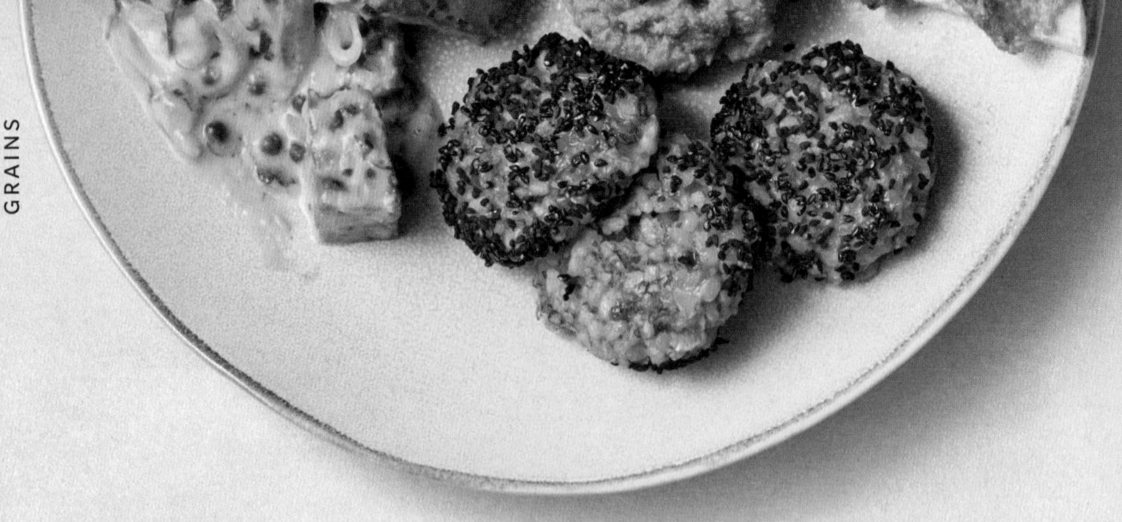

Baked curried rice rissoles

Serves 2

1 small onion, peeled | 1 tsp tomato purée | 5 sprigs of parsley | 2 tbsp yeast flakes | 1 tsp curry powder (see tip p.122) | 1 tsp cider vinegar | 1 tsp salt (or vegetable stock paste, see p.99) | pinch of freshly ground pepper | 200g (7oz) cooked brown rice (see p.136) | 1–2 tbsp wholemeal flour | 3 tbsp black sesame seeds | 1 tsp olive oil

Nutritional values per portion: 311 kcal | 40.4g carbohydrate | 11.6g fat | 11.5g protein | 5.2g fibre | 0.3g ALA | 504mg lysine | 156mg calcium | 1.5mg zinc | 4.6mg iron | 0.3mg B2 | < 0.1mg RE | 5μg iodine | 0.1g salt

Preheat the oven to 200°C (180°C fan/400°F/Gas 6). Finely chop the onion, add it to a pan with 1 tablespoon of water and fry over a high heat for 2–3 minutes until browning slightly. Add the tomato purée and fry for 30 seconds, then leave the onion mixture to cool.

Finely chop the parsley. Add the yeast flakes, curry powder, 2 tablespoons of water, vinegar, salt, and pepper to the onion mixture and stir well. Add the onion mixture and rice to a bowl and mix. Sprinkle over the flour and work this in by hand. Add the parsley and knead the mixture again by hand until it is slightly sticky and holding together well.

Mould the mixture with slightly damp hands to make 1.5cm (¾in) thick rissoles (4cm/1½in diameter). Press one side of the rissoles down onto the sesame seeds, then place them seed-side down on a baking tray lined with baking paper. Brush the tops with olive oil and bake in the oven (middle shelf) for 15 minutes until they are slightly crisp on the outside. Remove the cooked rissoles from the oven, leave to cool for 3 minutes and eat straight away, or enjoy them cold the following day.

VARIATION

These rissoles also work well if made with millet or quinoa.

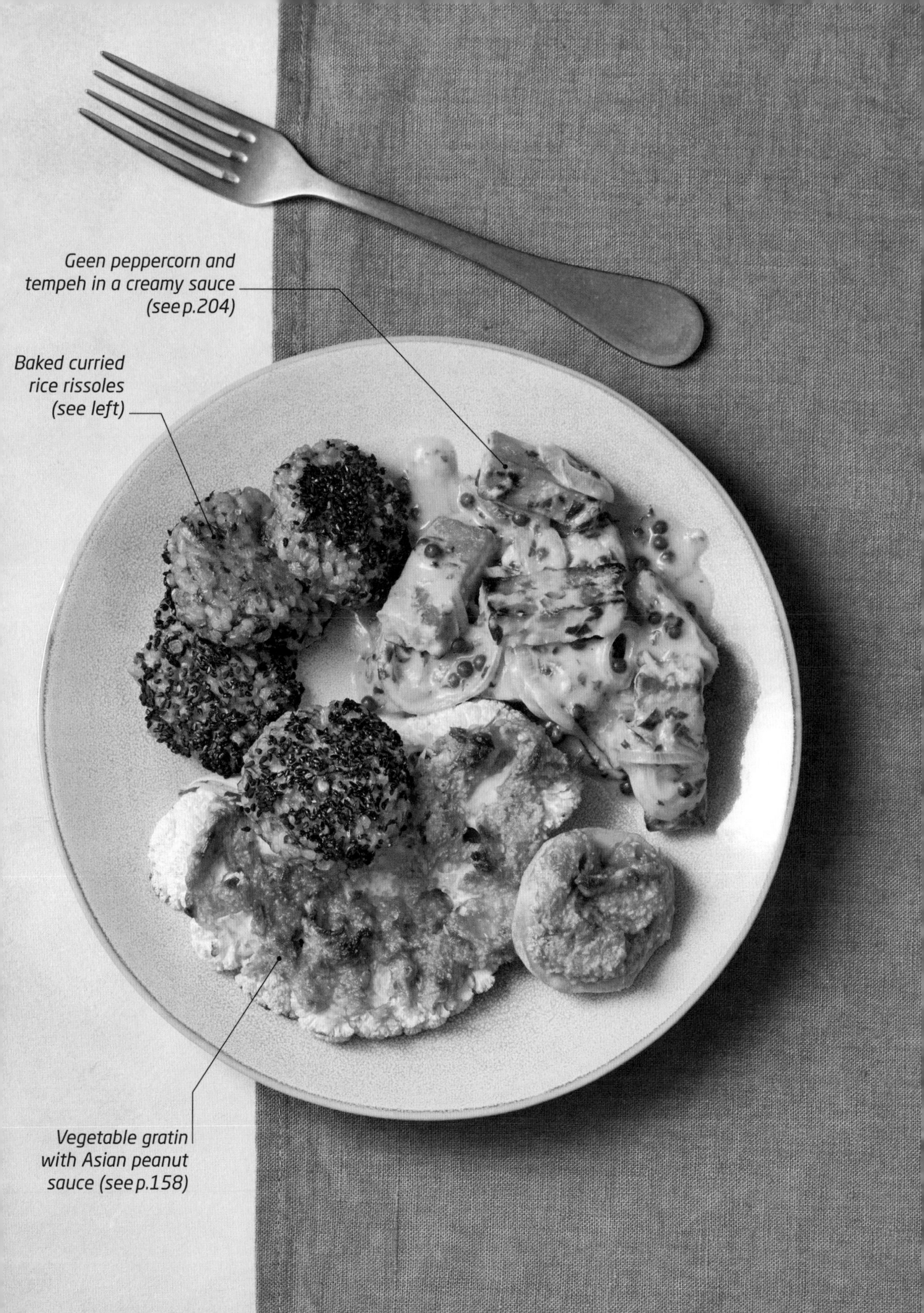

Geen peppercorn and tempeh in a creamy sauce (see p.204)
Baked curried rice rissoles (see left)
Vegetable gratin with Asian peanut sauce (see p.158)

Smoky millet polenta

Serves 2

1 onion, peeled | 2 garlic cloves, peeled | 1 tsp olive oil | 1 level tsp smoked paprika | 400ml (14fl oz) light vegetable stock | 200g (7oz) cooked millet (see p.135) | 2 tbsp shiro miso (or yeast flakes) | 1 tsp white almond nut butter (or cashew nut butter) | salt | freshly ground pepper | lemon juice | 1 small handful of rocket | 2 tbsp black olives, finely chopped

Nutritional values per portion: 289 kcal | 36.7g carbohydrate | 11.9g fat | 7.9g protein | 6.2g fibre | 0.2g ALA | 337mg lysine | 75mg calcium | 1mg zinc | 3.9mg iron | 0.1mg B2 | < 0.1mg RE | 4µg iodine | 2.8g salt

Finely chop the onion and garlic. Put a pan on a high heat, add the onion, garlic, and olive oil in that order and sauté until the onion and garlic are browning slightly. Add the smoked paprika and continue frying for 10 seconds. Deglaze the contents of the pan with the stock and loosen any bits that are stuck to the base.

Add the millet, miso, and nut butter. Bring to the boil and simmer gently over a low heat, stirring occasionally, until the consistency is like porridge. Season with salt, pepper, and lemon juice.

Wash, shake dry, and finely chop the rocket. Divide the millet polenta between two bowls and garnish with the rocket and chopped olives.

BASTI'S TIP

It is important to prepare the millet as described on p.135 to ensure the recipe works perfectly.

VARIATION

Spelt, pearl barley, couscous, rice, or quinoa also taste great here instead of millet.

Sushi rice onigiri with sesame seeds

Serves 2

1 piece of fresh root ginger (1cm/½in) | 1 tbsp date paste (see p.97) | 1 tsp cider vinegar | 1 tbsp organic soy sauce | 200g (7oz) cooked brown rice (see p.136) | 1 nori sheet | 1 tbsp sesame seeds, toasted

Nutritional values per portion: 171 kcal | 30.4g carbohydrate | 3.4g fat | 4.1g protein | 1.9g fibre | 0.1g ALA | 140mg lysine | 47mg calcium | 1.3mg zinc | 2.1mg iron | 0.1mg B2 | < 0.1mg RE | 54µg iodine | 0.7g salt

Peel and finely grate the ginger. Combine the date paste, vinegar, soy sauce, and ginger in a bowl. Use damp hands to shape four small balls from the cooked rice, then roll the balls until slightly longer in shape – twice as long as they are thick. Cut the nori sheet into four equal rectangles and fry in a hot pan for 5 seconds on each side, pressing them flat with a spatula.

Place one roll of rice in the centre of each nori sheet with the tapered ends pointing towards the corners. Brush some of the marinade over the rice. Pick up each of the corners facing the long side of the rice roll and fold them over the rice. Sprinkle some sesame seeds over the visible corners.

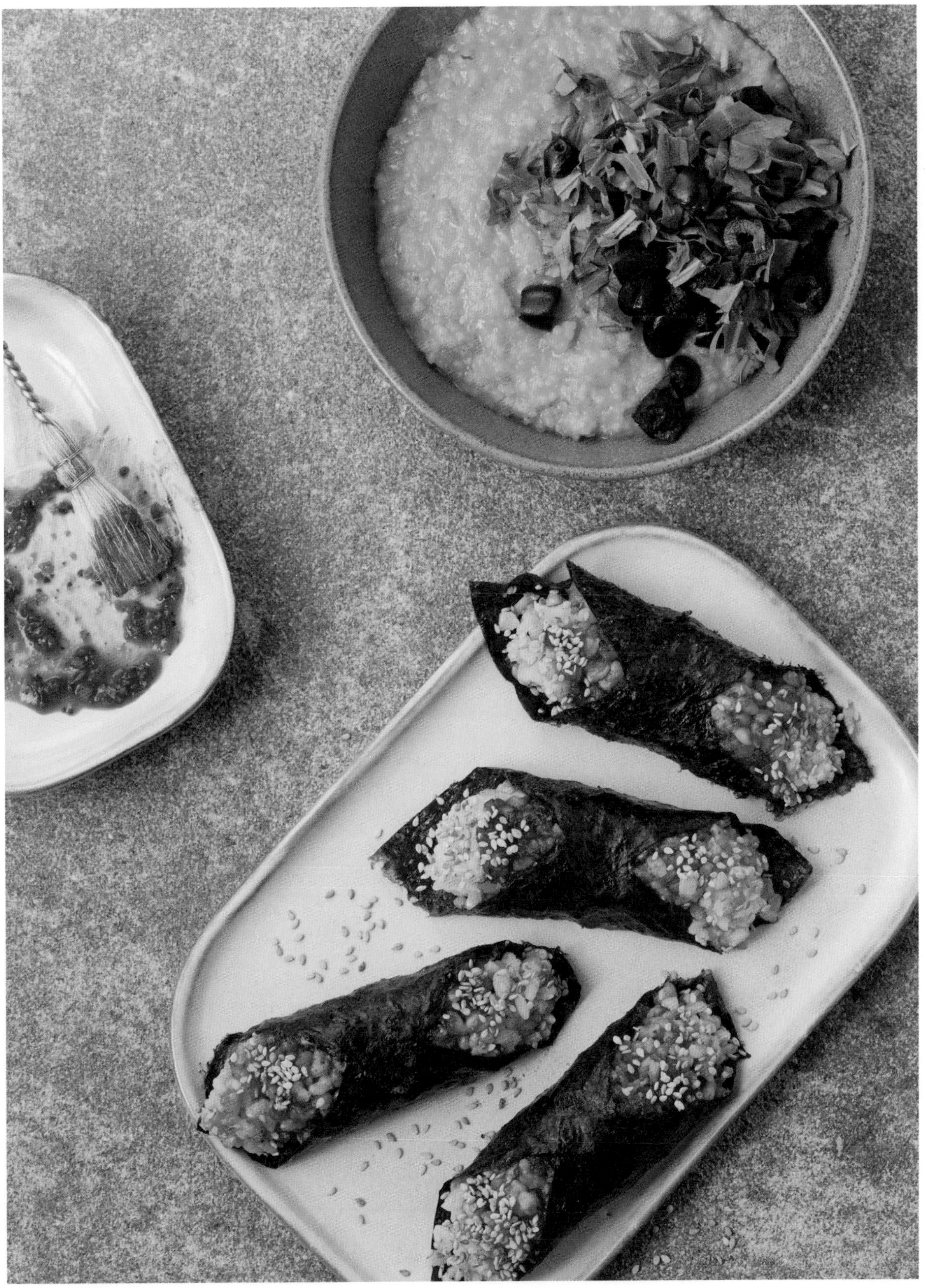

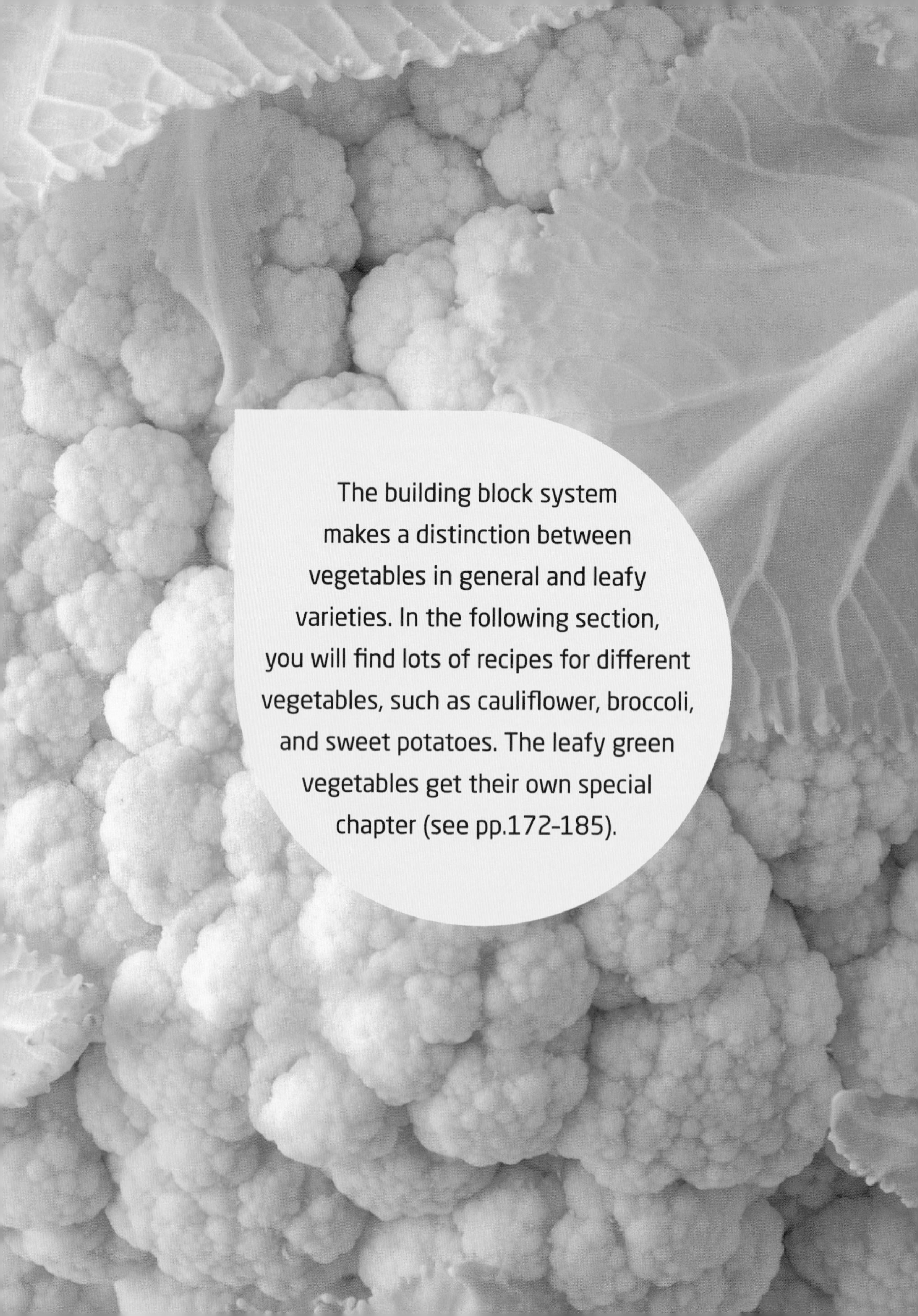

The building block system makes a distinction between vegetables in general and leafy varieties. In the following section, you will find lots of recipes for different vegetables, such as cauliflower, broccoli, and sweet potatoes. The leafy green vegetables get their own special chapter (see pp.172–185).

Vegetables

Building block basics: simple steamed vegetables and leafy vegetables

As we explained in the section describing the recipe building blocks (see from p.89), it is not always necessary to cook five gourmet components from the building block system in this book to create a nutritious meal. Three gourmet components, to ensure some complex flavours, plus two basic recipes that are easy to prepare will be quite enough. You can also choose to serve just three components (two gourmet and one basic). Here we will look at the basic vegetable components. You can steam vegetables in no time and this gentle cooking method ensures a good supply of nutrients. Steamed vegetables also taste delicious.

Take the vegetable of your choice, prepare and wash it, peeling it too if desired.

Add roughly 3cm (1in) of water to a saucepan and bring to the boil. Next, you need a steaming basket, bamboo steamer, or other steamer insert. Add the prepared vegetables. Close the lid and steam the vegetables for as long as required depending on how firm you like them and how small they have been chopped. Insert a sharp knife to test the vegetables occasionally and see how well they are cooked. Take care when removing the lid – the steam is extremely hot.

BASTI'S TIP

To preserve the maximum number of vitamins, vegetables are best steamed whole. This takes longer, but it is the best way to protect their nutritional content.

In general, very firm vegetables that contain less water (like celery, carrots, and parsnips) and vegetables that are high in starch (potatoes and some types of sweet potato) will need slightly longer to cook. The cooking time will be significantly shorter for vegetables with a high water content (like fennel, peppers, courgettes, and radishes) and for vegetables with a shape that allows the hot steam to permeate more easily (like cauliflower, broccoli, romanesco broccoli, sliced pointed cabbage, and red cabbage). Broccoli florets that are about 5cm (2in) in size can be steamed in a maximum of 3 minutes if you like your vegetables with a bit of bite.

If you want to steam different kinds of vegetables together, you will need to take their different cooking times into account and add them gradually to the steamer – starting with the variety with the longest cooking time.

The water used for steaming will absorb a certain amount of flavour and nutrients from the vegetables, so you should never throw it away – it makes a wonderful base for soups and sauces. The exception is potatoes, because they contain a toxin called solanine, which is released into the water and is heat-resistant, so it remains after cooking. Excess consumption of solanine can cause stomach ache, headaches, nausea, and diarrhoea.

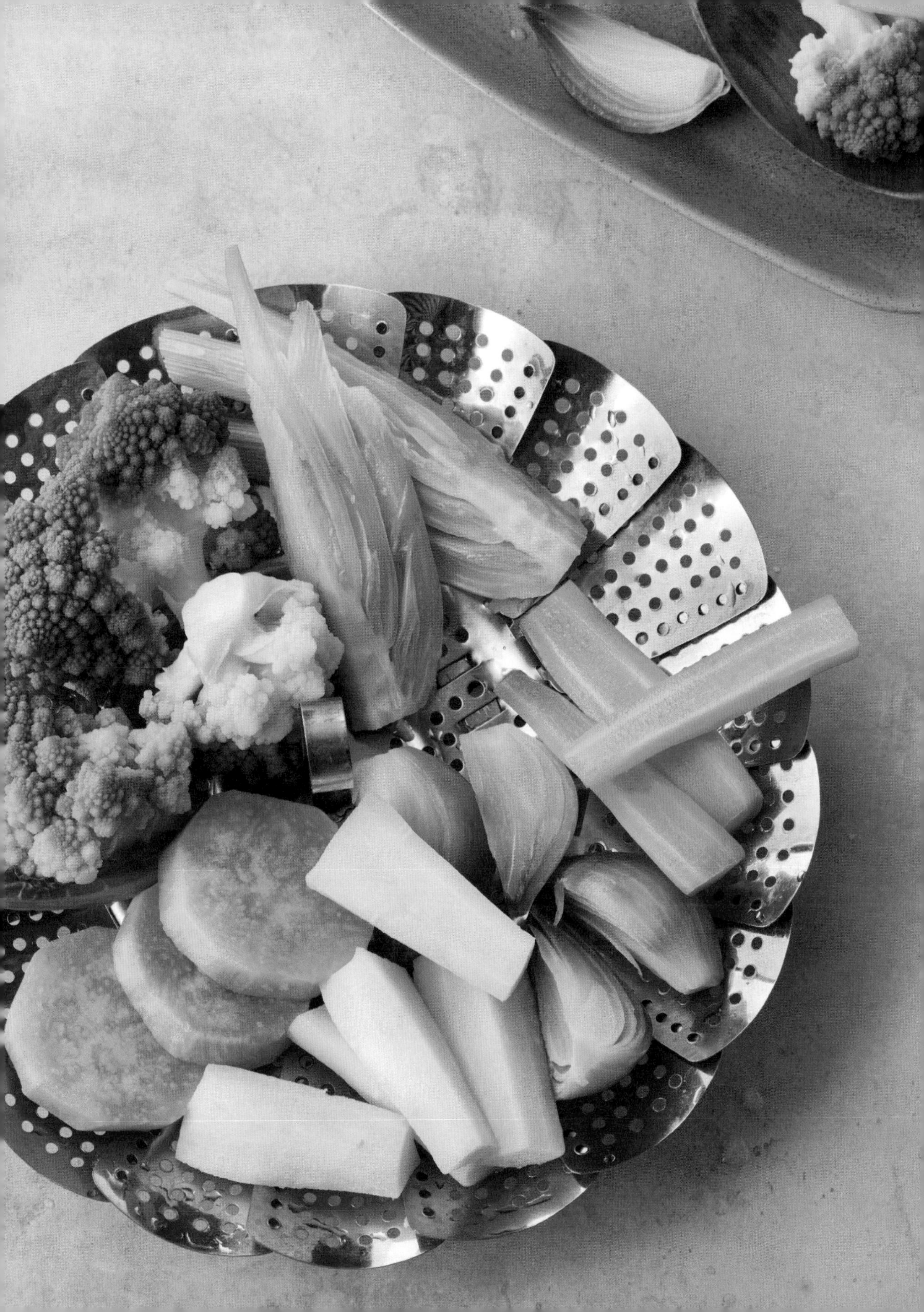

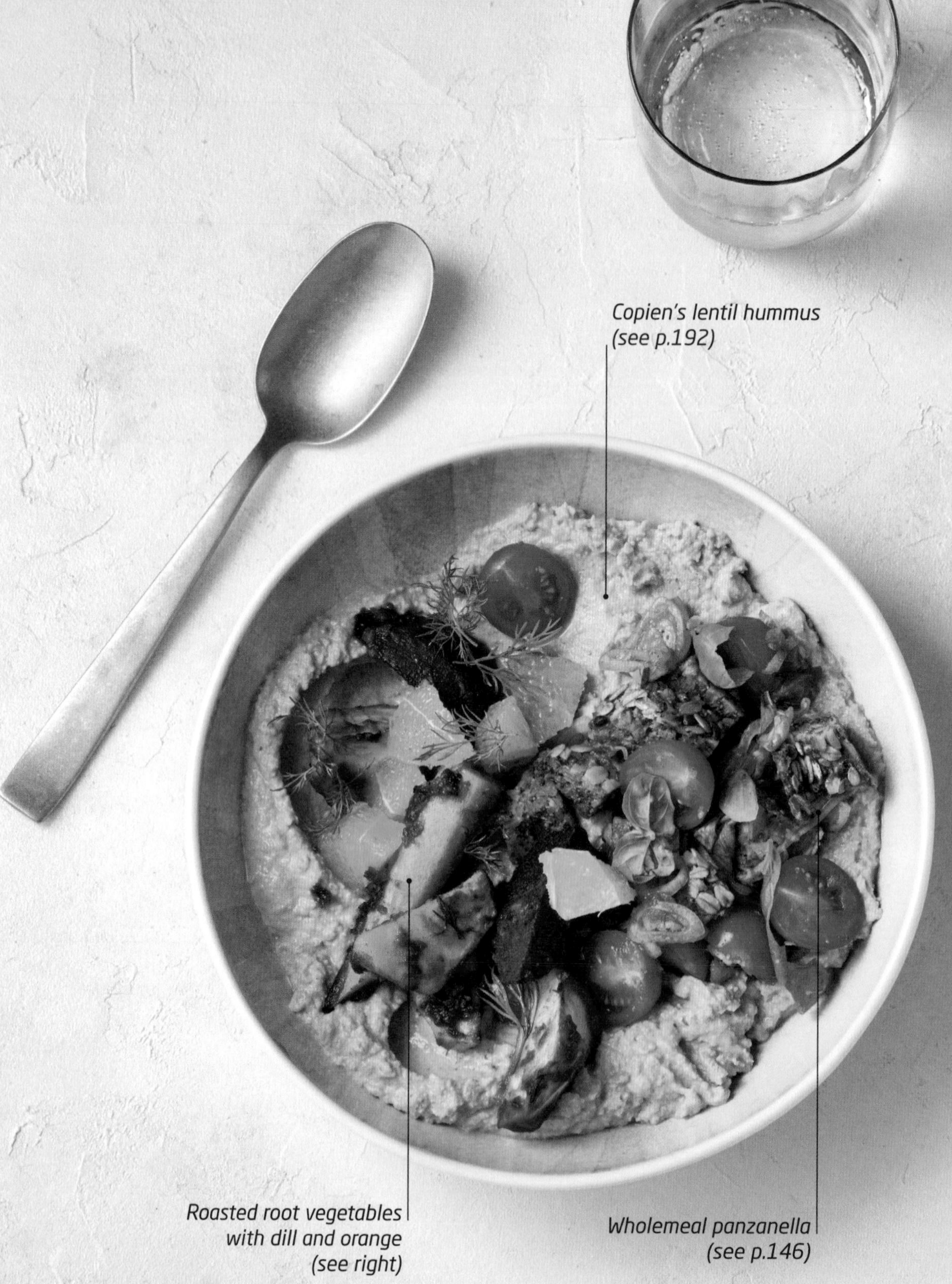
Copien's lentil hummus
(see p.192)
Roasted root vegetables
with dill and orange
(see right)
Wholemeal panzanella
(see p.146)

Roasted root vegetables with dill and orange

Serves 3

Vegetables: 400g (14oz) root vegetables, peeled (e.g. small red or yellow beetroot, turnips, carrots) | 1 large orange | 5 sprigs of dill
Marinade: 2 tbsp date paste (see p.97) | 1 tsp hot paprika | 1 tsp sweet paprika | ½ tsp ground cumin | small pinch of ground cloves | 1 tbsp olive oil | 1 tbsp shiro miso | 1½ tbsp organic soy sauce

Nutritional values per portion: 176 kcal | 25.4g carbohydrate | 5.8g fat | 3.9g protein | 7.1g fibre | 0.1g ALA | 212mg lysine | 73mg calcium | 0.6mg zinc | 1.7mg iron | 0.1mg B2 | < 0.1mg RE | 2μg iodine | 1.2g salt

Preheat the oven to 200°C (180°C fan/400°F/Gas 6). Slice the root vegetables into roughly 2cm (¾in) wedges. Combine the ingredients for the marinade in a bowl. Add the vegetables, toss them until well covered with the marinade, spread out on a baking tray lined with baking paper, and roast in the oven (middle shelf) for 10 minutes.

Meanwhile, use a sharp knife to remove the skin of the orange right down to the fruit, making sure no white pith remains. Then dice the orange into 1cm (½in) cubes. Finely slice the dill, including the stalks. During the final 6 minutes of the cooking time, turn on the grill to toast the vegetables, or place them under a separate grill. Remove the vegetables, which will be cooked al dente, add to a bowl with the orange, scatter with dill, and serve.

BASTI'S TIP

The quantity here is slightly larger because these oven-baked roots taste wonderful cold or eaten the following day.

If using fresh turnips, trim the greenery to about 2cm (¾in) in length. Clean well and slice the turnips so that each wedge includes a bit of green. Turnip leaves are edible and look really attractive.

VARIATION

Instead of the orange, you can use any ripe, juicy fruit and choose a different vegetable to replace the roots. Then chop the vegetables to an appropriate size for the cooking time.

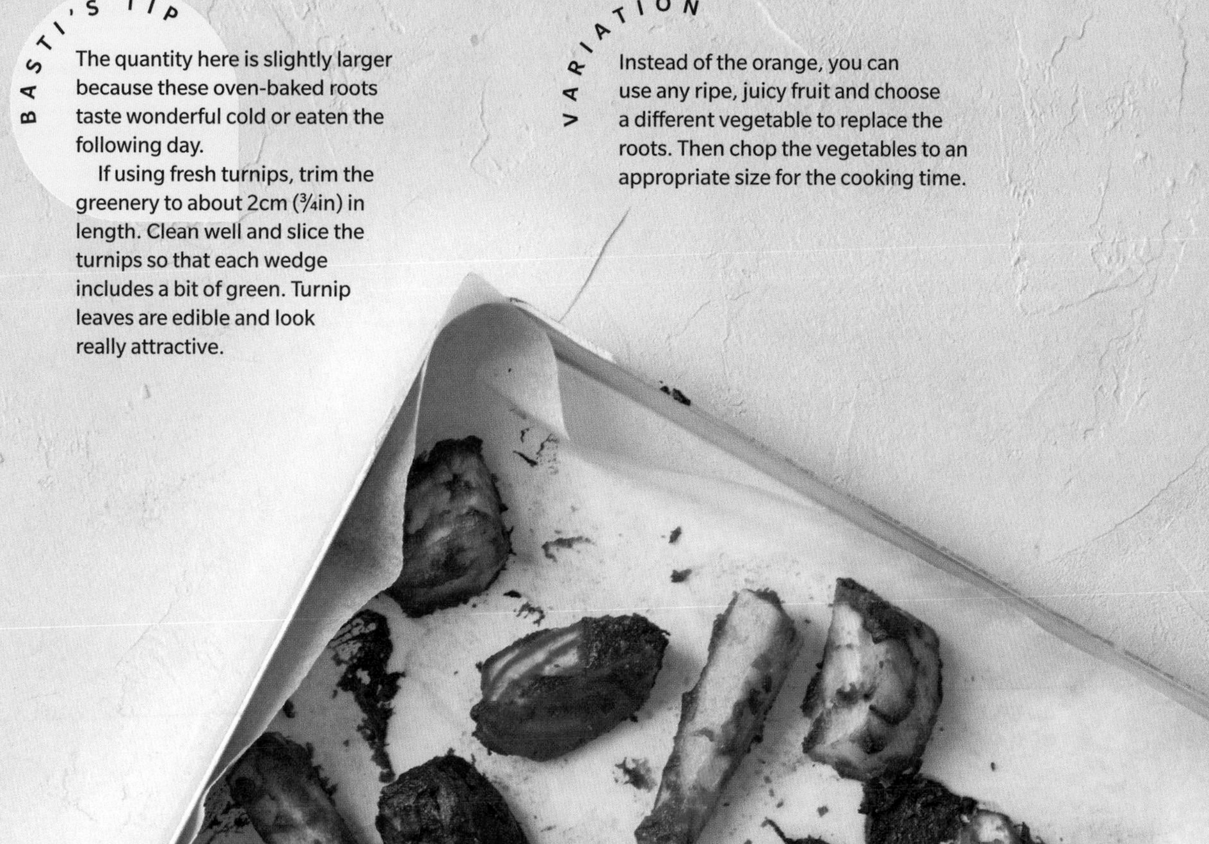

Risotto-style carrots

Serves 2

4 carrots (about 300g/10oz) | 1 small onion, peeled | 1 tsp olive oil | 1 tsp dried thyme | 150ml (5fl oz) soya milk with calcium (or other plant-based milk) | 8 basil leaves | 3 tbsp yeast flakes | 1 tbsp lemon juice | salt | freshly ground pepper

Nutritional values per portion: 155 kcal | 21.2g carbohydrate | 4.5g fat | 6.6g protein | 6.7g fibre | 0.2 g ALA | 374mg lysine | 153mg calcium | 1.2mg zinc | 2.2mg iron | 0.4mg B2 | 2.5mg RE | 6µg iodine | 0.2g salt

Wash the carrots, cut off a small section at the ends and slice into 2cm (¾in) pieces. Blitz these in the food processor until roughly the size of rice grains. Finely chop the onion.

Heat a small pan. Add the chopped onion, drizzle with oil, add the thyme, and sauté the onion until it is browning slightly. Stir in the carrot "rice" and sauté briefly. Deglaze the vegetables with the soya milk, bring to the boil briefly, then simmer the carrots, uncovered, over a moderate heat for 5 minutes until you have a creamy consistency, similar to a risotto.

Meanwhile, finely chop the basil. Season the risotto with yeast flakes, lemon juice, salt, and pepper. Serve the risotto on four plates, scatter with basil, and enjoy.

VARIATION

Any fairly firm vegetable can be used for this kind of risotto-style recipe: such as celeriac, beetroot, or parsley root. You can vary the spices depending on what you fancy – perhaps some curry paste or harissa.

Vegetable gratin with Asian peanut sauce

Serves 2

50g (1¾oz) peanut butter (or almond nut butter) | 1 small yellow banana (about 90g/3oz), peeled |1 tbsp organic soy sauce | ½ tsp hot paprika | 30g (1oz) desiccated coconut (or sesame seeds) | 2 thick slices of cauliflower (see p.160, Step 2) | juice of 1 lime | 3 tbsp finely chopped mint and finely chopped coriander (optional)

Nutritional values per portion: 330 kcal | 17.5g carbohydrate | 22.5g fat | 13g protein | 11.2g fibre | 0.3g ALA | 621mg lysine | 60mg calcium | 1.6mg zinc | 2.1mg iron | 0.3mg B2 | < 0.1mg RE | 6µg iodine | 0.7g salt

Preheat the oven to 200°C (180°C fan/400°F/Gas 6). Add the peanut butter, banana, soy sauce, and paprika to the food processor and blitz to a smooth, creamy consistency. Then stir in the desiccated coconut.

Place the cauliflower slices on a baking tray lined with baking paper, cover with the creamy sauce, and bake in the oven (middle shelf) for 15 minutes until the vegetables have turned nicely brown and are cooked, but still have a bit of bite. Arrange the cauliflower on two plates, drizzle with lime juice, and scatter with herbs before serving, if you like.

VARIATION

Instead of cauliflower you could use broccoli, 2cm (¾in) thick slices of sweet potato, squash, or kohlrabi, or even courgettes sliced in half lengthwise. Try replacing the banana with 3 soft dates and 1 tbsp of tomato purée, and the coconut with pine nuts, then sprinkle the vegetables with finely chopped basil for a Mediterranean feel.

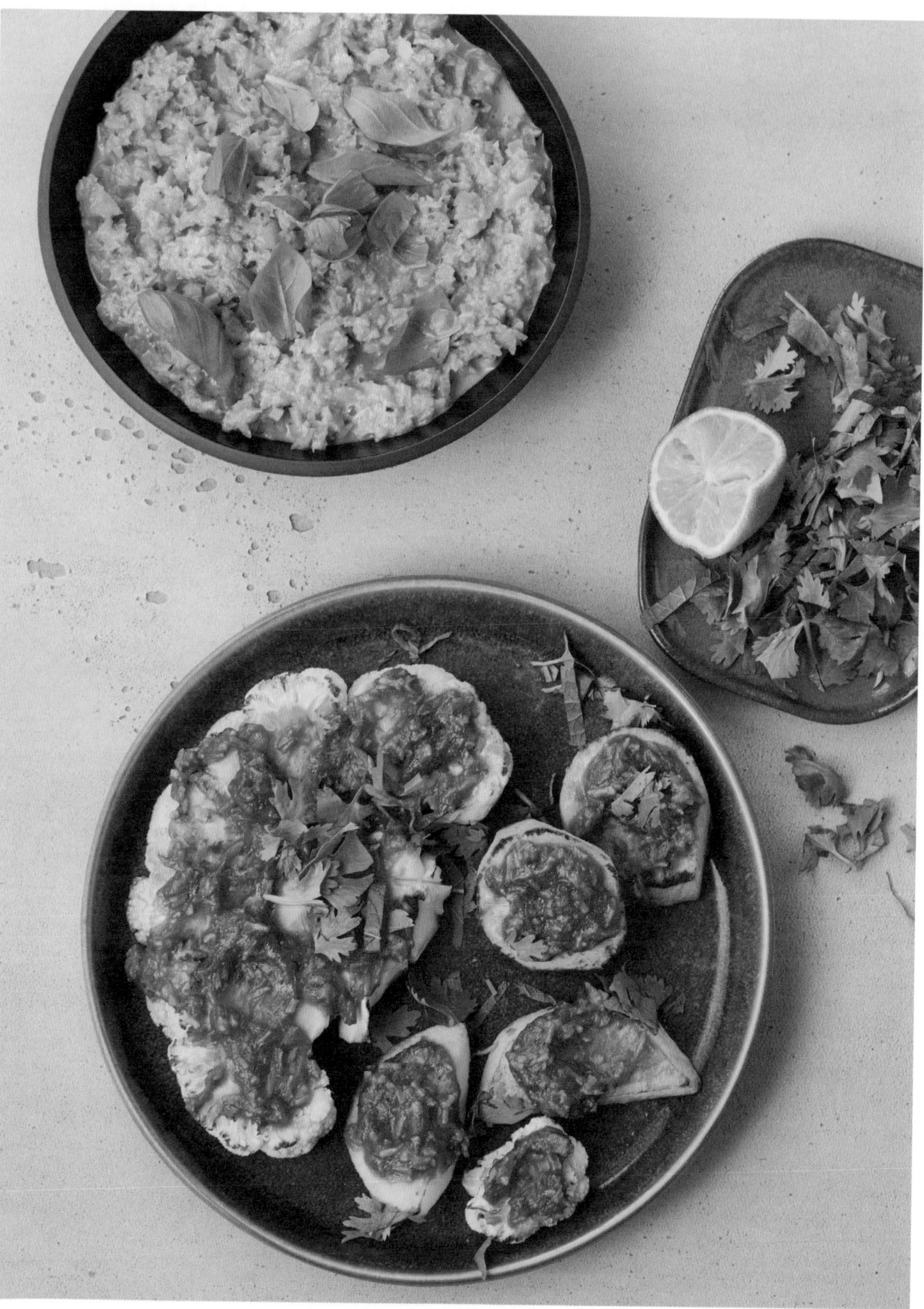

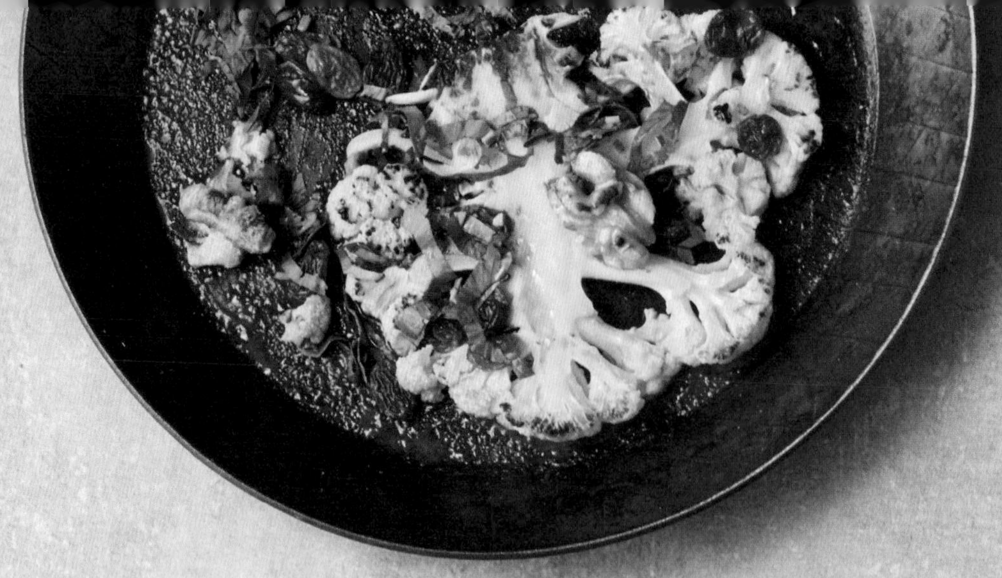

Cauliflower steak with a miso and citrus marinade

Serves 2

5 sprigs of coriander (or dill) | 1 organic orange | 20g (¾oz) raisins | 1 large cauliflower | 30g (1oz) walnuts | 1 tsp olive oil | 1 lemon | 2 tbsp shiro miso | 1 tsp organic soy sauce (or vegetable stock paste, see p.99)

Nutritional values per portion: 360 kcal | 35.6g carbohydrate | 16g fat | 12g protein | 14.8g fibre | 2g ALA | 634mg lysine | 156mg calcium | 1.4mg zinc | 2.9mg iron | 0.3mg B2 | < 0.1mg RE | 6µg iodine | 2g salt

Finely chop the fresh coriander. Wash the orange in hot water, dry it, and remove two strips of zest using a peeler. Add the raisins to a small pan with 100ml (3½fl oz) of water and the orange peel, bring to the boil, and simmer gently for 10 minutes over a low heat.

Meanwhile, wash the cauliflower and slice two roughly 2cm (¾in) thick slices, including the stalk, from the middle of the cauliflower head. Use the rest of the cauliflower in some other way, such as for the pickled vinegar and spice vegetables (see p.162).

Gently toast the walnuts in a dry pan for 3 minutes, stirring constantly, then tip them out onto a plate.

Use your hands to rub oil over the cauliflower slices, ensuring they have a very thin coating all over. Place the cauliflower slices in the hot pan and fry for 1 minute on each side. Continue cooking over a moderate heat, turning the slices occasionally, until they are cooked to your taste. They should be nicely browned.

Squeeze the orange and lemon, mix the juices with the miso paste and soy sauce in a bowl. Deglaze the cauliflower pan with the citrussy marinade. Turn the cauliflower and remove it from the hob. Arrange the cauliflower steaks on two plates and garnish with the rest of the sauce, raisins, coriander, and nuts.

BASTI'S TIP

The cauliflower is best when cooked but still with a bit of bite.

VARIATION

If you are short of time, a dash of organic soy sauce will also work as a steak marinade. In which case, a topping of fresh herbs, nuts, or fresh fruit is really important. These cauliflower steaks also taste fantastic with the apple and coriander topping (see p.216) or the smoky umami gomasio (see p.215). Thanks to their tree-like shape, broccoli, romanesco, and cauliflower all look particularly attractive as steaks, but large slices of kohlrabi, sweet potato, or celeriac work just as well.

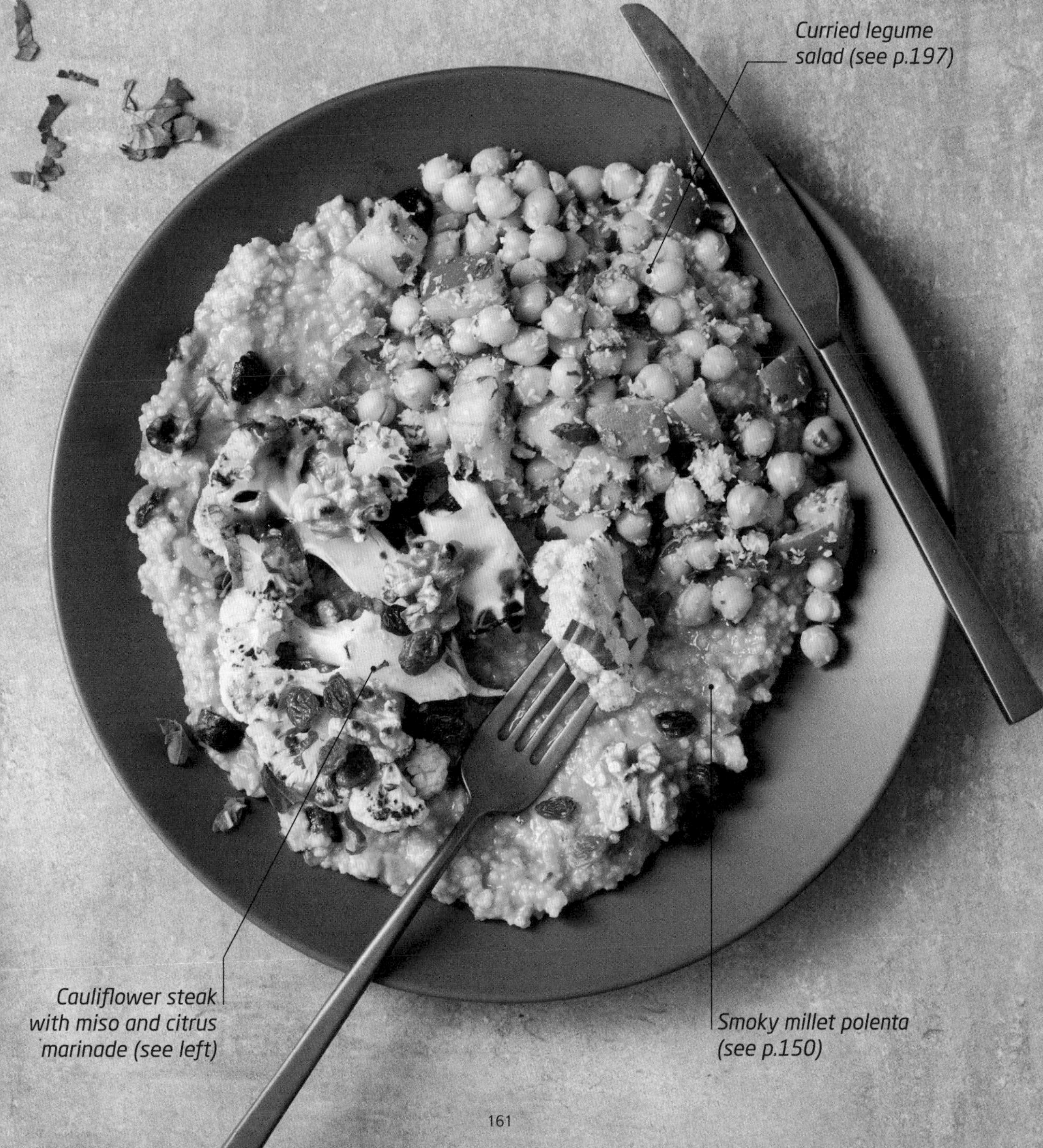

Vegetables pickled in vinegar and spice

Serves 2 (1 preserving jar with 750ml/1¼ pints capacity)

5 Deglet Noor dates, stones removed | 2 garlic cloves, peeled | 1 small red onion, peeled | 150ml (5fl oz) cider vinegar | 2 tbsp organic soy sauce | 2 tsp pink peppercorns | ½ tsp freshly ground pepper | ½ tsp ground turmeric | 250g (9oz) broccoli (about 1 small head) | 1 sprig of rosemary (or thyme)

Nutritional values per portion: 115 kcal | 20.8g carbohydrate | 0.5g fat | 5.9g protein | 6.6g fibre | 0.1g ALA | 247mg lysine | 100mg calcium | 0.8mg zinc | 1.7mg iron | 0.2mg B2 | 0.2mg RE | 20µg iodine | < 0.1g salt

Finely chop the dates and garlic and slice the onion into rings. Put 300ml (10fl oz) of water, vinegar, soy sauce, pink peppercorns, pepper, turmeric, the dates, garlic, and onion rings into a pan, bring to the boil, and cook for 2 minutes.

Wash the broccoli and slice into 4cm (1½in) florets. Peel the stalk and slice this into chunks, including the lovely leaves. Add the broccoli pieces and leaves plus the sprig of rosemary to the cooking liquid, cover, and boil for 5 minutes. While it is still boiling hot, transfer the broccoli and all the cooking liquid into a clean, sterilized jar and seal firmly. Turn the jar upside down and leave to cool. Then turn the jar the right way up and store in the fridge for at least 1 day to allow the flavours to develop.

BASTI'S TIP

Pickled vegetables will keep for at least 2 weeks if chilled and sealed. This is a quick, delicious vegetable side dish to have ready in your store cupboard.

VARIATION

This recipe is very flexible. In principle it works with lots of different vegetables – you just need to chop them into pieces the right size to cook in the specified time. Try the following options: small cauliflower florets, small romanesco broccoli florets, green beans, 1cm (½in) thick beetroot batons, sliced fennel, or sweet potato, 2cm (¾in) thick slices of kohlrabi or radish, 4cm (1½in) thick slices of courgette or cucumber – or why not use a mixture? You can also play around with the spices. The crucial thing is to get the correct ratio of water to vinegar and a certain amount of sweetness.

Photo see p. 164 top

Celery and mushroom ceviche with blueberries

Serves 2

1 red onion, peeled | 2 large celery sticks | 2 tomatoes | 8 sprigs of coriander | 1 orange | 3 limes | 1 mild fresh chilli | 3 tbsp blueberries (optional) | 2 tsp olive oil (or ½ ripe avocado, finely diced) | 200g (7oz) mushrooms (large firm button mushrooms or king oyster mushrooms) | 2 tsp organic soy sauce

Nutritional values per portion: 249 kcal | 25.3g carbohydrate | 9.2g fat | 9g protein | 11.4g fibre | 0.7g ALA | 368mg lysine | 121mg calcium | 1.1mg zinc | 2.8mg iron | 0.5mg B2 | 0.2mg RE | 23μg iodine | 0.4g salt

Slice the onion into very thin rings. Wash the celery. First slice the stalks lengthwise into thin strips, then dice finely. Wash the tomatoes and grate coarsely to create a tomato purée. Finely chop the coriander. Squeeze the orange and limes. Wash and finely chop the chilli. If using, wash the blueberries and leave to drain. Put the prepared ingredients into a bowl with the olive oil, mix, and leave to infuse.

Dry the mushrooms and remove the section at the stalk. Roughly break up the mushrooms by hand into uneven pieces about 3cm (1in) in size. Heat a pan over a very high heat. Add the mushrooms and use a pan lid to press them down on the base of the pan for 30 seconds until the mushrooms have browned. Turn the mushrooms, press down with the lid for another 30 seconds and fry. Add the mushrooms to the other ingredients in the bowl. Season the ceviche with soy sauce, leave to infuse for at least 5, ideally 20, minutes. Then serve on two plates and enjoy.

BASTI'S TIP

If you do not like the flavour of raw onion, just let the onion rings soak for 10 minutes in cold water with salt and a dash of cider vinegar. This makes the onions milder, but valuable oils are also lost.

VARIATION

Instead of mushrooms, you can also make this ceviche with sweet potato (adjust the cooking time), smoked tofu, courgettes, or watermelon. But do not fry the melon.

Photo see p. 164 bottom

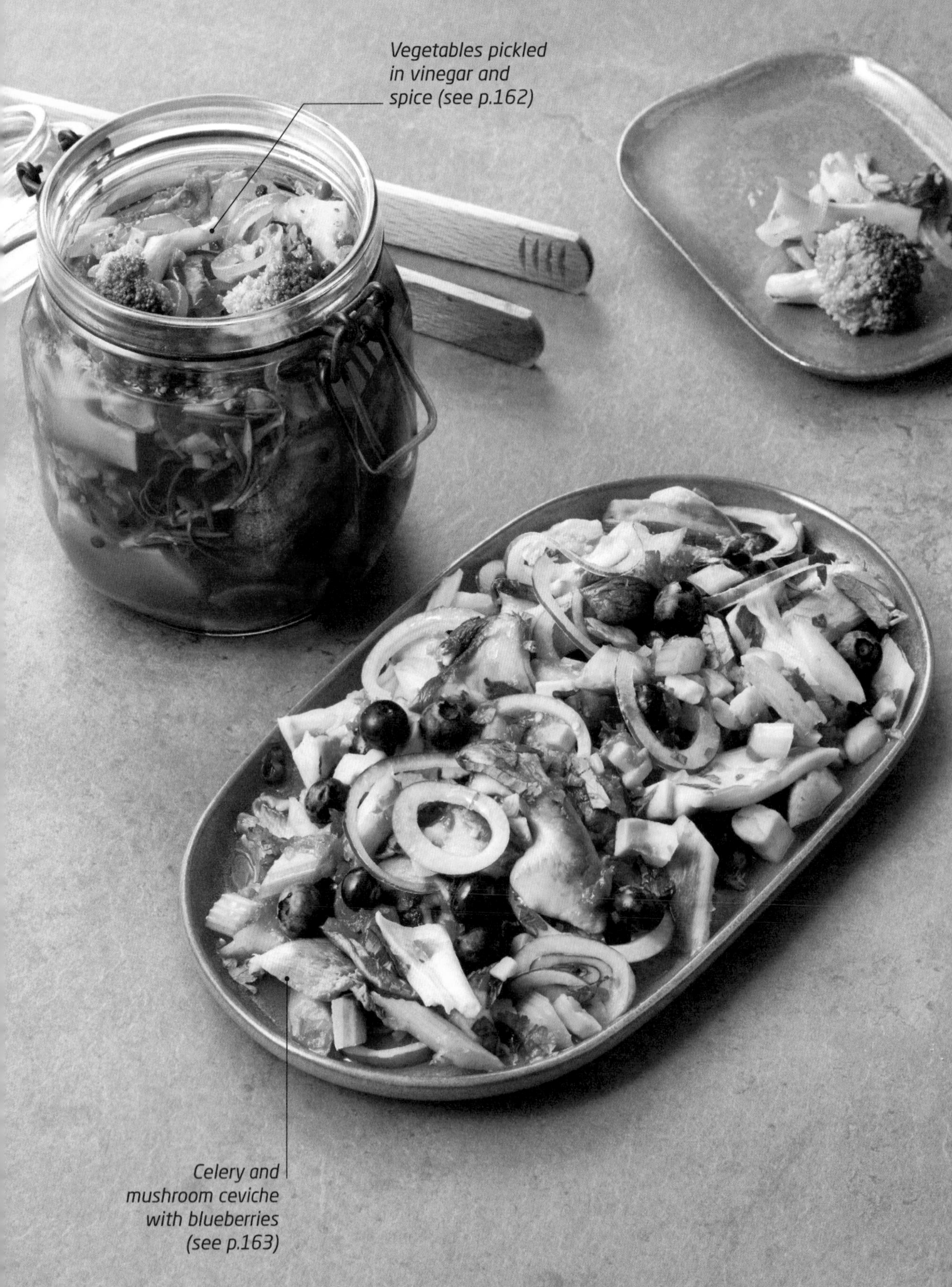

Vegetables pickled in vinegar and spice (see p.162)

Celery and mushroom ceviche with blueberries (see p.163)

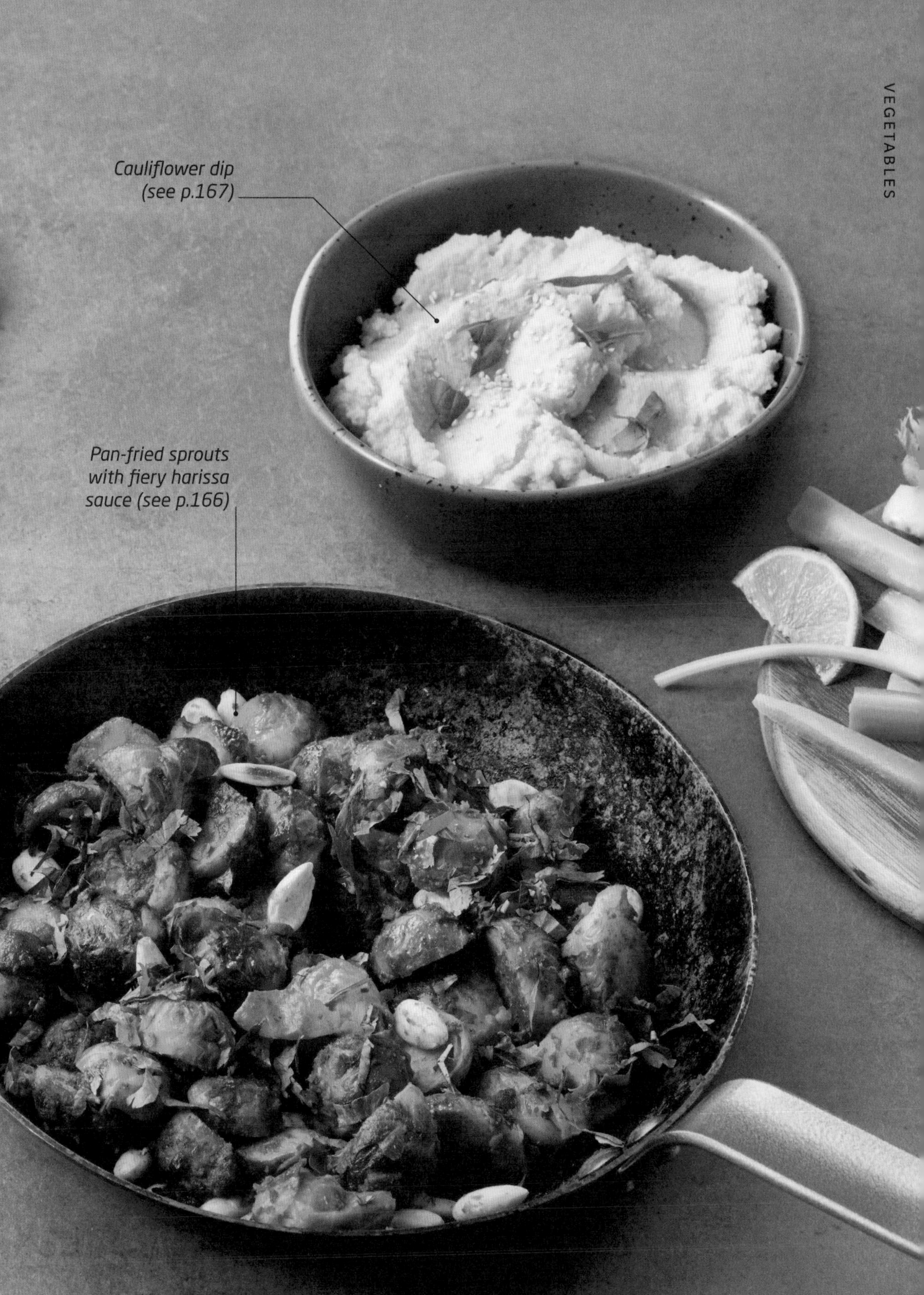

Cauliflower dip
(see p.167)

Pan-fried sprouts with fiery harissa sauce (see p.166)

Pan-fried sprouts with fiery harissa sauce

Serves 3

Sprouts: 400g (14oz) Brussels sprouts | 200ml (7fl oz) light vegetable stock | salt | 3 tbsp toasted almonds | 5 tbsp finely chopped fresh coriander
Sauce: 2 garlic cloves, peeled | 1 tsp olive oil | 1 tsp grated ginger | 4 Deglet Noor dates, stones removed | 1 tsp ground cumin | ½ tsp ground cinnamon | 2 tbsp pepper paste (or tomato purée) | 2 tsp hot paprika | 3 tbsp lime juice | 200ml (7fl oz) vegetable stock

Nutritional values per portion: 192 kcal | 14.4g carbohydrate | 10.4g fat | 9.7g protein | 9.5g fibre | 0.2g ALA | 448mg lysine | 105mg calcium | 1.5mg zinc | 2.3mg iron | 0.3mg B2 | 0.1mg RE | 2µg iodine | 1.1g salt

Wash the sprouts, remove any small stalks and wilting outer leaves, slice each sprout in half. Put a deep pan over a high heat, add the sprouts, and sauté vigorously without any fat. After 2 minutes, pour in the stock and simmer for 5 minutes.

Meanwhile, to make the sauce, put the garlic and other ingredients into a food processor and purée until smooth. Once the stock in the pan has virtually boiled away, pour in the sauce and cook over a high heat for 1–2 minutes until the sprouts are completely coated in the sauce. Season with salt before serving on three plates scattered with almonds and fresh coriander.

VARIATION

The Brussels sprouts can be replaced by green asparagus, kohlrabi, broccoli florets, cauliflower florets, or other vegetables.

BASTI'S TIP

You can also coat the sprouts with the sauce, spread them out on a baking tray lined with baking paper and roast for 15 minutes in an oven preheated to 180°C (160°C/350°F/Gas 4). For this recipe, the quantities are designed to be slightly more generous, but the sprouts taste great cold or eaten the following day.

Photo see p. 165 bottom

Cauliflower dip

Serves 3

360g (12oz) cauliflower | 200g (7oz) sweet potato (or celeriac) | 2 garlic cloves, peeled | small pinch of ground cloves | 2 tbsp shiro miso | 2 tsp white almond nut butter | 2 tsp olive oil | 1 tsp grated organic lemon zest | salt

Nutritional values per portion: 211 kcal | 25.2g carbohydrate | 8.9g fat | 6.6g protein | 7.7g fibre | 0.2g ALA | 361mg lysine | 72mg calcium | 0.5mg zinc | 1.6mg iron | 0.2mg B2 | 0.9mg RE | 3μg iodine | 0.9g salt

Wash the cauliflower and slice into small florets. Peel the sweet potato and cut into 1cm (½in) thick slices. Put roughly 3cm (1in) of water in a large pan and add a steamer insert. Bring the water to the boil. Put the vegetables in the steamer, cover, and steam over a high heat for about 8 minutes until soft. Alternatively, put water to a depth of roughly 2cm (¾in) in a pan, bring to the boil, and cook the vegetables directly in the water (with no steamer insert) for 8 minutes until soft.

Transfer the vegetables to the food processor with the rest of the ingredients and 4 tablespoons of the cooking water. Blend to a smooth purée. Season to taste with salt.

VARIATION

Instead of cauliflower, you could use broccoli or romanesco. Kohlrabi also works well; just add a bit more nut butter to get the right consistency.

BASTI'S TIP

Serve the dip in a pretty bowl with vegetable batons and bread as a starter, garnish with a handful of roasted diced sweet potato, toasted sesame seeds, a handful of torn basil leaves, and fresh lime slices. It's a good idea to make this in a slightly larger quantity because the dip still tastes delicious the next day.

Photo see p.165 top

Celeriac tagliatelle with lemon cream sauce

Serves 3

1 small onion, peeled | 300ml (10fl oz) light vegetable stock | 1 tbsp white almond nut butter (or cashew nut butter; about 30g/1oz) | 2 Deglet Noor dates, stones removed | 1 tsp dried thyme | 1 tbsp shiro miso | 3 tbsp lemon juice | 3 strips of organic lemon peel (about 4cm/1½in long) | ½ small celeriac (about 300g/10oz) | 5 tbsp finely chopped parsley | freshly ground pepper | 1 tbsp hazelnuts, toasted (optional)

Nutritional values per portion: 256 kcal | 20.2g carbohydrate | 15.7g fat | 8.3g protein | 10.8g fibre | 0.2g ALA | 373mg lysine | 174mg calcium | 1.mg zinc | 2.4mg iron | 0.3mg B2 | 0.1mg RE | 6µg iodine | 1.6g salt

Dice the onion. Heat a pan. Add the diced onion and drizzle with 1 tablespoon of water. When the onion begins to take on some colour, add it to the food processor along with the stock, almond butter, dates, thyme, miso, lemon juice and peel, and purée until smooth. Return the sauce to the pan and simmer gently over a moderate heat for 3 minutes.

Meanwhile, peel the celeriac and chop into 1cm (½in) thick slices. Use a peeler to create strips like tagliatelle from the celeriac slices. Alternatively, use a julienne peeler or spiralizer to create celeriac noodles.

Add the celeriac to the sauce and cook for 1–2 minutes over a high heat until nice and thick. Add the parsley and leave the flavours to develop briefly. Season the "pasta" with pepper, garnish with chopped hazelnuts, if you like, and enjoy.

VARIATION

You can freely substitute other vegetables here, too. This recipe is delicious made with radish or carrot tagliatelle. But you can also use a spiralizer to transform kohlrabi, beetroot, courgettes, or sweet potato into veggie pasta. Instead of nut butter, you could replace 150ml (5fl oz) of the stock with oat cream or soya cream.

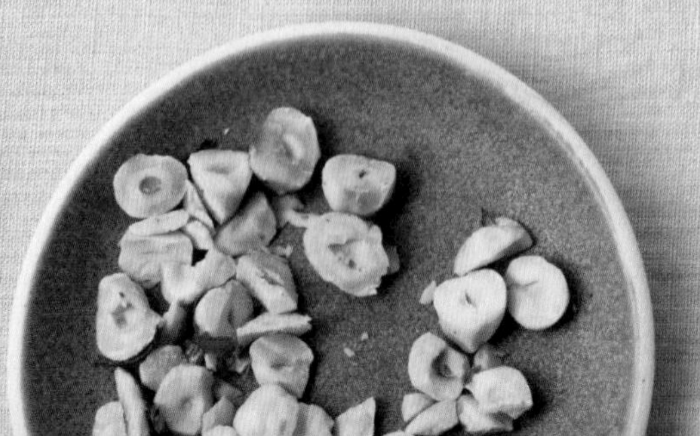

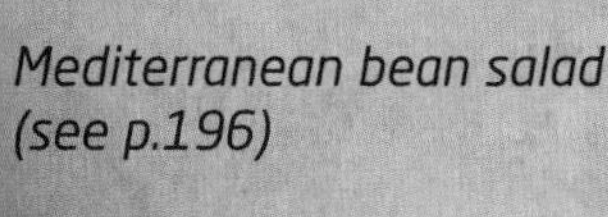

Mediterranean bean salad (see p.196)

Celeriac tagliatelle with lemon cream sauce (see left)

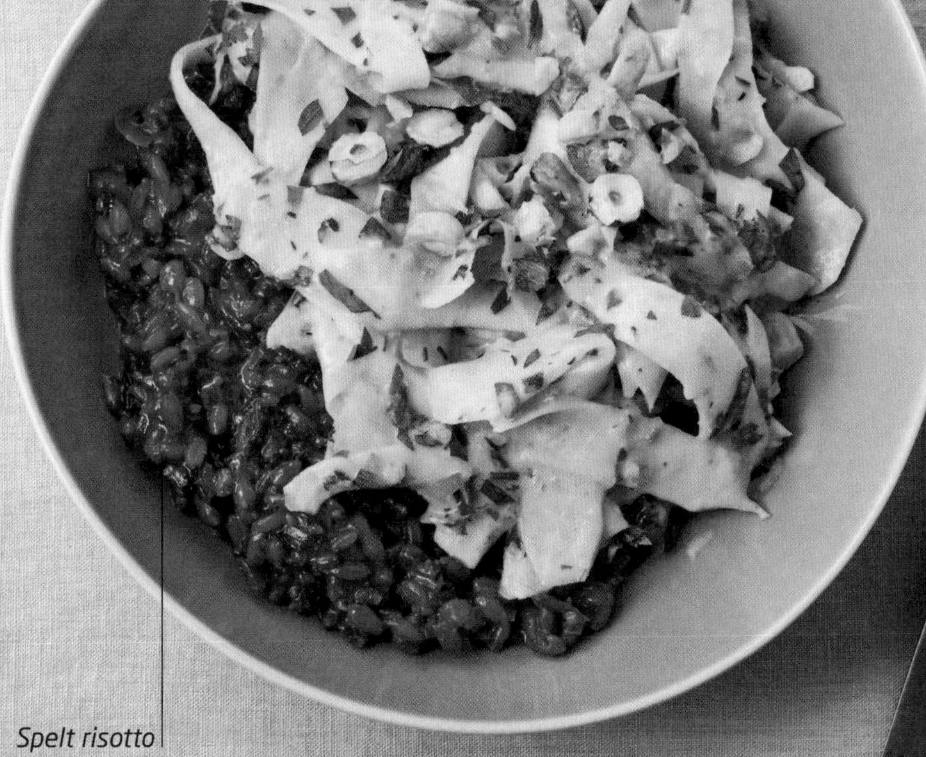

Spelt risotto (see p.145)

Roasted sweet potato purée with tahini salsa

Serves 3

Purée: 2 sweet potatoes (about 500g/1lb 2oz) | 1 tsp olive oil | 2 garlic cloves, peeled | ½ tsp ground turmeric | ½ tsp ground cumin
Salsa: 100ml (3½fl oz) vegetable stock | 1 tbsp shiro miso | 3 tbsp light tahini (sesame seed paste; see tip p.192) | 6 tbsp finely chopped herbs (e.g. rocket, basil, or parsley) | 3 tbsp lemon juice | salt | freshly ground pepper | 2 tbsp sesame seeds, toasted

Nutritional values per portion: 433 kcal | 49.9g carbohydrate | 20.7g fat | 9.9g protein | 7.6g fibre | 0.2g ALA | 376mg lysine | 234mg calcium | 2.4mg zinc | 2.8mg iron | 0.3mg B2 | 1.8mg RE | 5µg iodine | 0.6g salt

Preheat the oven to 180°C (350°F/Gas 4), not on a fan setting. Peel the sweet potatoes and chop into 3cm (1in) cubes. Put in a bowl with the oil, coat the cubes thinly all over. Add the garlic, turmeric, and cumin and mix again. Spread the sweet potato cubes out on a baking tray and roast in an oven (middle shelf) for 15–20 minutes until they are browning nicely.

Meanwhile, to make the salsa, put the stock, miso, tahini, herbs, and lemon juice in a bowl. Stir to make a thick sauce and season with salt and pepper. Put the sweet potato cubes and garlic in a bowl, mash roughly to make a purée, drizzle with the salsa, scatter with sesame seeds and enjoy.

BASTI'S TIP

Tahini can vary greatly in quality; read the tip for Copien's lentil hummus (see p.192). Feel free to make a larger quantity as this purée also tastes great cold.

VARIATION

Instead of sweet potato, you can also use any kind of squash, or even parsnips or celeriac: the preparation time is the same and the result just as delicious.

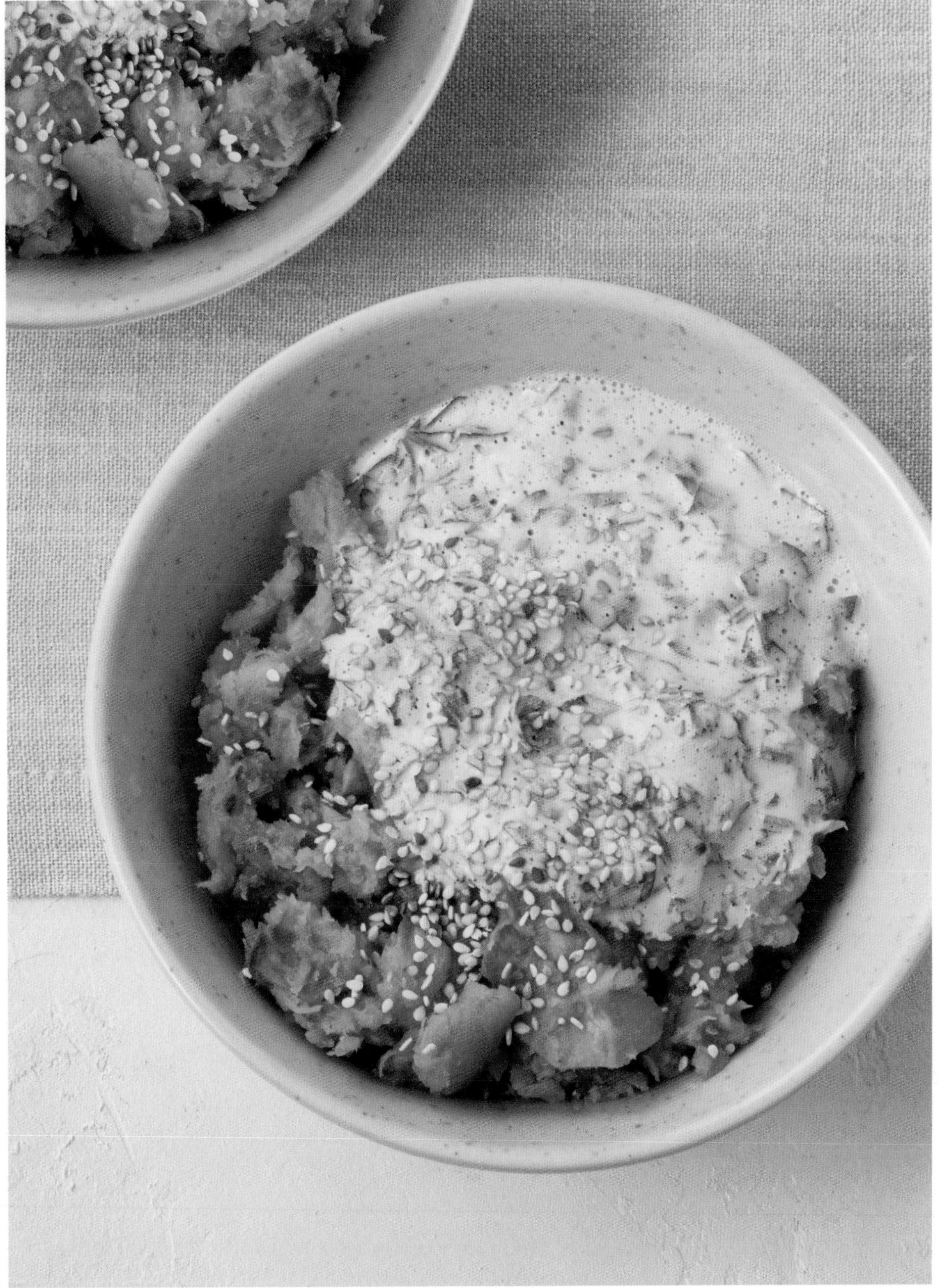

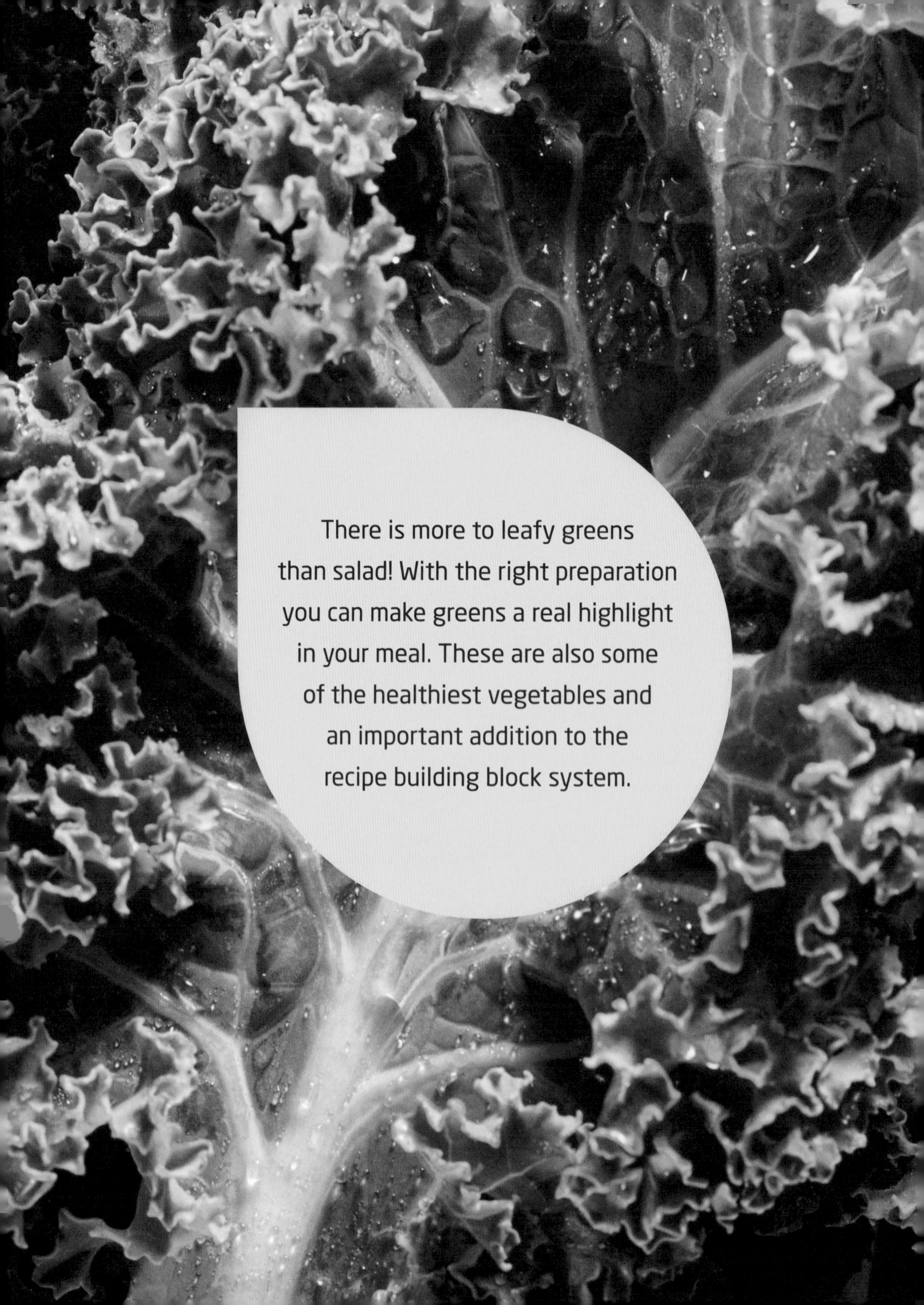

There is more to leafy greens than salad! With the right preparation you can make greens a real highlight in your meal. These are also some of the healthiest vegetables and an important addition to the recipe building block system.

Leafy vegetables

Tahini spinach

Serves 2

1 celery stick, with leaves | 1 small garlic clove, peeled | 2 tbsp raisins (or dried cranberries) | 200g (7oz) frozen or 170g (6oz) fresh spinach | juice of ½ orange | 1 tbsp light tahini (sesame seed paste; see p.192) | 1 tbsp lemon juice | pinch of salt | pinch of freshly ground pepper

Nutritional values per portion: 245 kcal | 27.9g carbohydrate | 8.5g fat | 11.2g protein | 14.1g fibre | 0.6g ALA | 380mg lysine | 496mg calcium | 1.9mg zinc | 4.7mg iron | 0.6mg B2 | 2.5mg RE | 16μg iodine | 0.5g salt

Wash the celery and chop very finely. Finely dice the garlic. Heat a pan over a high heat and brown the celery, garlic, and raisins without oil for 2 minutes. Add the spinach, deglaze with orange juice, cover, and simmer gently for 3 minutes. Meanwhile, put the tahini, 4 tablespoons of water, and the lemon juice in a bowl and stir to combine. Season the spinach with a pinch of salt and pepper, transfer to a bowl, and drizzle with the sauce.

Asian pan-fried leafy vegetables

Serves 2

Spicy sauce: 4 tbsp date paste (see p.97) | 1½ tbsp organic soy sauce | 2½ tbsp lemon juice | pinch of chilli powder
Vegetables: 150g (5½oz) firm leafy vegetables (e.g. Swiss chard, kale, wild broccoli, broccoli leaves, fresh kohlrabi leaves, large spinach leaves, turnip greens, beetroot leaves) | 1 piece of fresh root ginger (3cm/1in), peeled | 1 small garlic clove, peeled | 1 small onion, peeled | 1 tsp olive oil | 1½ tbsp sesame seeds

Nutritional values per portion: 155 kcal | 16g carbohydrate | 7.3g fat | 5.8g protein | 6.3g fibre | 0.3g ALA | 282mg lysine | 241mg calcium | 1mg zinc | 2.7mg iron | 0.2 mg B2 | 0.7mg RE | 6μg iodine | 1g salt

Add all the ingredients for the spicy sauce to a bowl with 4 tablespoons of water and combine.

Wash the leafy vegetables and, if possible, leave them in relatively large pieces. Chop the ginger and garlic very finely. Slice the onion into fine rings.

Heat a pan over a high heat. Add the ginger, onion rings, and garlic to the pan. Drizzle with oil and sauté for 20 seconds. Add the leafy vegetables on top and after 30 seconds combine everything. Sauté the vegetables for 1 minute then deglaze the pan with the spicy sauce. Mix the vegetables and sauce well and allow to simmer down, stirring constantly. If the vegetables are cooked to your taste, remove from the hob, otherwise let them continue cooking over a low heat. Divide the vegetables between two plates, sprinkle with sesame seeds, and serve.

BASTI'S TIP

You can vary the flavour by choosing different leafy vegetables. Newcomers to cooking with greens should start with mild varieties such as spinach, Swiss chard, or wild broccoli. Due to its strong flavour, kale is an acquired taste.

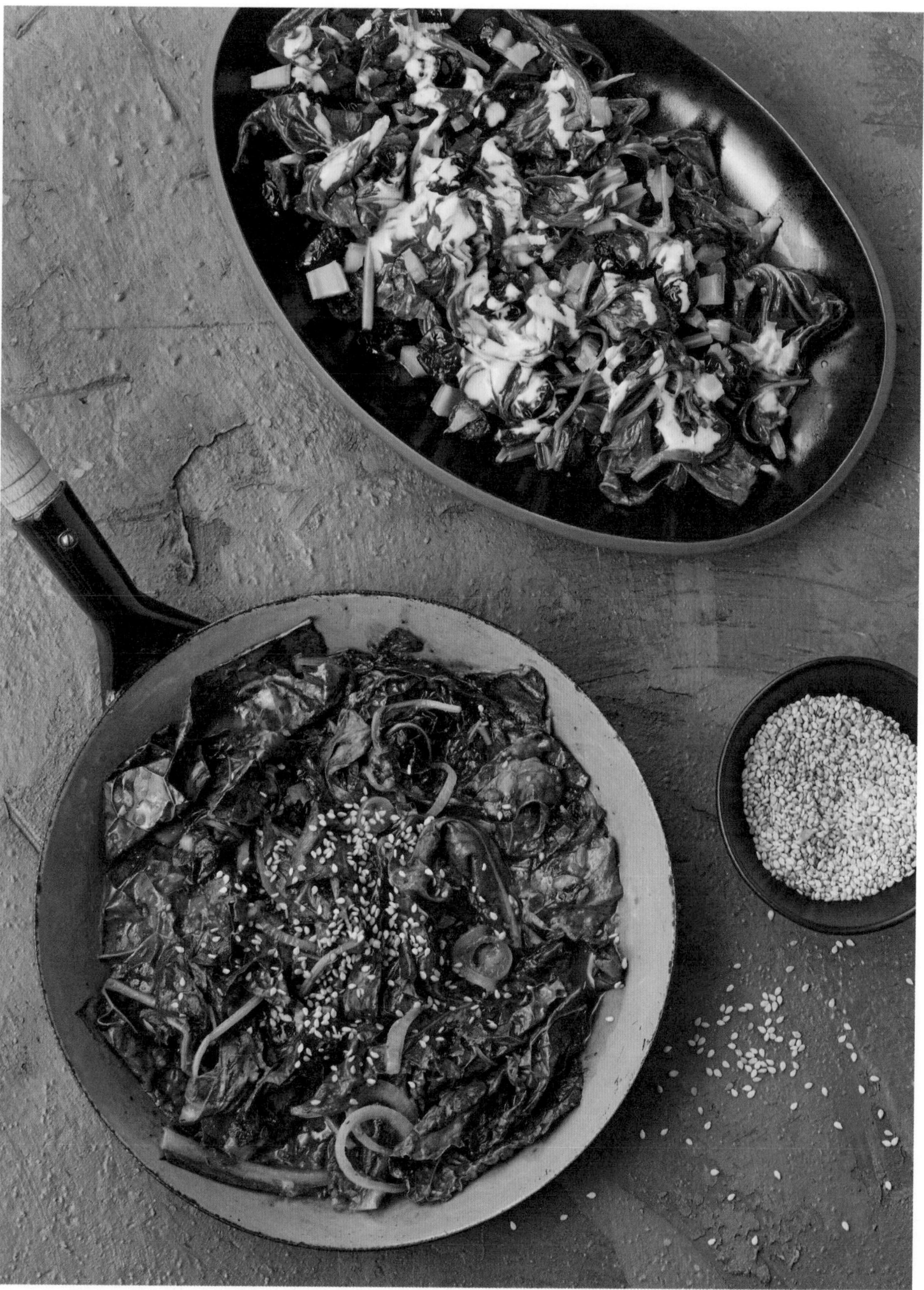

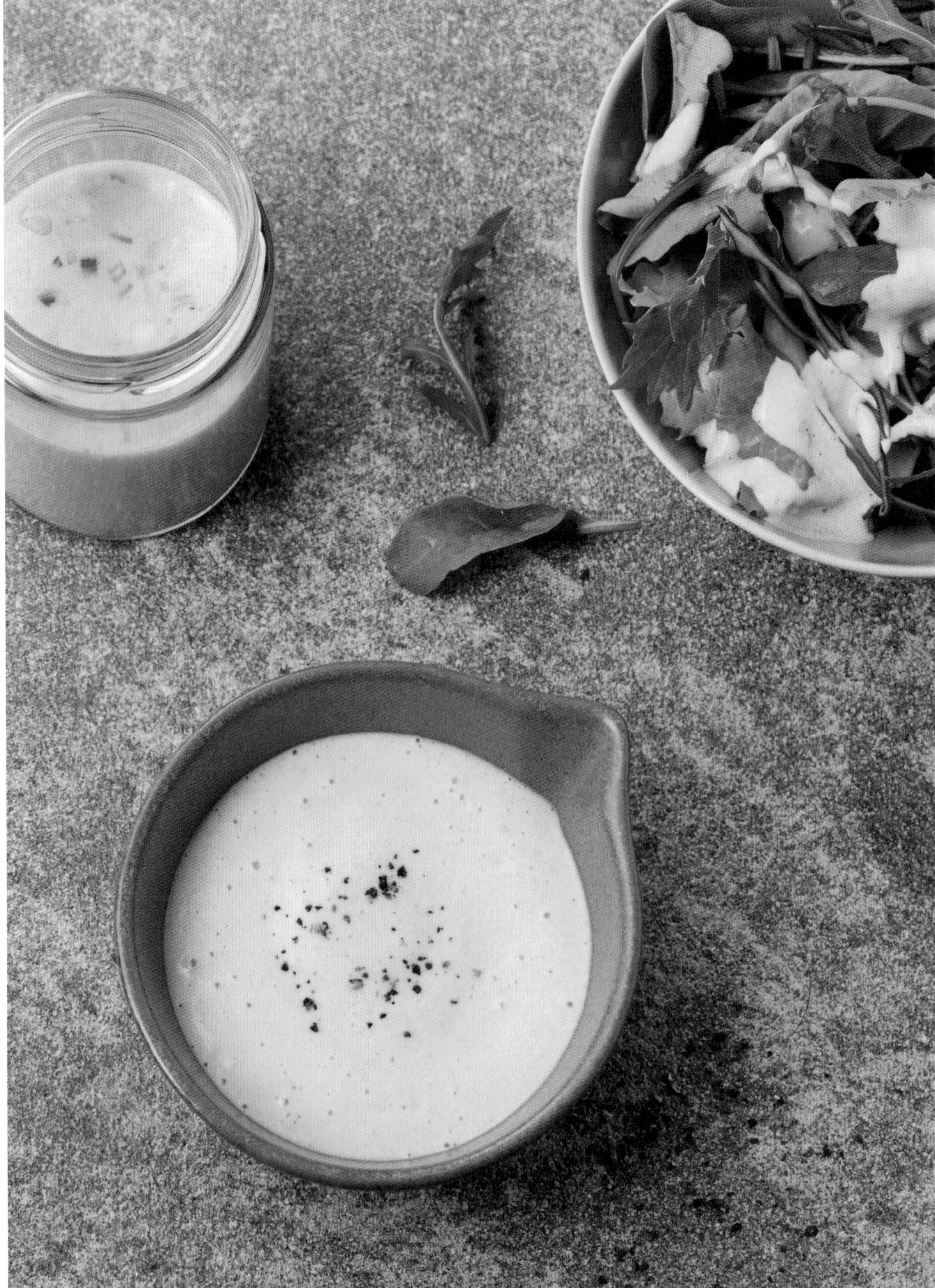

Green salad with date vinaigrette

Serves 6

Vinaigrette: 1 small shallot (or ½ small red onion), peeled | 6 tbsp cider vinegar | 2 Medjool dates, stones removed (or 2 tbsp date paste, see p.97) | 1½ tbsp olive oil | 1½ tbsp shiro miso | 2 tsp medium-hot mustard | 6 tbsp light vegetable stock | pinch of salt | pinch of freshly ground pepper
Salad: 6 handfuls of lettuce (or wild herb salad, rocket, or thinly sliced cabbage)

Nutritional values per portion: 61 kcal | 5.1g carbohydrate | 4.2g fat | 0.7g protein | 1.2g fibre | 0.1g ALA | 49mg lysine | 9mg calcium | 0.1mg zinc | 0.2mg iron | < 0.1mg B2 | < 0.1mg RE | < 1µg iodine | 0.6g salt

Finely chop the shallots for the vinaigrette. Put all the vinaigrette ingredients except the shallots into the food processor and blitz until smooth. Add the diced shallots and leave the vinaigrette to infuse for 3 minutes.

Wash and spin-dry the lettuce, transfer to a bowl, and toss the leaves in the dressing. Serve this salad alongside other components.

Green salad with yogurt dressing

Serves 6

Dressing: 100g (3½oz) soya yogurt (or coconut yogurt) | 1 tbsp white almond nut butter | 3 tbsp cider vinegar | 10 basil leaves | 1 tbsp shiro miso | ½ orange, peeled | pinch of salt | pinch of freshly ground pepper
Salad: 6 handfuls of lettuce (or wild herb salad, rocket, or thinly sliced cabbage)

Nutritional values per portion: 62 kcal | 4.9g carbohydrate | 3.5g fat | 2.6g protein | 1.5g fibre | 0.1g ALA | 134mg lysine | 31mg calcium | 0.2mg zinc | 0.5mg iron | 0.1mg B2 | < 0.1mg RE | 1µg iodine | 0.2g salt

Add all the ingredients for the dressing to the food processor and blitz until smooth.

Wash and spin-dry the lettuce, transfer to a bowl, and toss the leaves in the dressing. Serve this salad alongside other components.

VARIATION

Replace the basil with fresh coriander and use coconut milk instead of yogurt for a wonderful Asian-style green dressing.

BASTI'S TIP

The recipe makes 6 portions. Since the dressing will keep for a couple of days in the fridge, you can always make extra.

You will need 1–2 tbsp of dressing for each portion of salad.

Simple greens with chermoula

Serves 2

Chermoula: 1 small celery stick | 1 small mild chilli | 30g (1oz) flaked almonds | 2 tbsp raisins (or cranberries) | 2 tbsp capers | 5 mint leaves | 5 sprigs of parsley | 5 sprigs of fresh coriander | 1 organic orange | 3 tbsp lemon juice | 2 tsp olive oil | 1 tbsp vegetable stock paste (see p.99) | salt | freshly ground pepper
Vegetables: 250g (9oz) robust leafy vegetables (such as Swiss chard, kale, Savoy cabbage leaves, tenderstem broccoli, young kohlrabi leaves, spinach, beetroot leaves)

Nutritional values per portion: 316 kcal | 27.2g carbohydrate | 17.1g fat | 11.3g protein | 11.6g fibre | 0.6g ALA | 487mg lysine | 359mg calcium | 1mg zinc | 3.7mg iron | 0.5mg B2 | 1.1mg RE | 8µg iodine | 1.8g salt

To make the chermoula, first wash and finely dice the celery. Wash the chilli, slice in half lengthwise, remove the seeds and chop finely. Toast the almonds in a dry pan over a moderate heat until pale brown, stirring constantly. Chop the raisins, capers, and herbs very finely. Wash the orange in hot water and dry it, grate 1 tablespoon of zest and squeeze the juice. Put all the chermoula ingredients in a bowl, mix, and leave to infuse for 5 minutes.

Add 4cm (1½in) of water to a saucepan with a steamer insert and lid, then bring the water to the boil. Cook the leafy vegetables in the steamer with the lid on for 3 minutes. If you do not have a steamer, just add water to the pan so it is 5mm (¼in) deep, bring to the boil, and cook the leafy vegetables in this water with the lid on. Put the vegetables in a bowl, drizzle with chermoula, and serve immediately.

Vietnamese herb salad

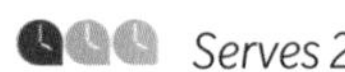

Serves 2

Salad: 1 pak choi (about 150g/5½oz) or Chinese cabbage or iceberg lettuce | 1 tsp olive oil | 8 sprigs each of dill and coriander | 8 mint and 8 basil leaves | 2 tbsp sesame seeds, toasted
Dressing: 1 piece of fresh root ginger (2cm/¾in) | 2 large organic limes | 1 tbsp organic soy sauce | 1 tsp olive oil | 3 tbsp date paste (see p.97) | 1 tsp medium-hot mustard

Nutritional values per portion: 182 kcal | 11.3g carbohydrate | 12.2g fat | 3.6g protein | 3.3g fibre | 0.4g ALA | 142mg lysine | 127mg calcium | 1.3mg zinc | 1.9mg iron | 0.1mg B2 | 0.1mg RE | 2µg iodine | 0.7g salt

Wash the pak choi and cut out the stalk so you can separate the leaves. Put a pan over a high heat, add the pak choi, and drizzle with oil. Fry the pak choi for 3 minutes until cooked but with a bit of bite, then set aside. Finely chop the dill and coriander. Roughly tear the mint and basil.

To make the dressing, peel and finely grate the ginger. Wash a lime in hot water, dry it and grate ½ teaspoon of zest. Squeeze the juice of both limes. Put the grated ginger, 5 tablespoons of lime juice, lime zest, soy sauce, olive oil, date paste, 2 tablespoons of water, and mustard in a salad bowl and stir to combine. Mix the warm pak choi with the dressing and scatter over the herbs and toasted sesame seeds to serve.

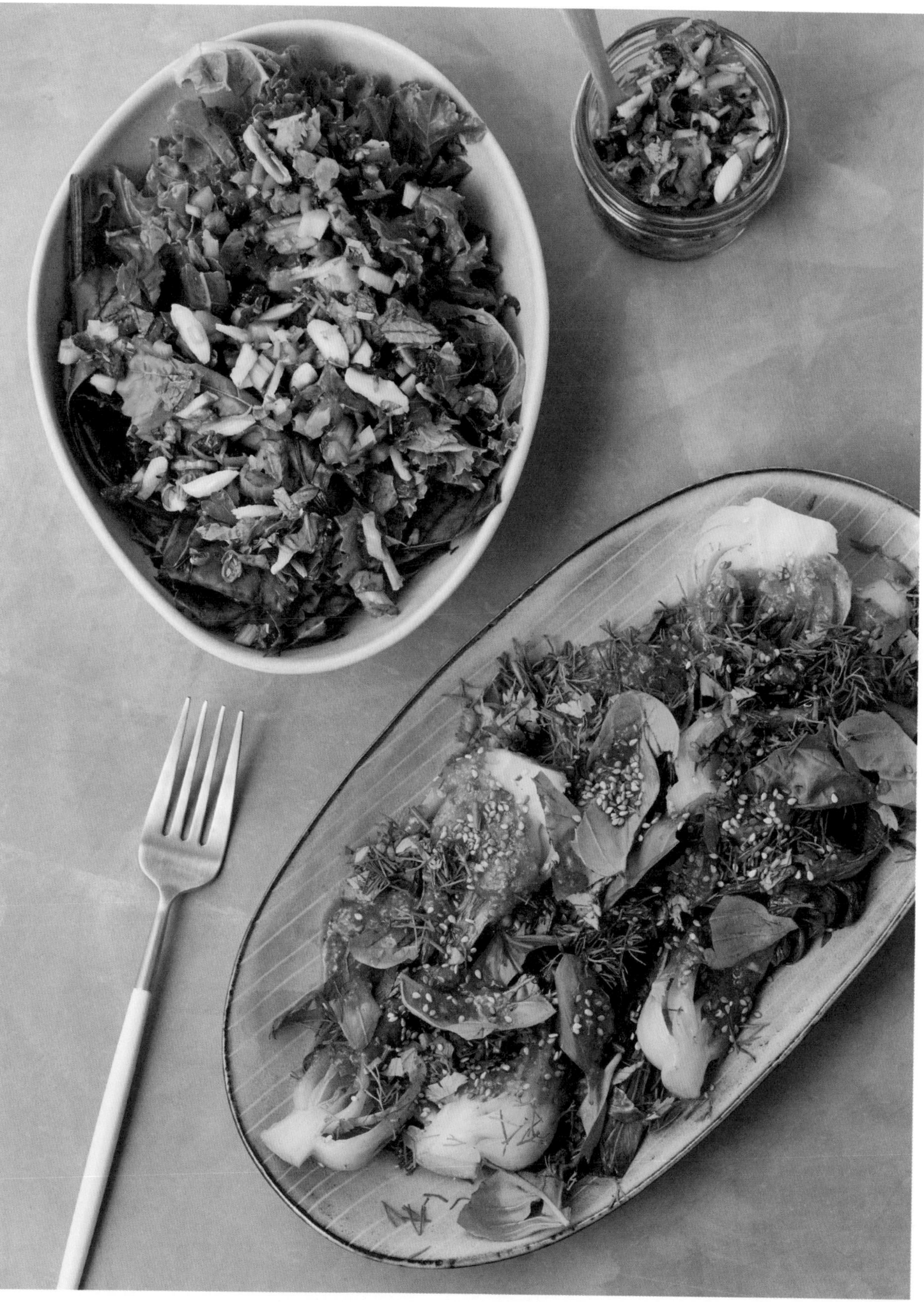

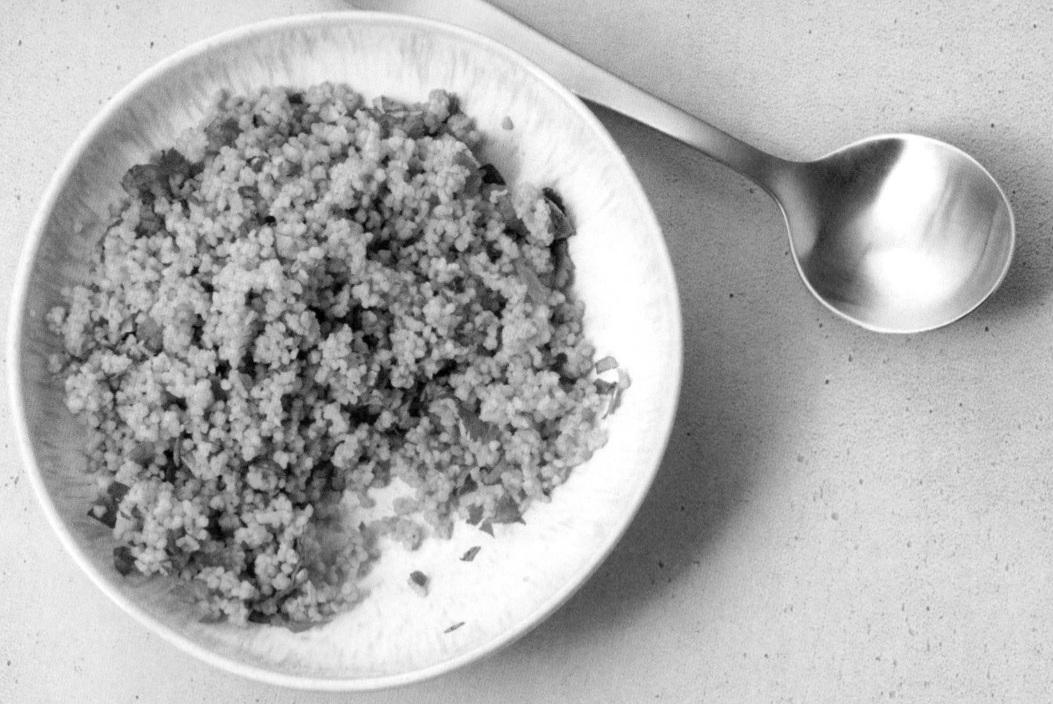

Greens with peas and a coriander and ginger sauce

Serves 2

Sauce: 6 sprigs of coriander | 50g (1¾oz) white almond nut butter | 150ml (5fl oz) light vegetable stock | ½ tsp ground turmeric | 1 piece of fresh root ginger (3cm/1in), peeled | 1 tbsp yeast flakes | 1 soft date, stone removed | 1 tbsp organic soy sauce | 1 tbsp lime juice
Vegetables: 120g (4oz) leafy vegetables (such as Swiss chard without stalks, spinach, Savoy cabbage leaves, lamb's lettuce, tenderstem broccoli) | 100g (3½oz) baby peas | salt | freshly ground pepper

Nutritional values per portion: 241 kcal | 15.7g carbohydrate | 15.4g fat | 10g protein | 5.3g fibre | 0.2g ALA | 550mg lysine | 151mg calcium | 1.5mg zinc | 3.9mg iron | 0.5mg B2 | 0.4mg RE | 3µg iodine | 1g salt

Add all the ingredients for the sauce to a powerful food processor and purée until smooth. Cook the sauce in a pan over a low to moderate heat until it has thickened slightly.

Wash the leafy vegetables and spin them dry. Add them to the sauce with the peas and continue cooking over a moderate heat until the leaves begin to wilt. Season the vegetables with salt and pepper and serve on two plates.

BASTI'S TIP

Choose different leafy vegetables to give this dish a milder or more intense flavour. Some leafy green vegetables, such as rocket, have more bitter flavours than milder varieties like spinach. Use whatever tastes best to you! The quality of the almond butter is also crucial for the flavour of the sauce.

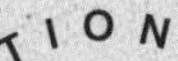

VARIATION

Instead of almond nut butter, use cashew nut butter or mix 100ml (3½fl oz) of stock with 100ml (3½fl oz) of soya or oat cream. Swap the coriander for basil and the ginger for capers for a Mediterranean feel.

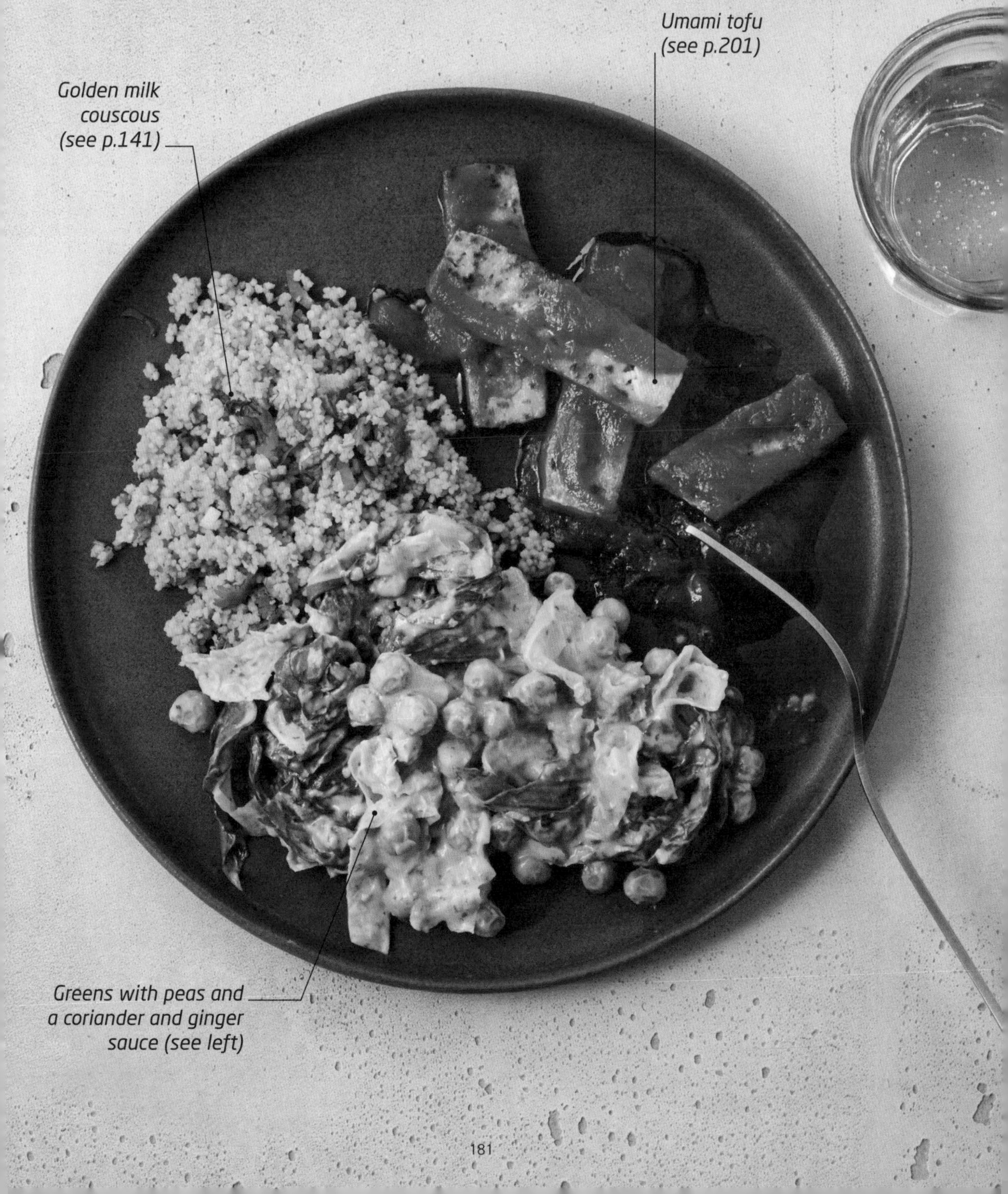

Umami tofu (see p.201)

Golden milk couscous (see p.141)

Greens with peas and a coriander and ginger sauce (see left)

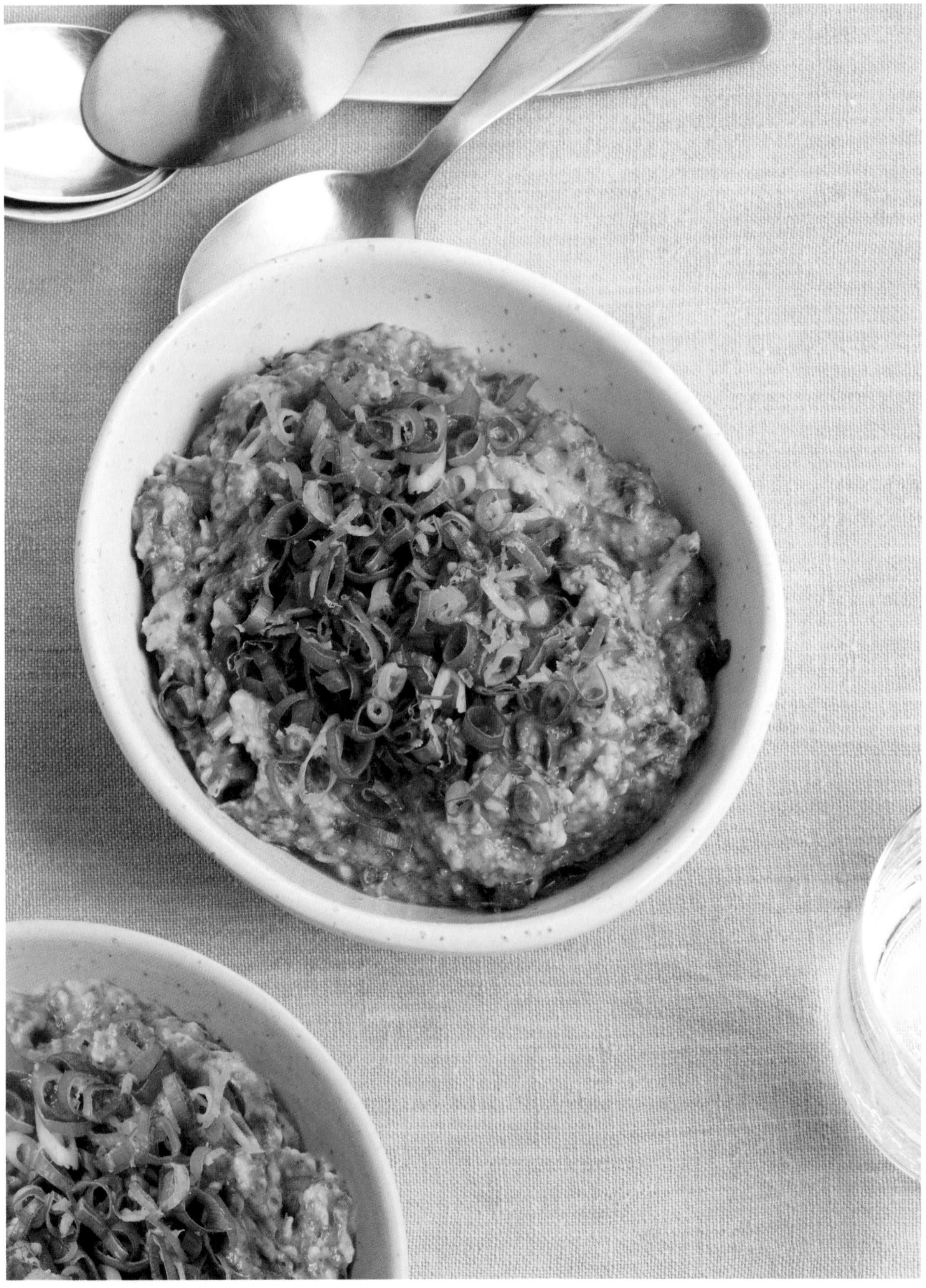

Chlorophyll guacamole

Serves 2

1 organic orange | 2 spring onions | 50g (1¾oz) spinach | 8 sprigs of parsley (or coriander) | 10 basil leaves | ½ small garlic clove, peeled | 1–2 tsp organic soy sauce | 1 tbsp shiro miso | 4 tbsp lime juice | 2 large ripe avocados (about 250g/9oz flesh)

Nutritional values per portion: 269 kcal | 22.6g carbohydrate | 16.9g fat | 5.5g protein | 11.1g fibre | 0.3g ALA | 361mg lysine | 130mg calcium | 1.4mg zinc | 2.6mg iron | 0.3mg B2 | 0.3mg RE | 9µg iodine | 1.7g salt

Wash the orange in hot water, dry it, and grate 1 tablespoon of zest. Wash the spring onions, slice the green section very thinly and use the whites in another recipe. Mix the onions and orange zest in a bowl and set aside.

Squeeze the juice of the orange. Finely chop the spinach and herbs. Add the orange juice, spinach, herbs, garlic, soy sauce, miso, and lime juice to the food processor and purée thoroughly. Halve the avocados, remove the stones, scoop out the flesh with a spoon and mash this in a bowl with a fork. Fold the mashed avocado into the spinach purée. Transfer the guacamole to a bowl and scatter with the spring onion and orange zest mixture.

VARIATION

You can really go wild and experiment with the herbs and leafy vegetables here.

BASTI'S TIP

If the quantity of spinach and herbs is too small for your food processor to handle, add half the avocado. But do mash the other half with a fork because the resulting texture always makes the avocado taste better than if it is all prepared in the food processor.

The avocados need to be perfectly ripe because the flavour of the guacamole depends on their quality.

Palak – spicy Indian spinach

Serves 2

2 tomatoes (or 120g/4oz passata) | 300g (10oz) frozen spinach (or 250g/9oz fresh spinach) | 200ml (7fl oz) soya milk with calcium (or other plant-based milk) | 1 small onion, peeled | 1 piece of fresh root ginger (2cm/¾in), peeled | 2 tsp olive oil | 1 tsp ground coriander | ½ tsp ground cumin | 1 tsp ground turmeric | ½ tsp hot paprika | salt

Nutritional values per portion: 178 kcal | 14.8g carbohydrate | 7.9g fat | 10.6g protein | 6.9g fibre | 0.4g ALA | 588mg lysine | 318mg calcium | 1.7mg zinc | 6.5mg iron | 0.4mg B2 | 1.4mg RE | 31µg iodine | 0.3g salt

Wash the tomatoes and remove the cores. Add the spinach, tomatoes, and soya milk to the food processor and purée until you have a slightly lumpy consistency. If the spinach is frozen, bring the soya milk to the boil and mix this with the frozen spinach. Separately, finely chop the onion and ginger.

Heat a small pan. Add the diced onion and oil and sauté for 2 minutes. Then add the spices and ginger and fry for 10 seconds. Add the spinach mixture, bring to the boil and simmer gently without a lid over a low heat for 10 minutes. Season the palak to taste with salt.

VARIATION

Instead of spinach, palak also works beautifully with Savoy cabbage or Swiss chard. And make full use of all the spices in your spice rack!

Kale curry

Serves 2

200g (7oz) fresh young kale (or 150g/5½oz frozen kale) | 1 small onion, peeled | 1 piece of fresh root ginger (2cm/¾in), peeled | 2 Deglet Noor dates, stones removed | 2 tbsp mild curry powder (see tip p.122) | 250g (9oz) coconut milk | 100ml (3½fl oz) light vegetable stock | 8 sprigs of coriander | 1 organic lemon | 1 tbsp organic soy sauce | freshly ground pepper

Nutritional values per portion: 364 kcal | 17.3g carbohydrate | 29.1g fat | 7.6g protein | 8g fibre | 0.5g ALA | 388mg lysine | 190mg calcium | 1.2mg zinc | 3.2mg iron | 0.2mg B2 | 0.7mg RE | 6µg iodine | 0.9 g salt

Wash the kale and separate the leaves from the stalks (frozen kale is already prepared for eating). Discard the stalks, wash the leaves once more. Finely chop the onion and ginger. Dice the dates.

Put a non-stick pan over a high heat. Add the chopped onion, dates, and ginger to the pan and fry without any oil for 1 minute. Add the curry powder and continue frying for 10 seconds, then deglaze the pan with coconut milk and stock, mix everything well, and bring to the boil. Add the kale, cover, and simmer gently over a low heat for 5 minutes.

Finely chop the coriander. Wash the lemon in hot water, then dry it, grate 1 tablespoon of zest and squeeze 3 tablespoons of juice. Add the coriander, lemon juice, and lemon zest to the kale, mix well, then simmer gently for 10 minutes. Season to taste with soy sauce, pepper, and more lemon juice before serving.

VARIATION

Instead of kale, you can use spinach, Savoy cabbage, red cabbage, or another leafy vegetable.

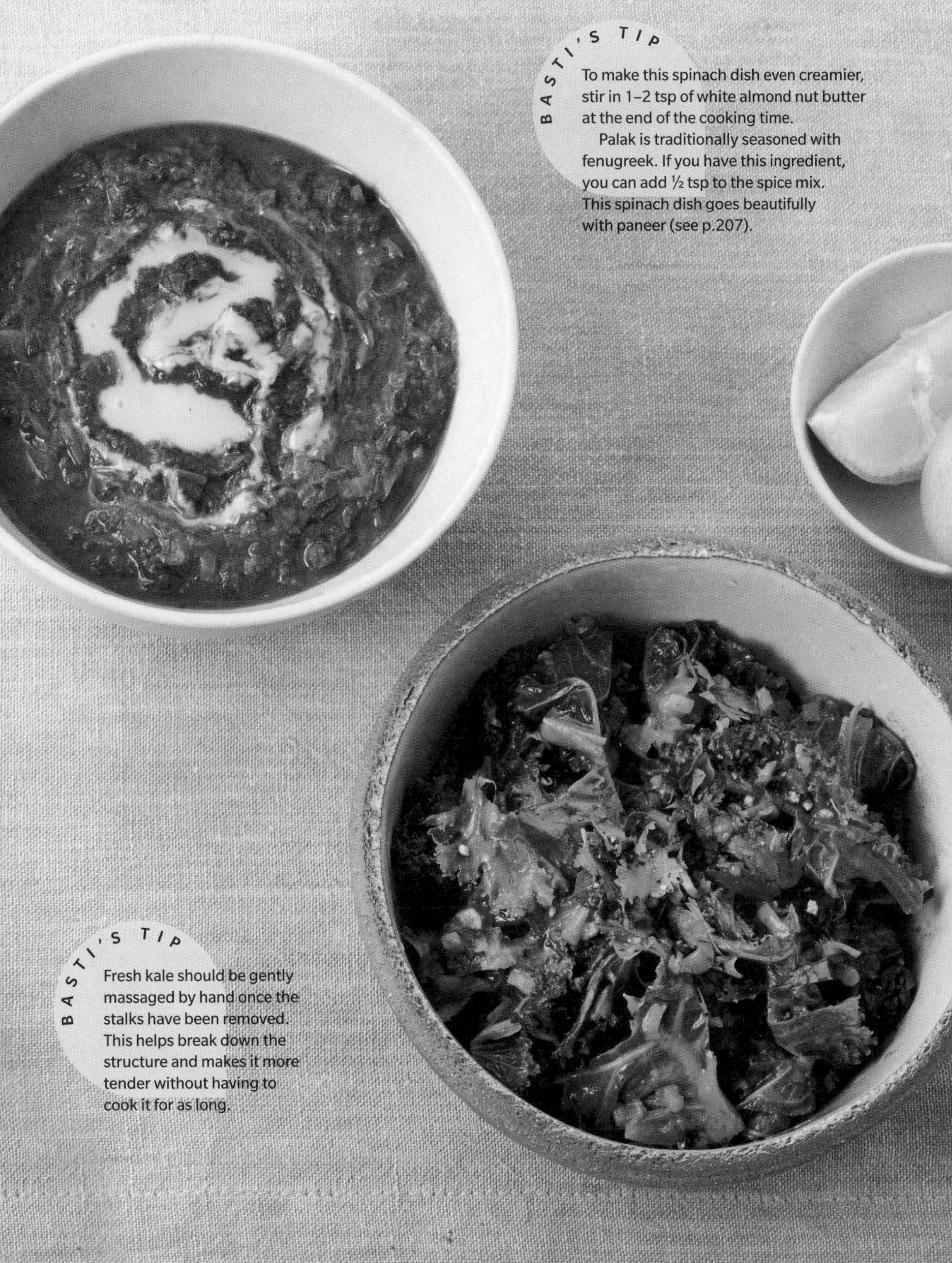

BASTI'S TIP

To make this spinach dish even creamier, stir in 1–2 tsp of white almond nut butter at the end of the cooking time.

Palak is traditionally seasoned with fenugreek. If you have this ingredient, you can add ½ tsp to the spice mix. This spinach dish goes beautifully with paneer (see p.207).

BASTI'S TIP

Fresh kale should be gently massaged by hand once the stalks have been removed. This helps break down the structure and makes it more tender without having to cook it for as long.

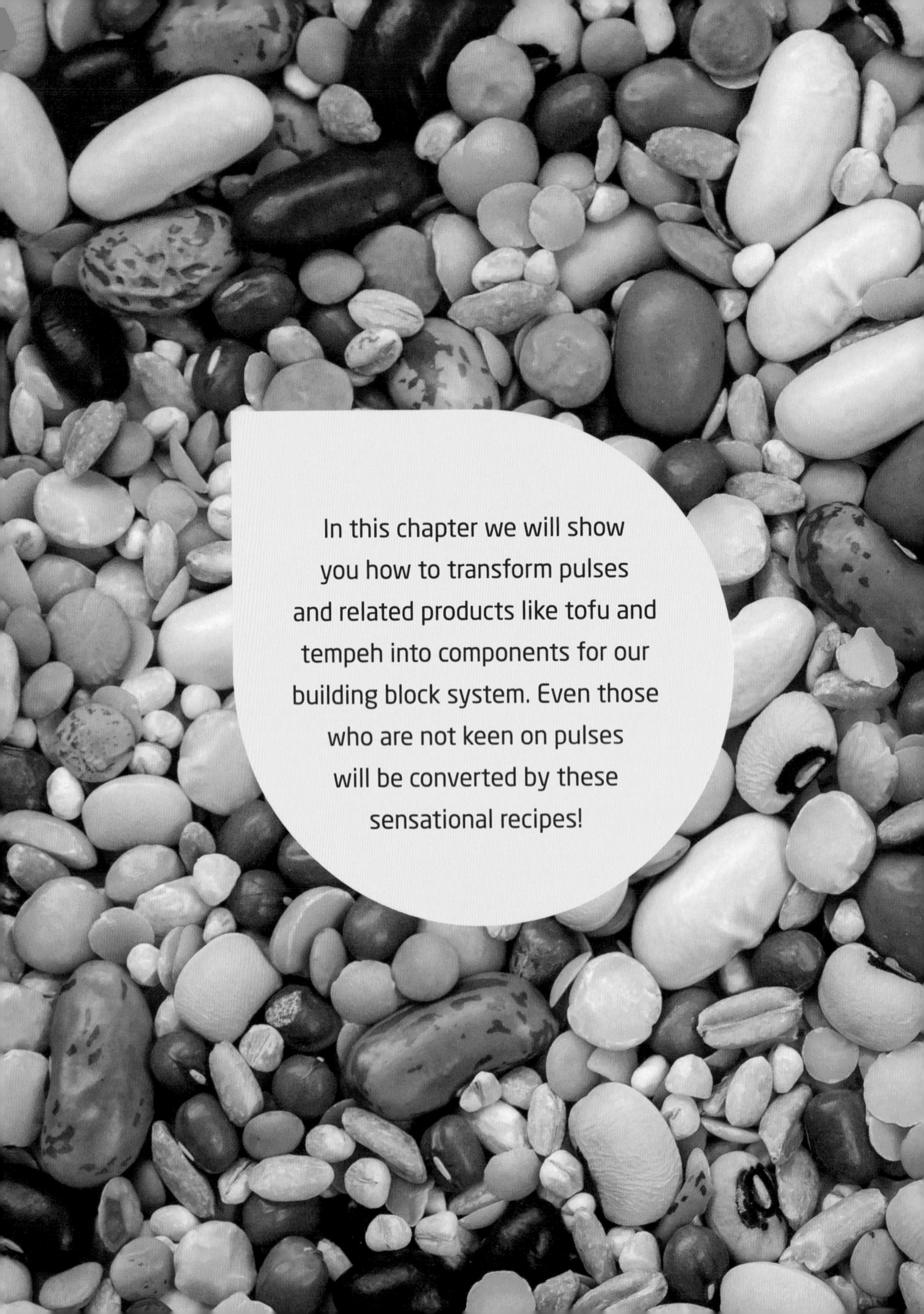

In this chapter we will show you how to transform pulses and related products like tofu and tempeh into components for our building block system. Even those who are not keen on pulses will be converted by these sensational recipes!

Pulses

Building block basics: pulses

Always store pulses in their cooking water to ensure a consistently high quality. Pulses will keep for about five days in the fridge if stored this way. Without the cooking water, pulses lose their flavour after just two to three days. The cooking water is extremely valuable in terms of flavour, umami, and nutritional content. Sebastian usually makes a simple soup from the final portion of pulses and cooking water – therapeutic and easy.

General tips

Multiply the dry weight of the pulses by 2.5. This lets you estimate the weight of the cooked beans, etc. For example, 100g (3½oz) of dried pulses equates to about 230–250g (8–9oz) once cooked.

Add vegetables and spices to the cooking water with beans or chickpeas to ensure a wonderful flavour and more delicious results than just using plain water. But of course, you can always just cook the pulses in water for the specified period.

We recommend soaking a packet of beans on Friday evening then cooking these as described the following day or on Sunday. This is an easy way to create a valuable, healthy source of protein for the coming week.

If you soak the beans for two days, remember to replace the soaking water two or three times during this period, and in summer keep the bowl refrigerated.

Soaking pulses helps reduce some of the substances that make them difficult to digest, so they are easier for the body to process. The rest of the substances that inhibit digestion are broken down during the subsequent cooking process. This is why pulses should never be eaten raw.

Cooking pulses correctly

Never add salt or acidic substances like lemon juice, vinegar, or tomatoes to the raw pulses while cooking. These foods can harden the cell structure in the pulses, drastically increasing their cooking time.

It is vital not to boil pulses rapidly over a high heat as this can cause them to split open. The cooking liquid should bubble as gently as possible and no more. Complete dishes with pulses in will need to be seasoned again the next day because they absorb lots of the spices.

Shelf life

Dried pulses and beans can be kept for many years. Don't throw them away just because the expiry date has passed. You can stick a ten-year-old bean into the ground and it is highly likely to grow into a plant.

Cooking lentils

Makes about 1.25kg (2¾lb) cooked lentils

500g (1lb 2oz) lentils

Wash the lentils well and either cook them straight away or, if desired, you can soak them (see table below – this makes them easier to digest, but it is not essential in the way that it is for beans and chickpeas, and lentils taste great even without soaking).

In either case, put the lentils in a pan with 3 litres (5¼ pints) water and bring to a rapid boil. Skim off the foam with a spoon. Immediately reduce the heat so the lentils continue cooking very gently – this is important. Simmer the lentils gently over a low heat, uncovered, for the cooking time specified in the table until they are soft but with a bit of bite inside and still intact on the outside.

VARIATION

For added flavour, put 1 sprig of rosemary, 3 sage leaves, 1 tsp caraway seeds, ground cumin, or ground turmeric in the cooking water.

For batch cooking – to store

Remove the cooked lentils from the hob, drain in a sieve (retaining the cooking water), and leave to cool. Immerse the lentils in cold water in the sieve to stop them cooking further. Remember, pulses retain heat very effectively, which is why it is important to lower the temperature of delicate lentils as soon as they have finished cooking. Put the cooled cooking water and lentils into a clean, sealable container (e.g. 2-litre/3½-pint capacity Kilner jars). Then you can keep the lentils in the fridge for 4–5 days. Exception: red lentils are the only pulse that should not be stored in their cooking liquid as they are too fragile and will go soft quickly. This variety should be stored dry in the fridge. For all other lentil varieties, storing in their cooking water works beautifully. Or you can use the lentils straight away.

Cooking and soaking times for lentils

Variety	Soaking time	Cooking time for soaked beans	Cooking time without soaking
Red lentils	about 2 hours	simmer gently for about 5 minutes. Important: do not boil vigourously, just gently simmer.	about 7 minutes
Beluga lentils	about 2 hours	simmer gently for about 15 minutes	20–25 minutes
Brown and green lentils	about 2 hours	simmer gently for 20–25 minutes	35–45 minutes

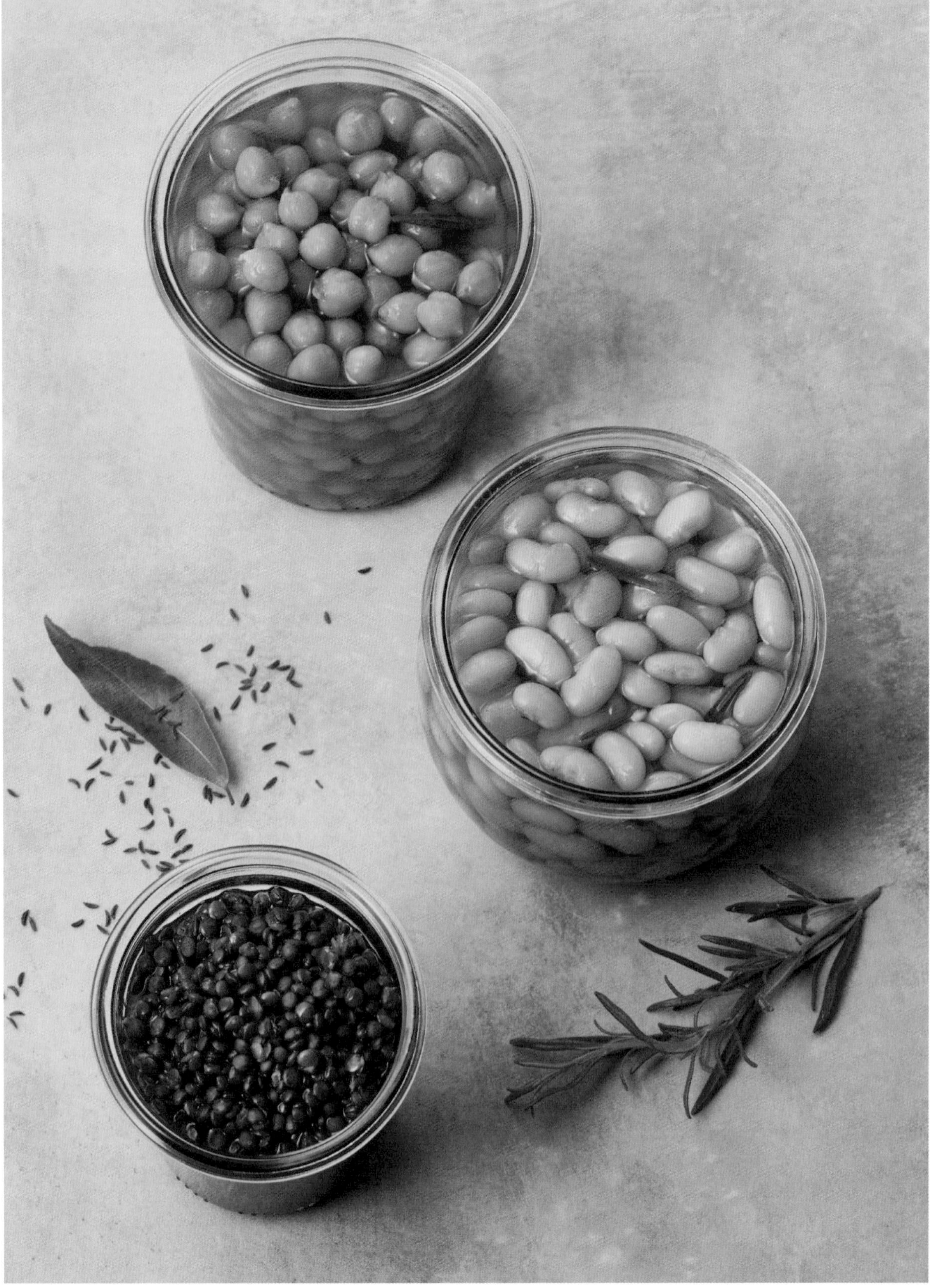

Cooking beans and chickpeas

Makes about 1.25kg (2¾lb) cooked beans or chickpeas

500g (1lb 2oz) beans (or chickpeas) | 1 onion, peeled | 2 garlic cloves, peeled | 100g (3½oz) celeriac, diced | 3 bay leaves | 1 sprig of rosemary | 1 tsp bicarbonate of soda

Soak the beans overnight in six times their volume of water. Drain the soaked beans in a sieve, rinse, and discard the soaking liquid.

Heat a pan. Halve the onion, place it in the pan with the cut surface facing down and fry until brown. Add the remaining ingredients and 3 litres (5¼ pints) of water, bring the contents of the pan to a rapid boil, skimming off any foam with a spoon. Then lower the heat significantly and simmer the beans gently, uncovered, over a low heat for about 1½ hours. Test a bean to see if it is nicely soft and creamy. If it still has a bit of bite, continue cooking until the beans are creamy inside but the outer skin is still intact. The bicarbonate of soda shortens the cooking time and ensures the beans cook more evenly.

For batch cooking – to store

Remove the cooked beans from the hob. Fill a basin with about 10cm (4in) of cold water. Put the pan in the water and leave the beans and their cooking liquid to cool.

Then transfer the beans and their cooking liquid (but not any vegetables, if used) to a clean, sealable container (e.g. 2-litre/3½-pint capacity Kilner jars). Then you can keep the beans in the fridge for 4–5 days (see tip). Alternatively, you can use the beans or chickpeas straight away.

Cooking and soaking times for beans and chickpeas

Variety	Soaking time	Cooking time for soaked beans
Pulses (like chickpeas, borlotti beans, kidney beans, white beans, unpeeled mung beans, adzuki beans, black beans, etc.)	about 12 hours	simmer gently for about 1½hours. Important: do not boil vigorously, simmer gently.
White giant beans (gigantes)	about 12 hours	simmer gently for 1 hour 40 minutes – 2 hours. Important: do not boil vigorously, simmer gently.

BASTI'S TIP

When soaking pulses and beans, always use a container with room for another third between the top of the water and the rim. This allows the beans to absorb sufficient liquid and swell to their maximum potential.

If you run out of time to cook the beans the next day, just rinse and cover them again with fresh water. Alternatively, you can freeze the soaked beans without any water. When you are ready, add them to the cooking water and follow the cooking instructions.

Copien's lentil hummus

Serves 3

150g (5½oz) red lentils | 60g (2oz) light tahini (sesame seed paste; see tip) | 50g (1¾oz) ice cubes (3–4 cubes) | ½ tsp salt (or vegetable stock paste, see p.99) | 2 tsp grated organic lemon zest | 1 tsp ground cumin

Nutritional values per portion: 271 kcal | 28.9g carbohydrate | 10.3g fat | 8.9g protein | 6.3g fibre | 0.1g ALA | 969mg lysine | 120mg calcium | 2.7mg zinc | 4.3mg iron | 0.2mg B2 | < 0.1mg RE | 1µg iodine | 0.2g salt

Wash the red lentils thoroughly, add to a pan with three times their volume of water, bring to the boil, cover, and simmer over a low heat until almost disintegrating. Drain the lentils in a sieve, wash briefly in cold water until they are just lukewarm, then leave to drain thoroughly.

Use a food processor or hand-held blender to purée the lentils and other ingredients to a smooth, creamy consistency.

BASTI'S TIP

Tahini (i.e. sesame seed paste) is essential for hummus and it should be made from hulled sesame seeds. You can tell it is the right variety because it is very pale. It should be almost liquid and not taste bitter. It is available in most supermarkets. Always blend the ingredients for hummus for 2–3 minutes on a moderate setting until you have a smooth consistency. Good hummus takes time, so you should never blitz it on the highest setting in your food processor.

This is the traditional preparation method (apart from the lentils) and it always works. The most important thing here is to mix slowly, use ice cubes and find a high-quality tahini. This gives the hummus a mild flavour without any other strong seasonings. If I'm serving the hummus with fresh bread, I top the dip with more flavoursome ingredients, such as the quick gremolata (see p.211), Asian pan-fried leafy vegetables (see p.174), or the apple and coriander topping (see p.216).

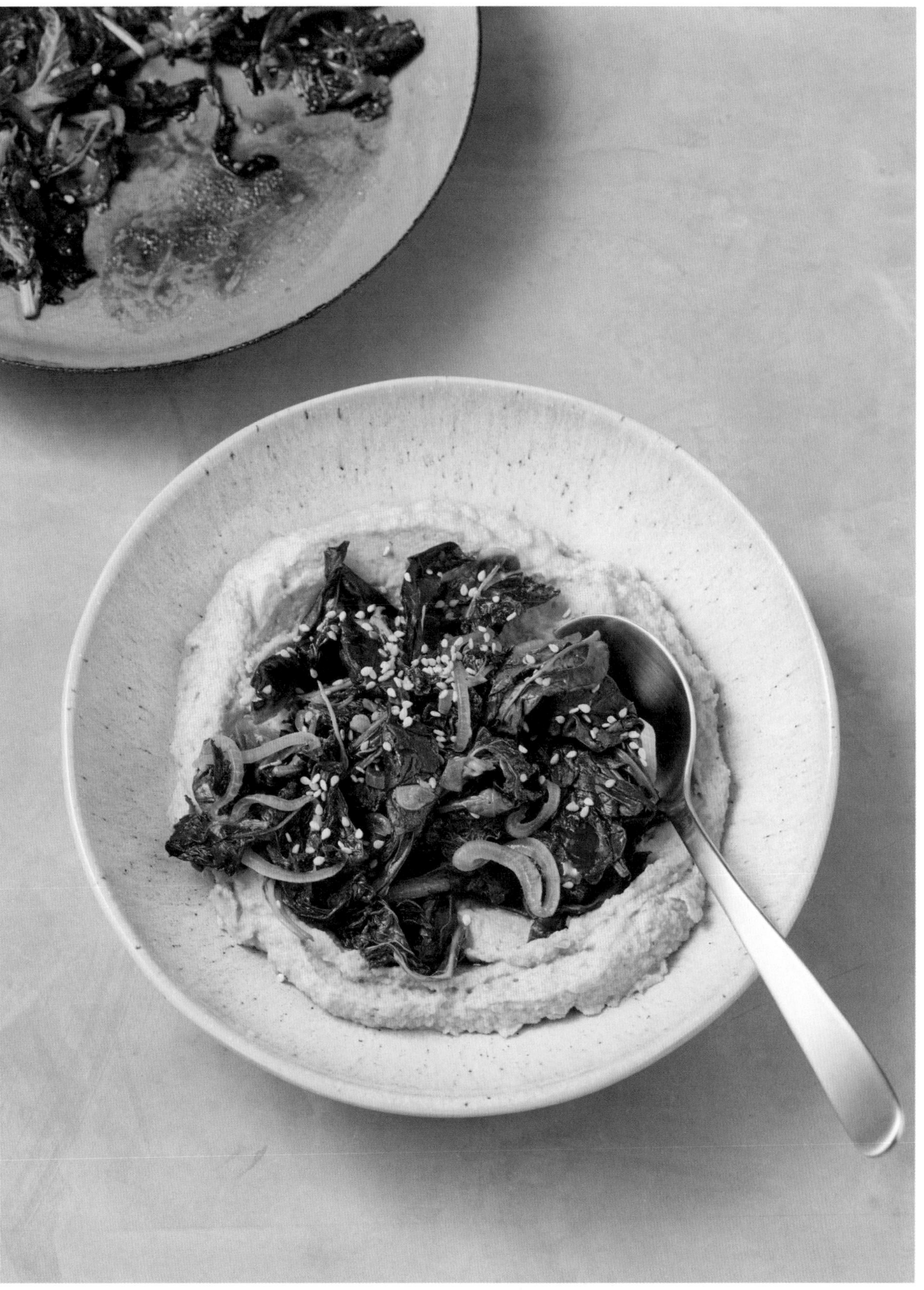

Easy tofu mince

Serves 2

250g (9oz) organic tofu | 1 small onion, peeled | 4 sprigs of parsley | 100ml (3½fl oz) light vegetable stock | 1 tbsp cider vinegar | 2 tbsp organic soy sauce | 2 tsp olive oil | 1–2 tbsp tomato purée | salt | freshly ground pepper

Nutritional values per portion: 216 kcal | 6.5g carbohydrate | 12.2g fat | 20.1g protein | 2.5g fibre | 0.7g ALA | 1247mg lysine | 245mg calcium | 2mg zinc | 3.7mg iron | 0.1mg B2 | < 0.1mg RE | 9µg iodine | 1.5g salt

Crumble the tofu by hand. Finely chop the onion. Finely chop the parsley. Combine the stock, vinegar, and soy sauce in a bowl.

Put a non-stick pan over a high heat. Tip in the crumbled tofu and drizzle over the olive oil. Fry the tofu for 3–4 minutes until brown. Add the diced onion and fry for 2–3 minutes until the onion and tofu have browned. Add the tomato purée and fry for 30 seconds. Deglaze the tofu pan with the vinegar mixture, add the parsley, mix well, and cook off the liquid over a high heat. Sauté the tofu again briefly then season with salt and pepper.

BASTI'S TIP

This tofu mince is a very basic recipe that lends itself to all sorts of different uses. It is quick to make and works great in any veggie bowl. It's also delicious served with steamed vegetables and salad or fried potatoes.

Once again it is the toasted flavour that really makes this dish special. Don't be afraid to cook it vigorously, you can always have some stock on hand (red wine also works here) to deglaze the pan if the tofu starts browning too quickly.

VARIATION

Pasta: add 1 tbsp of finely chopped capers and olives or juicy dried tomatoes to the tofu mince and combine with wholewheat pasta and a dash of non-dairy cream. Delicious!

Masala-style: add 1 tbsp of curry powder (see tip p. 122) or garam masala along with the tomato purée, sauté the spices with the tofu for 30 seconds, then deglaze with coconut milk instead of stock. Season the masala mince with a dash of lime juice plus salt and pepper. Serve with rice or baked sweet potatoes.

Roulade: mix the cooked mince, as per the recipe, with 100g (3½oz) of finely chopped kimchi, then add 1–2 tbsp of breadcrumbs so you can mould the mixture. Stuff cabbage leaves with the mix and sauté these in a pan. Serve with sweet potato purée (see p. 170) and a yogurt & garlic sauce (see p. 211).

Masala-style minced tofu (see variation)

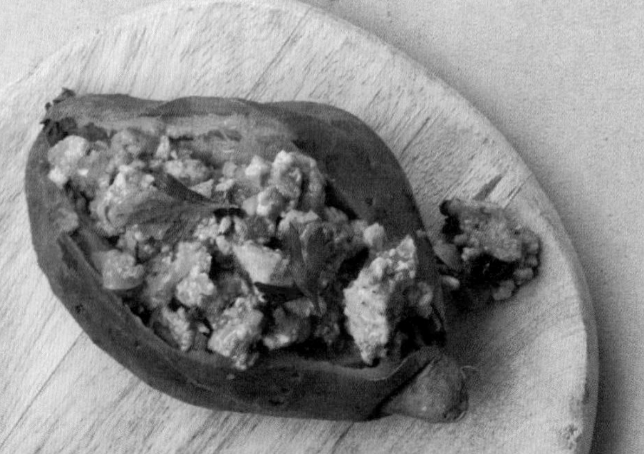

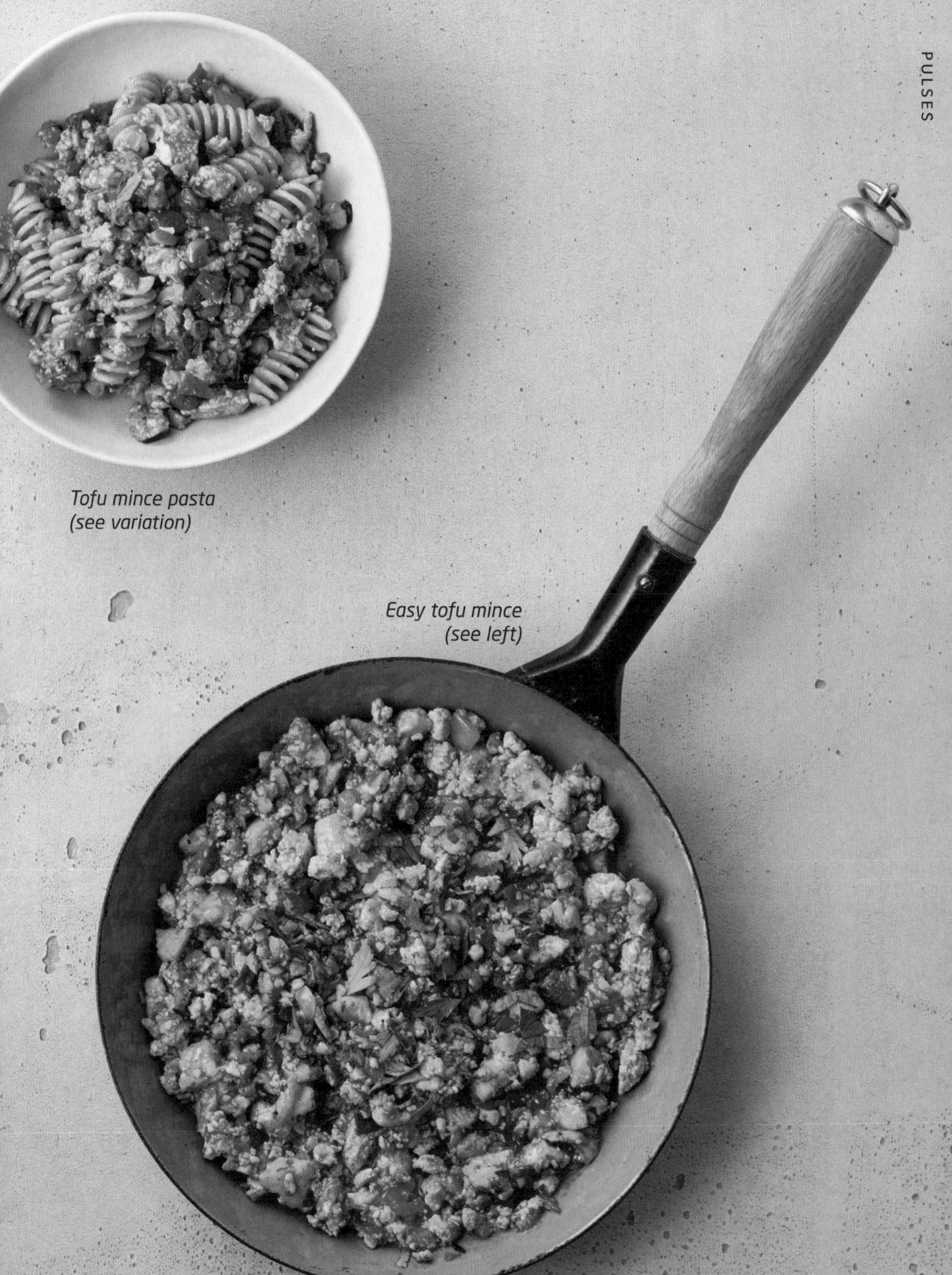

Tofu mince pasta
(see variation)

Easy tofu mince
(see left)

Mediterranean bean salad

Serves 2

1 red onion, peeled | salt | 1 large ripe tomato | ½ ripe avocado | 8 tbsp lemon juice (about 1 large lemon) | 1 tbsp yeast flakes | ½ tsp coarsely ground pepper | 10 olives, stoned and halved | 200g (7oz) cucumber | handful of basil leaves | 6 mint leaves | 200g (7oz) watermelon | 250g (9oz) cooked beans (see p. 191)

Nutritional values per portion: 344 kcal | 39.6g carbohydrate | 11g fat | 17.2g protein | 19.4g fibre | 0.6g ALA | 1214mg lysine | 139mg calcium | 2.3mg zinc | 5.4mg iron | 0.3mg B2 | 0.3mg RE | 11µg iodine | 0.4g salt

Slice the onion into fine rings and cover with water in a bowl. Add 1 teaspoon of salt and leave to stand for 10 minutes to make the onion flavour milder. Wash the tomato and remove the core. Remove the stone from the avocado and scoop out the flesh with a spoon. Grate the tomato and avocado to create a purée and combine with the lemon juice, yeast flakes, pepper, and olives in a bowl.

Wash the cucumber and slice into 2cm (¾in) cubes. Roughly tear the basil and finely chop the mint. Peel the watermelon and chop the fruit into 2cm (¾in) chunks. Add the cucumber, herbs, melon, and beans to the lemony dressing and mix. Season the salad with salt and pepper. Drain the salt water from the onion, rinse, and add to the salad.

BASTI'S TIP

As with all bean salads, this dish is best if the flavours are left to infuse for at least 1 hour. Adjust the seasoning with more lemon juice and salt, because beans are so absorbent they may taste as if they haven't been seasoned at all.

VARIATION

It's pasta time: double the quantity of avocado, stir 200g (7oz) of freshly cooked, warm wholewheat pasta into the salad and season with lemon juice, salt, and pepper. A delicious pasta salad served at room temperature for a summer's day.

Photo see p. 198 bottom

Curried legume salad

Serves 2

1 shallot, peeled | 100g (3½oz) peach (1–2 peaches or apples) | 8 sprigs of coriander | 2 tsp olive oil | 1 tsp ground turmeric | 1 tsp ground cumin | ½ tsp ground cinnamon | 8 tbsp lime juice (about 3 limes) | 2 tsp finely grated ginger | 2 tbsp desiccated coconut (or coconut chips) | 250g (9oz) cooked cold pulses (e.g. chickpeas or red lentils, see from p. 189) | salt | freshly ground pepper

Nutritional values per portion: 252 kcal | 20.1g carbohydrate | 12g fat | 10.7g protein | 11.1g fibre | 0.8g ALA | 796mg lysine | 65mg calcium | 1.8mg zinc | 3.2mg iron | 0.1mg B2 | 0.1mg RE | 3µg iodine | < 0.1g salt

Finely chop the shallot. Wash the peach, remove the stone, and chop into 1cm (½in) cubes. Finely chop the coriander.

Heat a small pan, add the olive oil, turmeric, cumin, and cinnamon, mix well with a wooden spoon and fry for 10 seconds. Deglaze the spices immediately with lime juice and ideally scrape into a bowl with a spatula. Add the grated ginger and coconut and leave the marinade to infuse for about 1 minute. Then stir in the pulses, shallot, and diced peach, season with salt and pepper, and serve.

VARIATION

You can use any kind of vegetable or salad ingredients in this dish and substitute your fruit of choice.

BASTI'S TIP

This salad tastes great fresh but is still excellent up to three days later. If you want to save it, leave out the shallot as this can make it bitter.

Photo see p. 198 top

Curried legume salad
(see p.197)

Mediterranean bean salad *(see p.196)*

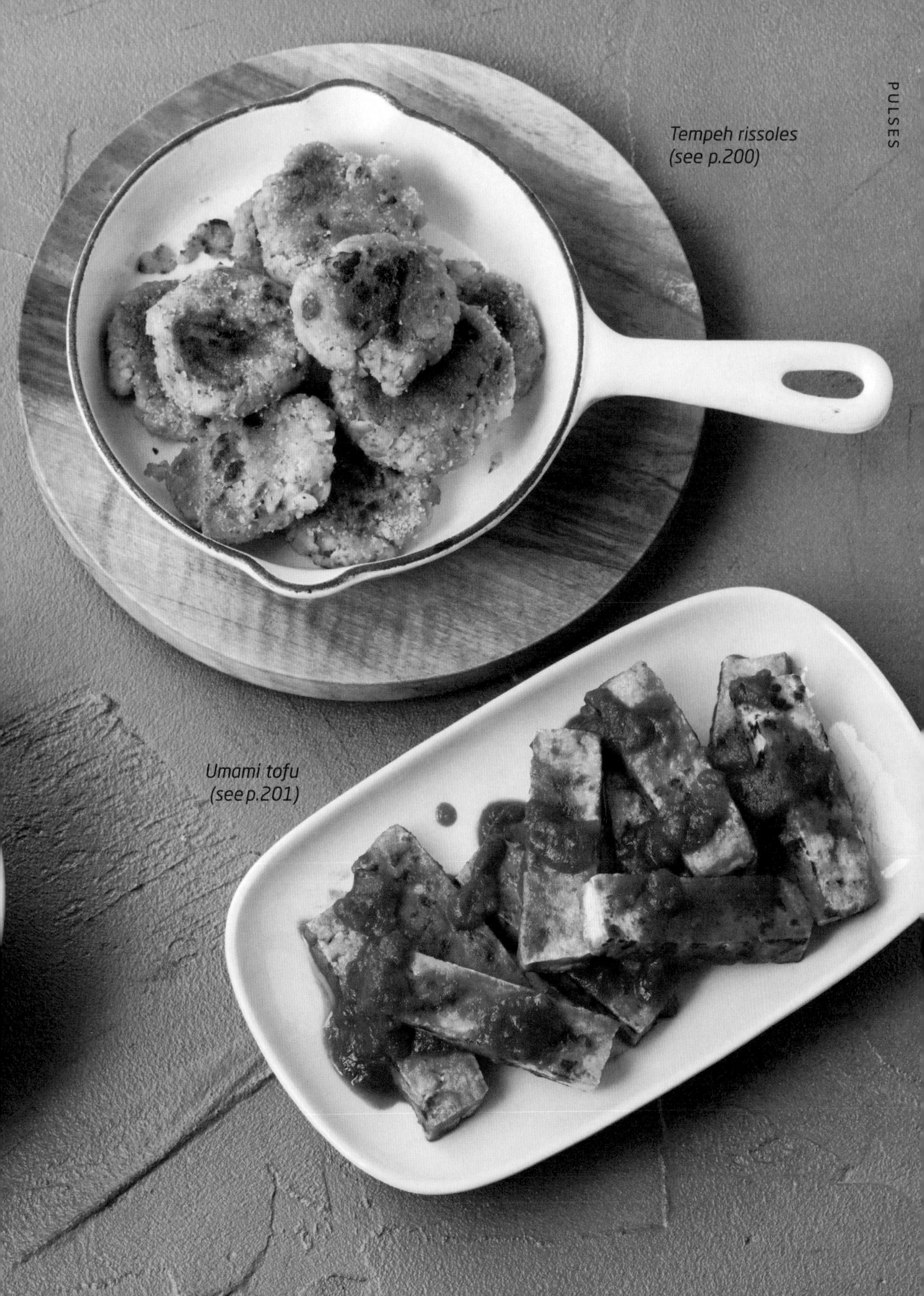

Tempeh rissoles *(see p.200)*

Umami tofu *(see p.201)*

Tempeh rissoles

 *Serves 2*

1 small onion, peeled | 200g (7oz) tempeh (made from soya, beans, or lupin – from an organic tempeh producer) | 35g (1oz) breadcrumbs (wholemeal or gluten-free) | 1 tbsp wholemeal flour | 1 tsp salt (or vegetable stock paste, see p.99) | 1 tsp dried thyme | 1 tbsp organic soy sauce (tamari) | 1 tbsp olive oil

Nutritional values per portion: 321 kcal | 22.1g carbohydrate | 15.9g fat | 22.3g protein | 9.1g fibre | 0.6g ALA | 1180mg lysine | 167mg calcium | 4.3mg zinc | 5.6mg iron | 0.7mg B2 | < 0.1mg RE | 4µg iodine | 3.2g salt

Finely chop the onion. Heat a pan, add the onion and 1 tablespoon of water and fry the onion until translucent. Use a fork to mash the tempeh into crumbs. Put the onion into a bowl with the tempeh, two-thirds of the breadcrumbs, flour, 2 tablespoons of water, salt, thyme, and soy sauce and mix until combined. Season to taste.

Use slightly damp hands to make eight small rissoles from this mixture and toss them to coat in the remaining breadcrumbs. Heat a non-stick pan, add the rissoles, drizzle with olive oil, and fry on both sides until crisp and brown. Leave to rest for 5 minutes then serve on two plates.

VARIATION

Try adding 1 tbsp of curry powder or a Mediterranean spice blend to the tempeh mixture to give these rissoles a different flavour. You can also finely grate 100g (3½oz) of sweet potato and work this into the tempeh mixture.

BASTI'S TIP

Tempeh freezes very well. Just buy a larger quantity to make a ready supply of these delicious protein bombs in your kitchen. For tempeh newbies, the seasoned products are particularly suitable because plain tempeh has its own distinct flavour that takes some getting used to. These rissoles taste amazing the next day served in a bread roll with a dash of mustard and a gherkin relish.

Photo see p.199 top

Umami tofu

Serves 2

50g (1¾oz) passata | 2 tbsp date paste (see p.97) | 2 tbsp organic soy sauce | 1 small garlic clove (optional), peeled | ¼ tsp hot paprika | ¼ tsp smoked paprika | 250g (9oz) tofu | 2 tsp olive oil

Nutritional values per portion: 228 kcal | 9.8g carbohydrate | 12.2g fat | 19.9g protein | 2.6g fibre | 0.7g ALA | 1216mg lysine | 238mg calcium | 2mg zinc | 3.8mg iron | 0.1mg B2 | < 0.1mg RE | 8µg iodine | 1.3g salt

Put all the ingredients except the tofu and olive oil into a high-sided container and process to a smooth consistency with a hand blender. Cut the tofu into 5mm (¼in) thick slices.

Heat a large non-stick pan until nice and hot then add the slices of tofu. Lower the heat, drizzle the oil over the tofu, shake the pan a bit to distribute the oil, and fry the sliced tofu over a moderate heat for 6–7 minutes on both sides until crisp and brown. This is very important: the tofu must be nicely browned and crisp. Most people do not fry the tofu long enough and it ends up being too pale and still soft! Remove the pan from the heat, add the sauce to the tofu, mix, and serve immediately. This is important for the combination of spicy marinade and crisp tofu to work.

BASTI'S TIP

When buying tofu, you need to look for good quality. This product is made using traditional methods, and the specific ingredients and production process have a huge impact on the final result. Particularly if tofu is not part of your cultural heritage, products may vary widely in quality.

VARIATION

Sweet and sour lemon tofu: once the tofu is cooked, add a marinade made from 6 tbsp of lemon juice, 2 tbsp of date paste (see p.97), 1 finely grated garlic clove, 1 tsp of salt, and 4 finely chopped basil leaves and cook off all the liquid. Fry the tofu again briefly and it's ready to serve!

Instead of tofu, you could also fry up some tempeh or beans and deglaze the pan with one of the two suggested marinades.

Photo see p.199 bottom

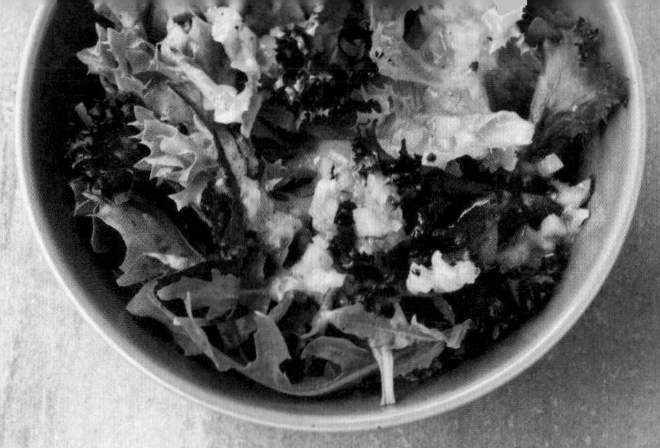

Green salad with date vinaigrette (see p.177)

Umami bean stew

Serves 3

2 tbsp shiitake mushroom powder (see tip p.144) | 1 tsp smoked paprika | 1 tbsp sweet paprika | 1 tsp dried thyme | 1 tsp freshly ground pepper | 2 tsp grated organic lemon zest | ½ tsp ground cinnamon | 100g (3½oz) smoked tofu | 1 celery stick | 1 onion, peeled | 2 garlic cloves, peeled | 2 tsp olive oil | 150ml (5fl oz) vegetable stock | 150ml (5fl oz) cooking water from beans (see p.191) | 2 tbsp cider vinegar | 250g (9oz) cooked white giant beans (see p.191) | 5 sprigs of parsley | organic soy sauce

Nutritional values per portion: 185 kcal | 16.8g carbohydrate | 7g fat | 14.1g protein | 9.5g fibre | 0.5g ALA | 1050mg lysine | 135mg calcium | 1.8mg zinc | 3.5mg iron | 0.1mg B2 | < 0.1mg RE | 6µg iodine | 0.8g salt

Combine the mushroom powder, paprikas, thyme, pepper, lemon zest, and cinnamon in a cup. Slice the smoked tofu into 5mm (¼in) cubes. Wash the celery then finely chop it with the onion and garlic.

Heat a pan to a high temperature. Add the smoked tofu to the pan and drizzle with olive oil. Fry the tofu for 5 minutes until crisp and brown. Add the onion, celery, and garlic and sauté for 3 minutes until brown. Add the spice mix, fry for 10 seconds, deglaze immediately with the vegetable stock, and loosen any residue on the base of the pan.

Add the cooking water from the beans, the vinegar, and the beans themselves and simmer gently over a low heat for 5 minutes. Meanwhile, finely chop the parsley. Add this to the pan and use a wooden spoon to crush 10–15 beans so everything binds together nicely. Mix all the bean stew ingredients once more then season to taste with vinegar, pepper, and soy sauce.

BASTI'S TIP

Ideally make double quantities the day before and allow the flavours to develop overnight in the fridge. This bean stew tastes best the following day, although it is still delicious if eaten straight away.

Using the cooking water from the beans gives the dish a fabulous texture and added umami flavour.

To make this dish even creamier, just stir 1–2 tsp of white almond nut butter into the bean mixture once it is cooked.

VARIATION

You can swap the giant beans for another variety of cooked bean.

Millet (see p.135)

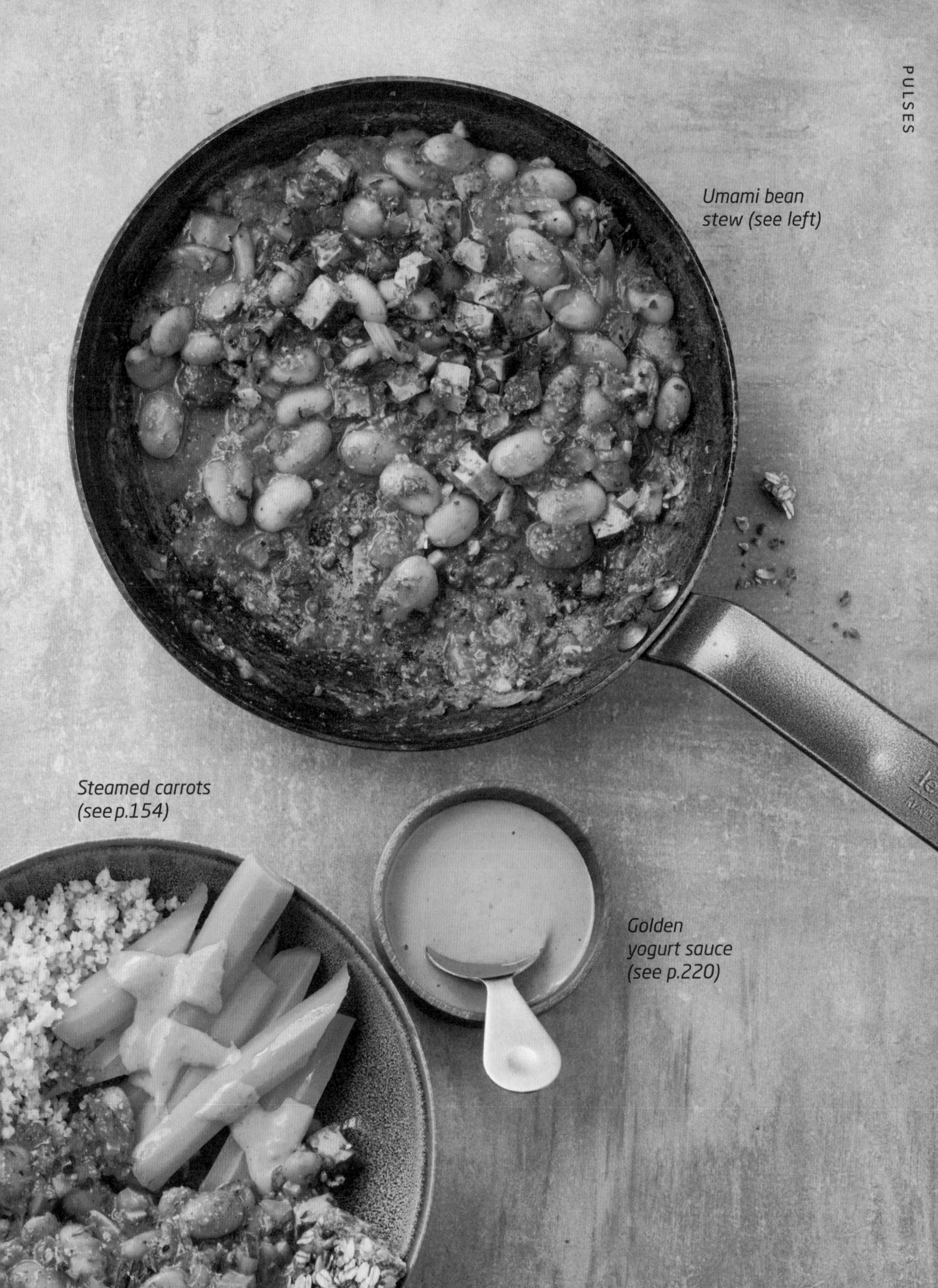
Umami bean
stew (see left)
Steamed carrots
(see p.154)
Golden
yogurt sauce
(see p.220)

Sour smoked tofu salad

Serves 2

200g (7oz) smoked tofu | ½ red pepper, deseeded | 60g (2oz) gherkin | 7 tbsp cider vinegar | 2 tbsp date paste (see p.97) | 1 tbsp shiro miso | 1 tbsp olive oil | 1 tbsp Dijon mustard | 1 small red onion, peeled and diced | salt | freshly ground pepper | 4 tbsp chopped chives

Nutritional values per portion: 339 kcal | 14.5g carbohydrate | 18.2g fat | 22.7g protein | 7.6g fibre | 0.9g ALA | 1680mg lysine | 335mg calcium | 2.8mg zinc | 7.3mg iron | 0.2mg B2 | 0.2mg RE | 14µg iodine | 2.9g salt

Slice the smoked tofu and pepper into very thin strips. Finely dice the gherkin. Combine these in a bowl with the remaining ingredients except the chives. Season the salad with salt and pepper, leave the flavours to infuse for 1–3 hours in the fridge, then adjust the seasoning with extra vinegar, salt, and pepper. Scatter the salad with chives to serve.

BASTI'S TIP

I think it is very important to give this dish time to infuse because this creates a more intense flavour. Of course, there is nothing stopping you eating the salad straight away.

VARIATION

Al pomodoro: prepare the salad as described in the recipe. Fry 5 cherry tomatoes in a pan over a high heat for 2–3 minutes until the skin has browned slightly. Before serving, mix a small handful of rocket and 6 basil leaves into the salad, then scatter the fried cherry tomatoes on top.

Green peppercorn and tempeh in a creamy sauce

Serves 2

200g (7oz) tempeh (made from soya, beans, or lupin) | 1 onion, peeled | 2 tsp olive oil | 3 sprigs of parsley | 200ml (7fl oz) vegetable stock | 1 tbsp white almond nut butter |1 tbsp shiro miso | 1 tbsp lemon juice | 1–2 tsp pickled green peppercorns (from a jar) | salt (optional)

Nutritional values per portion: 340 kcal | 11.5g carbohydrate | 22.4g fat | 23.1g protein | 9.2g fibre | 0.7g ALA | 1258mg lysine | 206mg calcium | 4.4mg zinc | 6mg iron | 0.8mg B2 | < 0.1mg RE | 4µg iodine | 1.2g salt

Slice the tempeh into 3cm (1in) long, 5mm (¼in) wide chunks or roughly crumble it by hand. Slice the onion into rings. Put a non-stick pan over a high heat. Add the onion and tempeh. Drizzle with oil and fry the tempeh mixture over a moderate heat for 6 minutes until nicely browned. Meanwhile, roughly chop the parsley. Add this to a food processor along with the stock, almond nut butter, miso, lemon juice, and purée to make a green sauce. Add this to the tempeh with the peppercorns and simmer gently for 4 minutes until the sauce has thickened nicely. Season with salt, if desired, and tuck in!

BASTI'S TIP

Note the tip about tempeh for the tempeh rissoles (see p.200).

VARIATION

Instead of tempeh, you can use mushrooms or tofu, or even cooked pulses – in which case, only add these to the pan at the stage where you add the peppercorns.

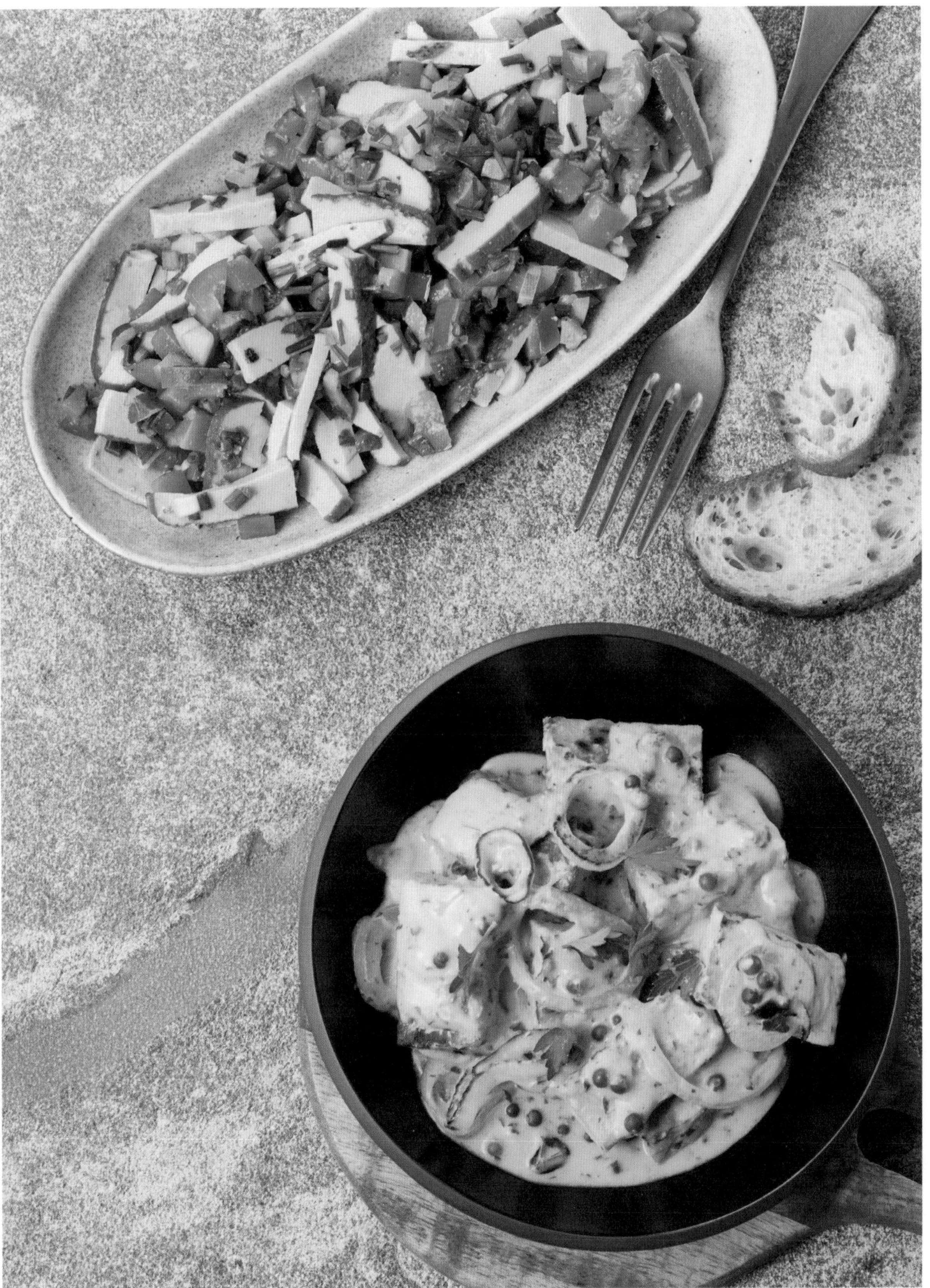

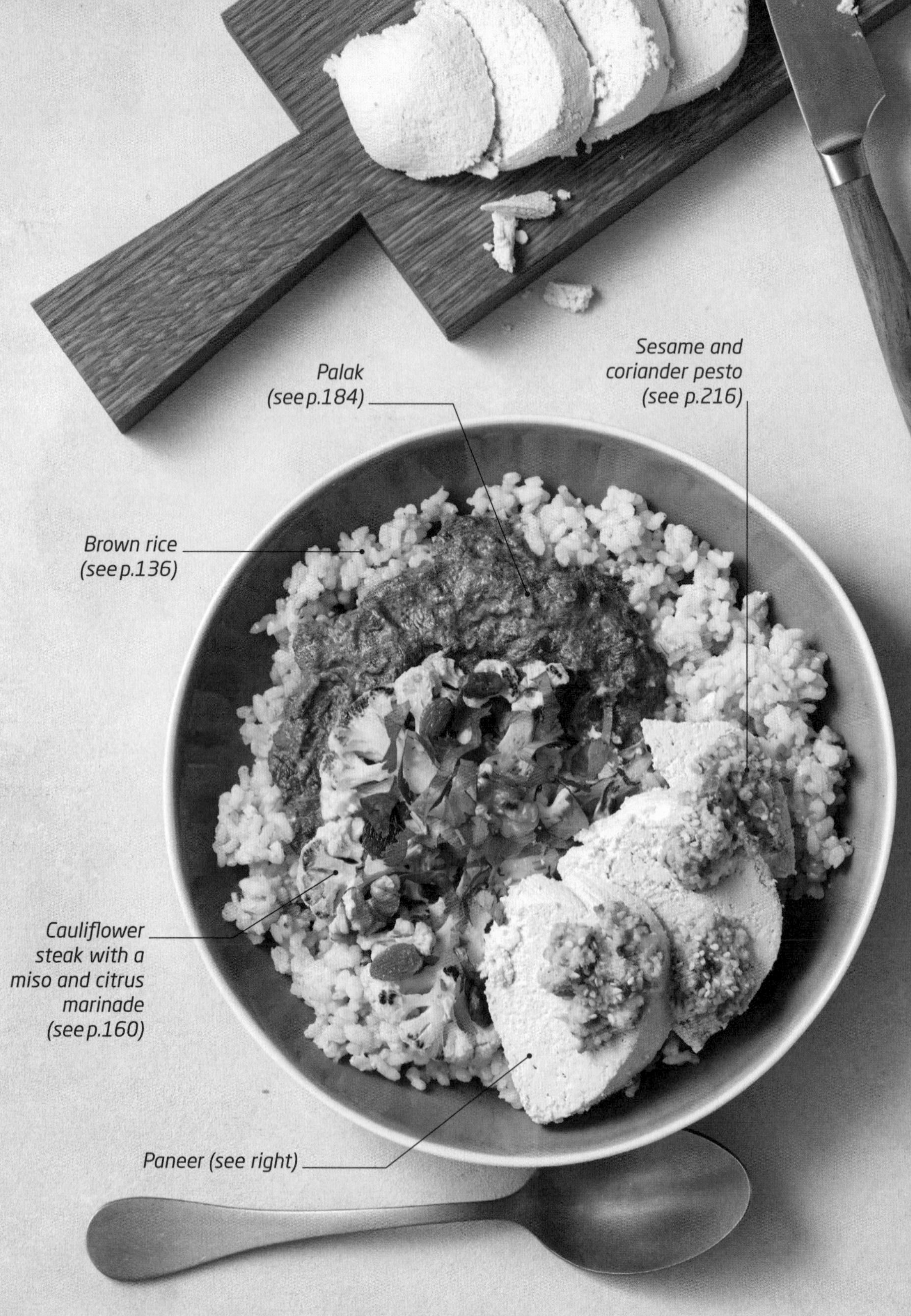
Palak
(see p.184)
Sesame and
coriander pesto
(see p.216)
Brown rice
(see p.136)
Cauliflower
steak with a
miso and citrus
marinade
(see p.160)
Paneer (see right)

Paneer – soya cheese

 *Serves 3*

2 litres (3½ pints) organic soya milk with calcium (ideally Provamel) | 6 tbsp lemon juice | 4 tbsp cider vinegar

Nutritional values per portion: 353 kcal | 38.4g carbohydrate | 12.3g fat | 23.3g protein | 4g fibre | 0.7g ALA | 1333mg lysine | 800mg calcium | 2.6mg zinc | 5.3mg iron | 0.3mg B2 | 0mg RE | 73µg iodine | 1g salt

Put the soya milk in a pan and bring to the boil. Be careful, soya milk burns easily. Stir in the lemon juice and vinegar and continue cooking for 2 minutes, stirring gently. Turn off the hob and allow the mixture to rest for 2 minutes. Line a fine sieve with a clean tea towel and suspend over a bowl to catch the whey.

Pour the curdled soya mixture into the sieve with the towel, mix everything slightly with a spoon to allow the whey to strain through nicely. Then twist the cloth together at the top and gently squeeze out some whey. Weigh down the paneer with a small pan and gently twist the towel again every 2 minutes. Repeat this process two to three times until you have a firm, compact residue. Slice the paneer into pieces and eat immediately or use in a recipe.

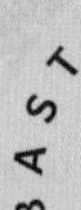

BASTI'S TIP

We have tested various kinds of soya milk for making paneer and some are not suitable for this recipe. Provamel's soya milk with calcium is the best choice for home-made paneer. If the soya milk fails to form clumps after it has been boiled and the acidic ingredients have been added, just help it on its way with another 1 tbsp of cider vinegar.

Traditionally paneer is made from cow's milk and is used in Indian cuisine. It works beautifully in spicy sauces or curries because it does not have a strong flavour itself and provides the perfect mild contrast.

It will keep for 3–4 days in an airtight container in the fridge. If you want to make paneer regularly, it is worth investing in a tofu press with cloth. This will press the soya curds into a nice rectangular shape, which is easier to cut into cubes.

Dice the paneer and use it in palak (see p. 184), scattered over a salad, or as a protein component in a bowl. The paneer is also excellent if grilled briefly then seasoned with garlic and soy sauce.

VARIATION

Adding 100ml (3½fl oz) of beetroot juice to the soya milk creates a beautiful purple paneer.

Add spices to the soya curds in the towel and work this into the paneer mixture.

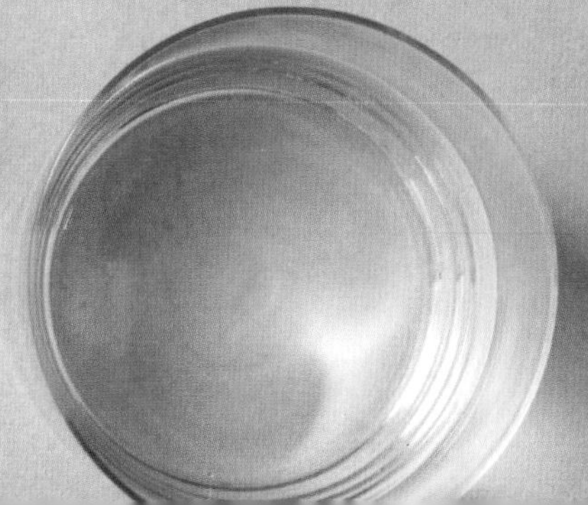

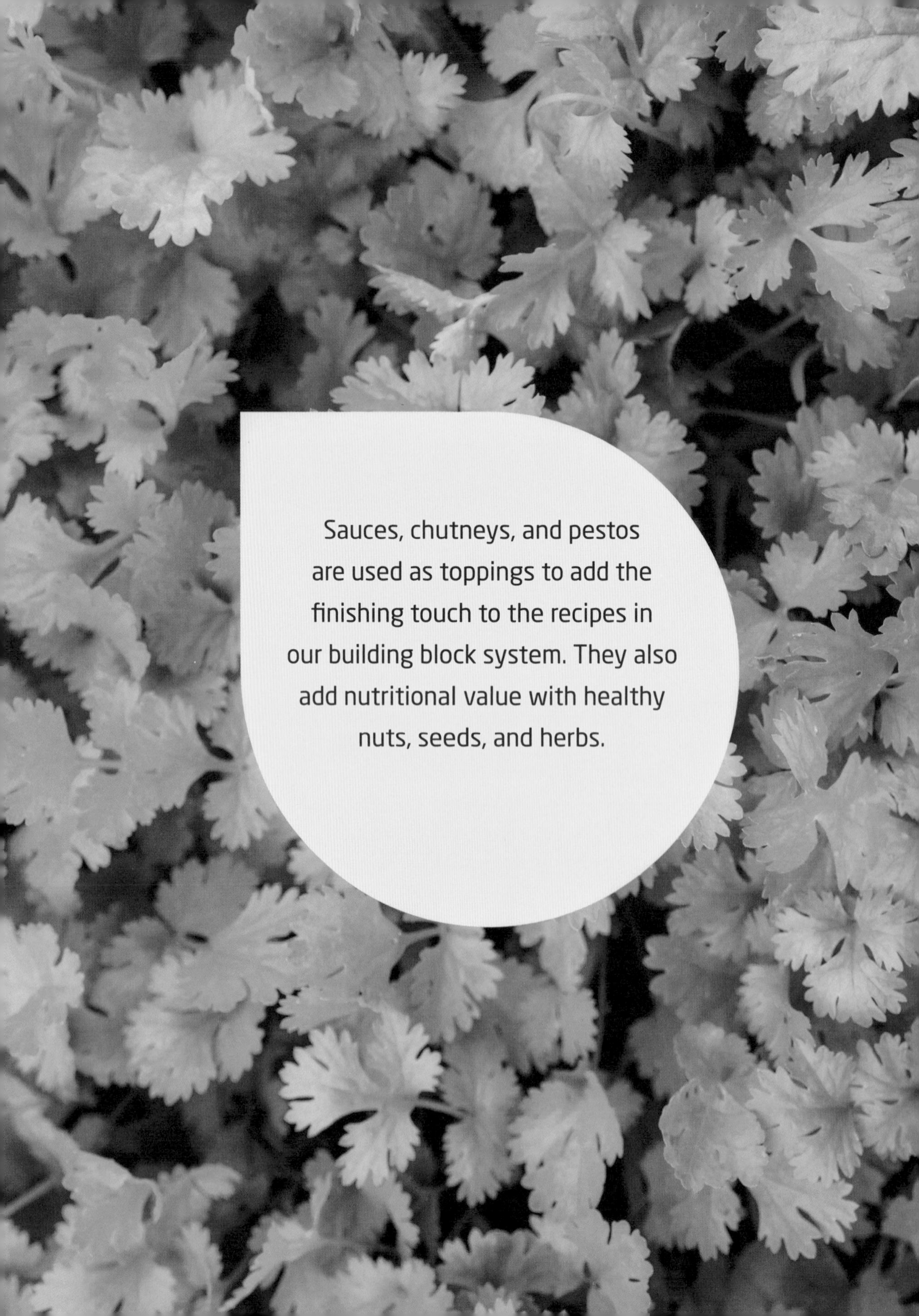

Sauces, chutneys, and pestos are used as toppings to add the finishing touch to the recipes in our building block system. They also add nutritional value with healthy nuts, seeds, and herbs.

Toppings

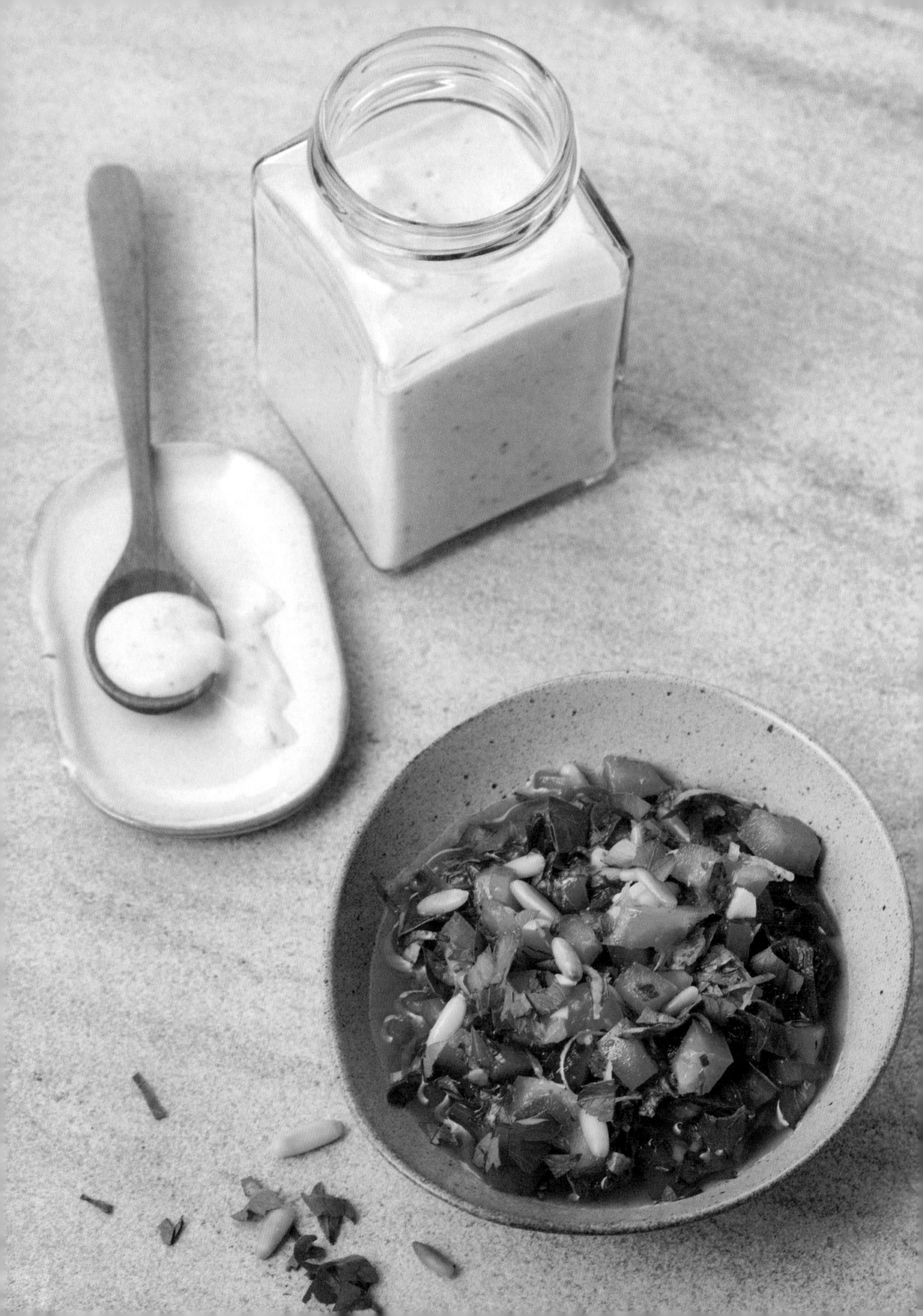

Yogurt and garlic sauce

Serves 3

1 garlic clove, peeled | 400g (14oz) organic soya yogurt | 60g (2oz) white almond nut butter | 10g (¼oz) celery greens (or parsley) | 30g (1oz) shiro miso | 3 tsp cider vinegar | pinch of salt

Nutritional values per portion: 187 kcal | 8.6g carbohydrate | 13.2g fat | 8.4g protein | 2.8g fibre | 0.2g ALA | 436mg lysine | 78mg calcium | 0.5mg zinc | 1.7mg iron | 0.2mg B2 | < 0.1mg RE | 3µg iodine | 0.8g salt

Add all the ingredients to the food processor and blend until you have a smooth sauce.

VARIATION

Use 3 dried tomatoes instead of garlic in the sauce. Try replacing the almond nut butter with light tahini (sesame seed paste, see tip p.192) or cashew nut butter and just use whatever herbs you have available, such as parsley, basil, or mint.

Quick gremolata

Serves 3

2 organic lemons | 1 garlic clove, peeled | 1 bunch of flat-leaf parsley | 1 small red pepper | 1 small, mild fresh chilli | 3 tbsp pine nuts | 3 tbsp date paste (see p.97) | 2 tsp olive oil | salt | freshly ground pepper

Nutritional values per portion: 213 kcal | 16g carbohydrate | 11.8g fat | 5.5g protein | 5.8g fibre | 0.3g ALA | 270mg lysine | 66mg calcium | 1mg zinc | 2.8mg iron | 0.2mg B2 | 0.4mg RE | 4µg iodine | < 0.1g salt

Wash the lemons in hot water and dry them. Finely grate the zest of both lemons and squeeze the juice from 1 lemon, adding this to the zest. Crush and add the garlic clove. Chop the parsley very finely. Wash the pepper and chilli, remove the seeds, and dice very finely. Gently toast the pine nuts in a dry pan, stirring constantly. Put all the ingredients in a bowl and season with salt and pepper.

BASTI'S TIP

This reduced-oil gremolata recipe goes beautifully with all sorts of vegetables, tofu, or pulses.

VARIATION

Instead of parsley, you could use basil, coriander, or dill. Or replace the red pepper with cherry tomatoes, yellow peppers, or kohlrabi and swap the pine nuts for other nuts or seeds.

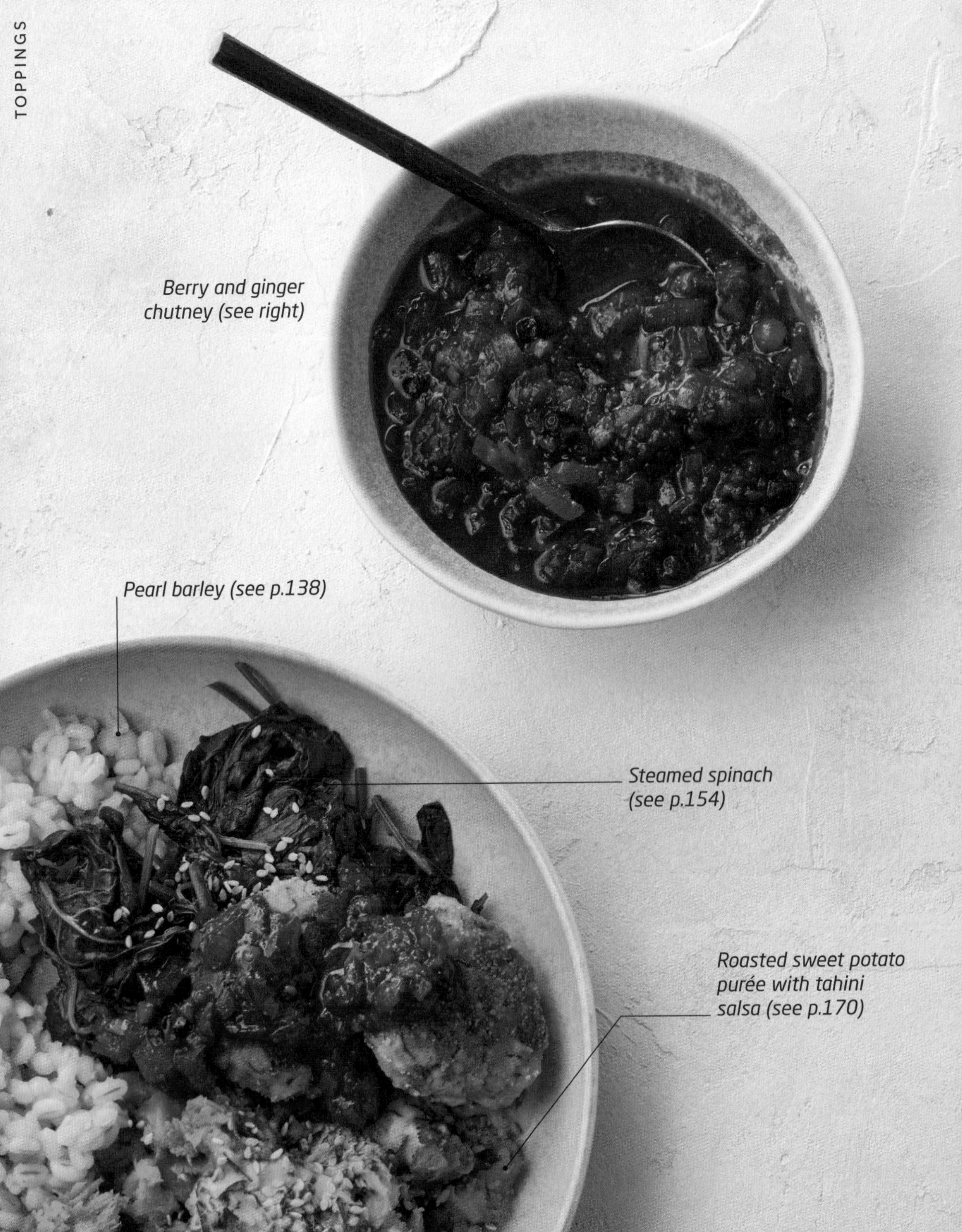
Berry and ginger chutney (see right)
Pearl barley (see p.138)
Steamed spinach (see p.154)
Roasted sweet potato purée with tahini salsa (see p.170)

Berry and ginger chutney

Serves 3

1 red onion, peeled | piece of fresh root ginger (2cm/¾in), peeled | ½ tsp ground coriander | good pinch of ground cloves | 2 tsp olive oil | juice of 1 large lemon | 3 tbsp date paste (see p.97) | 150g (5½oz) frozen berries | ½ tsp freshly ground pepper | 1 tbsp shiro miso

Nutritional values per portion: 124 kcal | 15g carbohydrate | 4.6g fat | 2.2g protein | 5.1g fibre | 0.2g ALA | 131mg lysine | 33mg calcium | 0.3mg zinc | 1mg iron | < 0.1mg B2 | < 0.1mg RE | 3µg iodine | 0.5g salt

Finely chop the onion and ginger. Heat a small pan. Add the diced onion and ginger, coriander, and cloves, and drizzle with olive oil. Sauté everything until the onion is beginning to take on some colour.

Deglaze the onion and spice mixture with the lemon juice and date paste and add two-thirds of the berries. Cover and simmer the chutney for 10 minutes over a moderate heat. Then add the remaining berries and the pepper. Turn off the hob, leave the chutney to stand for 10 minutes, then season with miso.

BASTI'S TIP

If stored in an airtight container, the chutney will keep for 3–4 days in the fridge and it tastes excellent with rice, steamed sweet potatoes, and crispy tofu.

VARIATION

Instead of berries, you could use diced mango, peach, or melon.

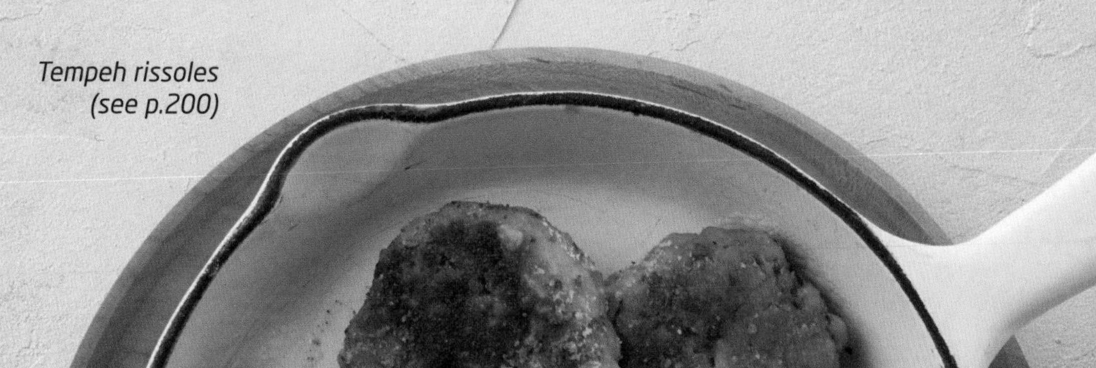

Tempeh rissoles (see p.200)

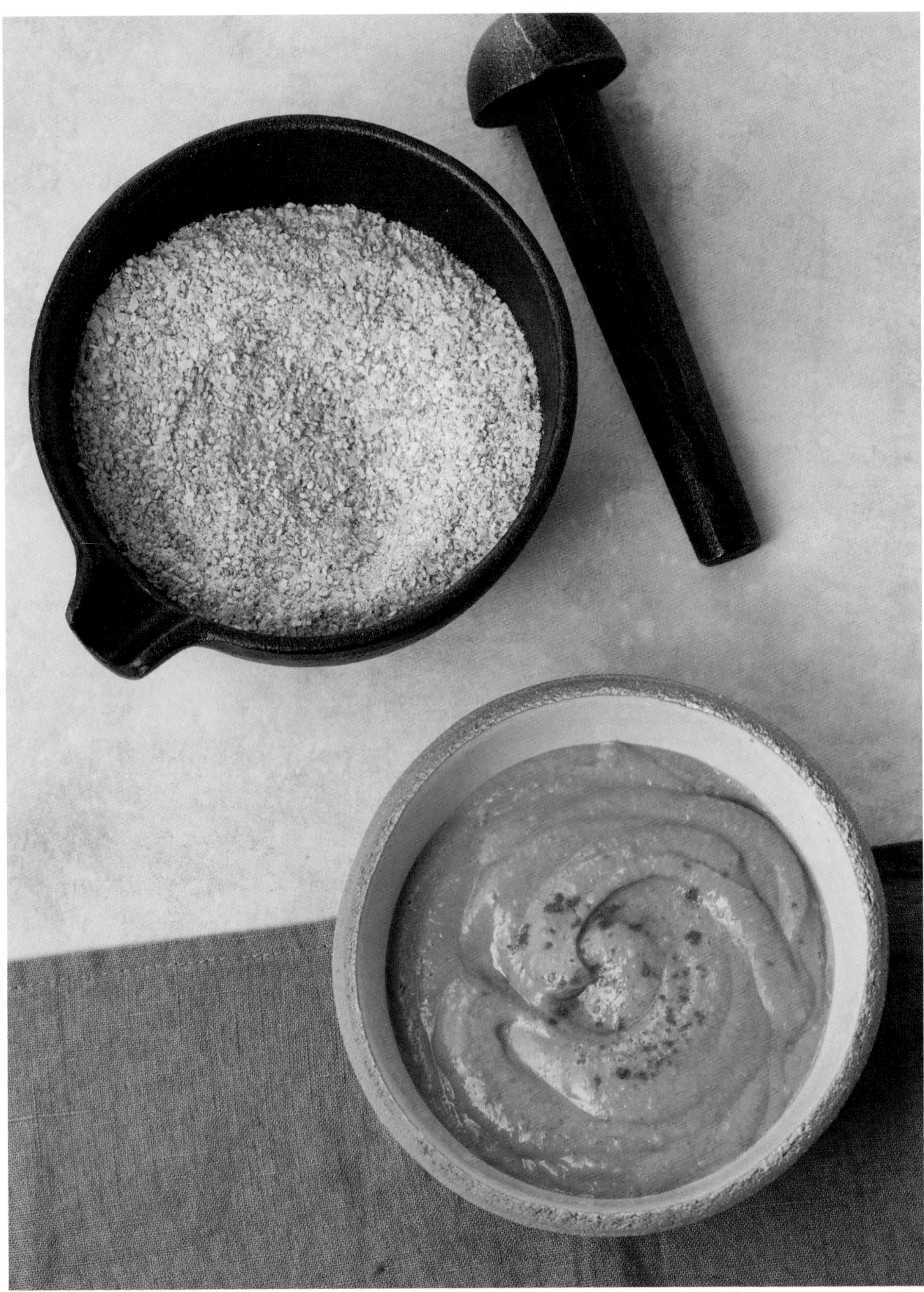

Smoky umami gomasio

Serves about 10

120g (4oz) sesame seeds | 8 tbsp yeast flakes | 1 tsp smoked paprika | 2 tsp salt | 1 tsp freshly ground pepper

Nutritional values per portion: 84 kcal | 2.9g carbohydrate | 6.3g fat | 4.6g protein | 1.7g fibre | 0.2g ALA | 218mg lysine | 104mg calcium | 1.3mg zinc | 2mg iron | 0.2mg B2 | < 0.1mg RE | 1µg iodine | 0.9g salt

Lightly toast the sesame seeds in a dry pan for 3 minutes, stirring constantly. Transfer to a food processor and gently process with the remaining ingredients until the sesame seeds have been broken up slightly. This also works well in a pestle and mortar. Leave the spice mix to cool and store in a clean jar.

BASTI'S TIP

This recipe makes a good quantity because gomasio keeps very well for a couple of weeks. The classic way to use gomasio is as a low-salt seasoning. In this recipe, additional umami flavours are introduced by using yeast flakes and the smoked spice.

VARIATION

Instead of sesame seeds, use pumpkin seeds or almond slivers. Or try substituting curry powder instead of the paprika, and miso paste instead of the yeast flakes. However, if you use miso paste rather than yeast flakes, you will need to dry out the gomasio for 30 minutes at 60°C (140°F) in the oven.

Banana and hoisin sauce

Serves 3

4 tbsp organic soy sauce (about 40ml/1fl oz) | 100g (3½oz) crunchy peanut butter | flesh of 1 small, ripe avocado | 50g (2oz) banana (½ small), peeled | ½ garlic clove, peeled | 5 tsp cider vinegar | 1 tsp hot paprika | pinch of ground cloves

Nutritional values per portion: 251 kcal | 8.1g carbohydrate | 20.4g fat | 9.4g protein | 4.4g fibre | 0.2g ALA | 395mg lysine | 18mg calcium | 1.1mg zinc | 0.8mg iron | 0.1mg B2 | < 0.1mg RE | 6µg iodine | 1.7g salt

Put all the ingredients in a food processor with 70ml (2½fl oz) water and purée until smooth.

BASTI'S TIP

This sauce is a great addition to Asian recipes with rice and a fruity salsa.

VARIATION

If you do not want to use soy sauce, a soy-free spicy sauce such as Coco Aminos from Big Tree Farms is a wonderful alternative.

Mango or peach tastes great in the sauce instead of banana, and the peanut butter can be replaced with light tahini (sesame seed paste, see tip p.192) or white almond nut butter.

Apple and coriander topping

Serves 3

1 large slightly tart apple | ½ bunch of coriander | 1 mild chilli | 4 tbsp black sesame seeds (or white sesame seeds) | 2 organic limes

Nutritional values per portion: 155 kcal | 11.9g carbohydrate | 8g fat | 3.3g protein | 3.4g fibre | 0.3g ALA | 115mg lysine | 115mg calcium | 1.1mg zinc | 1.6mg iron | < 0.1mg B2 | < 0.1mg RE | 2µg iodine | < 0.1g salt

Wash the apple. Place it on a board with the stalk upwards and work from the outside to cut thin slices from one side until you reach the core. Do the same on the opposite side, then on the two remaining narrow sides. Discard the core. Stack the slices of apple and cut into thin batons. This process is essential for a nice delicate topping.

Chop the coriander very finely. Wash and deseed the chilli, then dice very finely.

Gently toast the sesame seeds in a dry pan over a moderate heat, stirring constantly. Wash the limes in hot water and dry them. Grate 1 teaspoon of zest and squeeze the juice of both limes. Put all the ingredients in a bowl and mix gently.

VARIATION

Instead of coriander, you can easily use basil, parsley, or dill. And the apple can be replaced with pear or slightly unripe mango.

Sesame and coriander pesto

Serves 3

70g (2½oz) sesame seeds | 1 small bunch of coriander (about 25g/scant 1oz) | 1 apple | 2 tbsp lemon juice | 20g (¾oz) shiro miso | date paste (see p.97), to taste

Nutritional values per portion: 199 kcal | 13.6g carbohydrate | 12.1g fat | 5.6g protein | 4.6g fibre | 0.2g ALA | 202 mg lysine | 191 mg calcium | 1.9 mg zinc | 2.6 mg iron | 0.1 mg B2 | < 0.1 mg RE | 3 µg iodine | 0.3g salt

Gently toast the sesame seeds in a dry pan for 3 minutes, stirring constantly. Chop the coriander very finely. Wash, quarter, and core the apple.

Add all the ingredients to the food processor and blitz until you have a slightly lumpy pesto. Depending on how large and sweet your apple is, you may need to season the pesto to taste with some additional lemon juice or date paste. The pesto should be slightly spicy with a hint of bitterness and a fresh flavour.

BASTI'S TIP

This pesto tastes fantastic with any steamed vegetables or beans, but it does not work with pasta.

VARIATION

If you do not like coriander, just use basil or parsley. Instead of sesame seeds, you can use any kind of nuts or seeds.

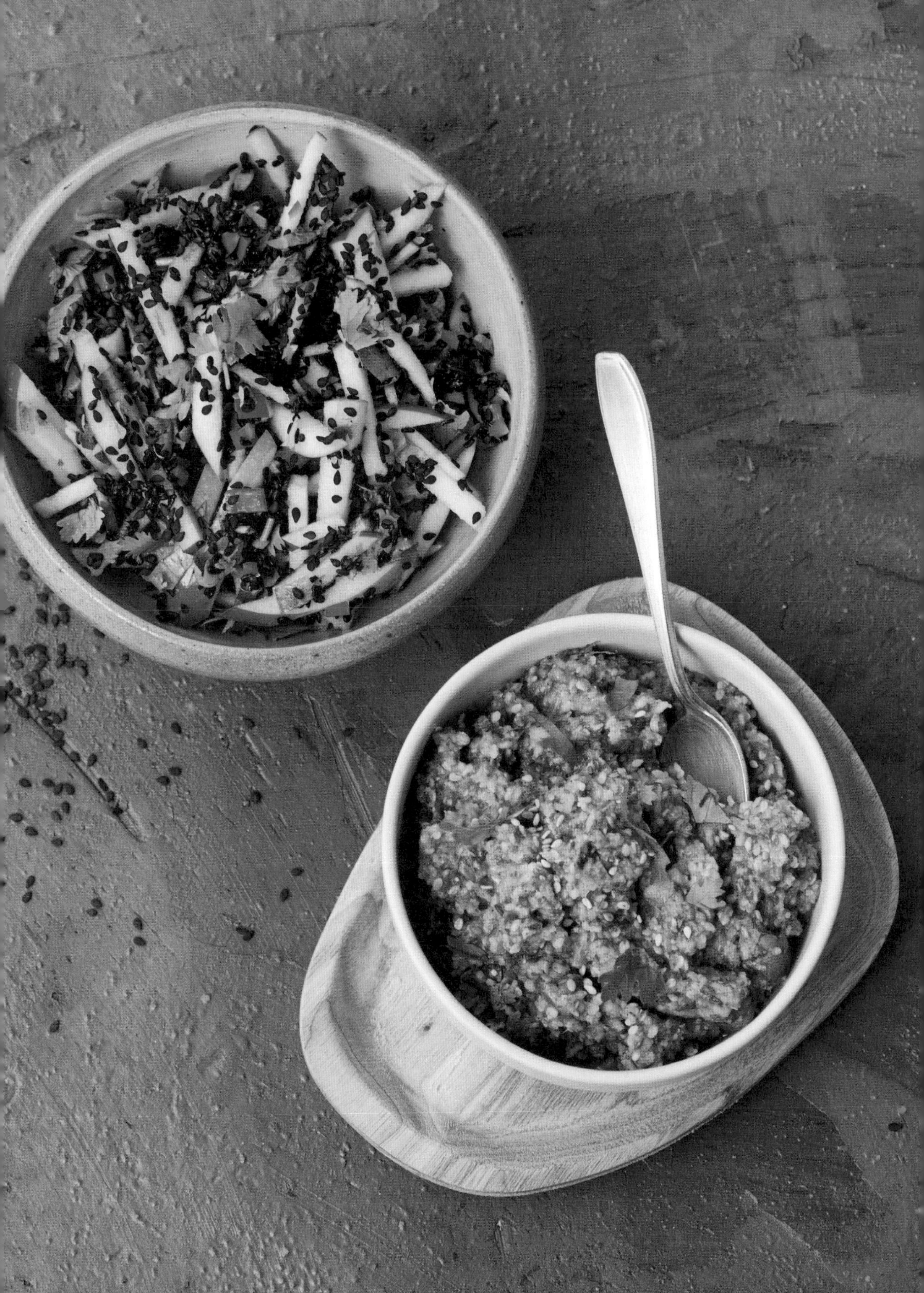

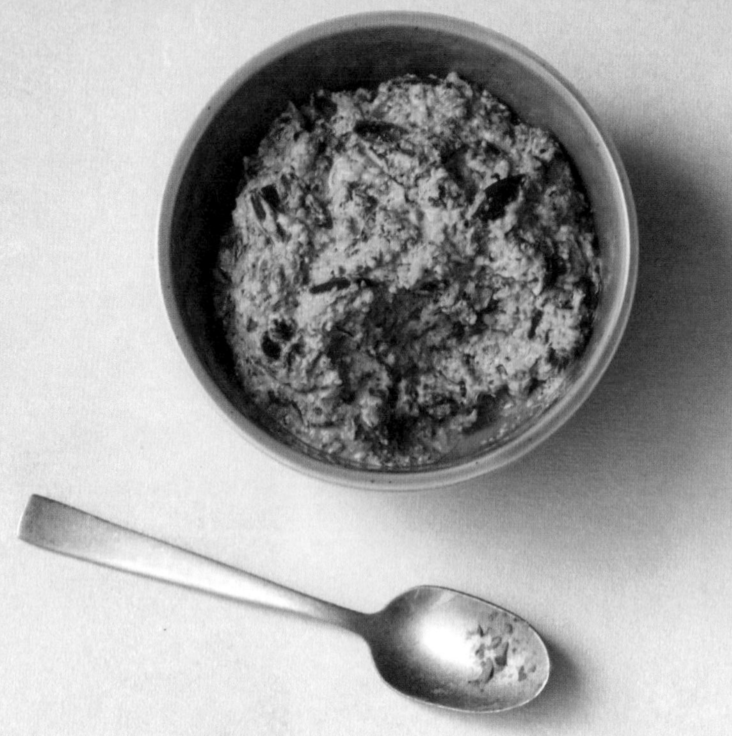

Cheesy pumpkin seed pesto

Serves 3

70g (2½oz) pumpkin seeds | 20g (¾oz) basil leaves | 1 garlic clove, peeled (optional) | 3–4 tbsp yeast flakes | 1 tbsp organic soy sauce | 2 tsp cider vinegar | salt (optional) | 1 tsp freshly ground pepper

Nutritional values per portion: 157 kcal | 3.4g carbohydrate | 11.2g fat | 11.5g protein | 2.7g fibre | 0.2g ALA | 752mg lysine | 33mg calcium | 2mg zinc | 2.6mg iron | 0.2mg B2 | < 0.1mg RE | 1µg iodine | 0.4g salt

Gently toast the pumpkin seeds in a dry pan over a moderate heat for 3 minutes, stirring constantly. Chop the basil very finely.

Add all the pesto ingredients to the food processor and blend until you have slightly lumpy pesto. Season the pesto to taste with salt and pepper.

BASTI'S TIP

Ideally, make bigger quantities of this pesto. It is delicious and will easily keep for 3–4 days in an airtight container in the fridge. It tastes great with wholewheat pasta or stewed tomatoes.

VARIATION

Feel free to swap the pumpkin seeds for other seeds or nuts, or replace the basil with other herbs, and if you don't like yeast flakes, season the pesto with miso paste.

You can add 100g (3½oz) of cooked vegetables to the pesto to create a purée. Sweet potatoes, celeriac, or beetroot work well here.

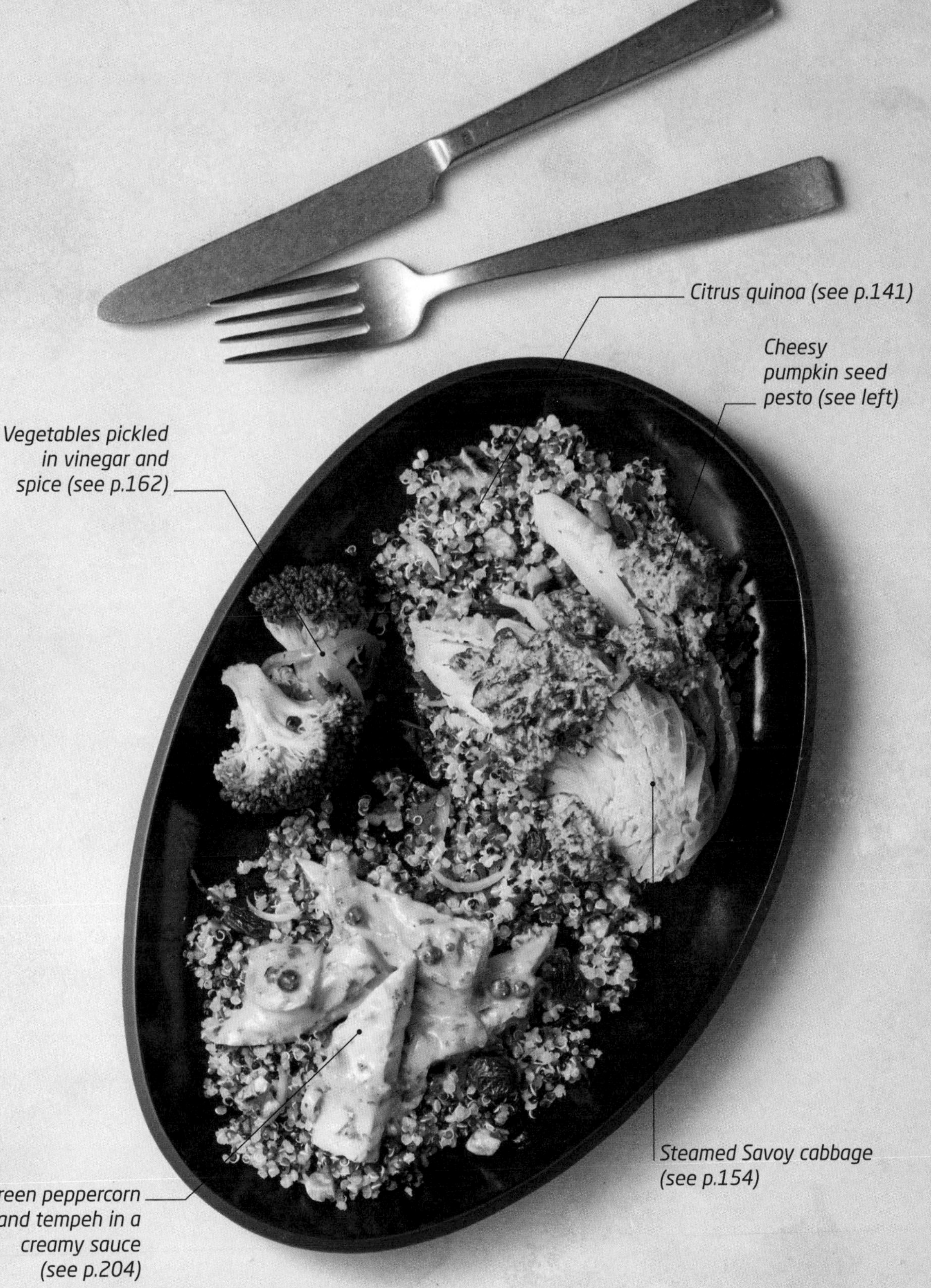
Citrus quinoa (see p.141)
Cheesy pumpkin seed pesto (see left)
Vegetables pickled in vinegar and spice (see p.162)
Steamed Savoy cabbage (see p.154)
Green peppercorn and tempeh in a creamy sauce (see p.204)

Golden yogurt sauce

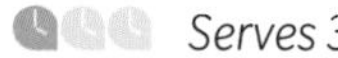

Serves 3

2 tsp ground turmeric | ½ tsp ground cinnamon | ¼ tsp ground cloves | ½ tsp freshly ground pepper | 1 tbsp finely grated ginger | 4 tbsp organic soya milk with calcium (or other plant-based milk) | 1 tbsp date paste (see p.97) | 2 tbsp white almond nut butter | 200g (7oz) organic soya yogurt | ½ orange, peeled | 1 tbsp organic soy sauce | salt | lemon juice

Nutritional values per portion: 187 kcal | 11.6g carbohydrate | 12.7g fat | 6.5g protein | 2.4g fibre | 0.2g ALA | 284mg lysine | 100mg calcium | 0.6mg zinc | 1.4mg iron | 0.2mg B2 | < 0.1mg RE | 3µg iodine | 0.4g salt

Heat a small non-stick pan and toast the turmeric, cinnamon, cloves, pepper, and ginger for 10 seconds. Deglaze the spices with the soya milk and briefly bring to the boil.

Put the spiced milk into the food processor with the other ingredients except the salt and lemon juice and purée until smooth. Season with salt and lemon and decant into a screwtop jar.

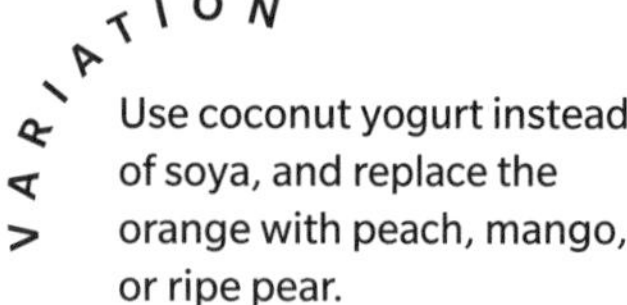

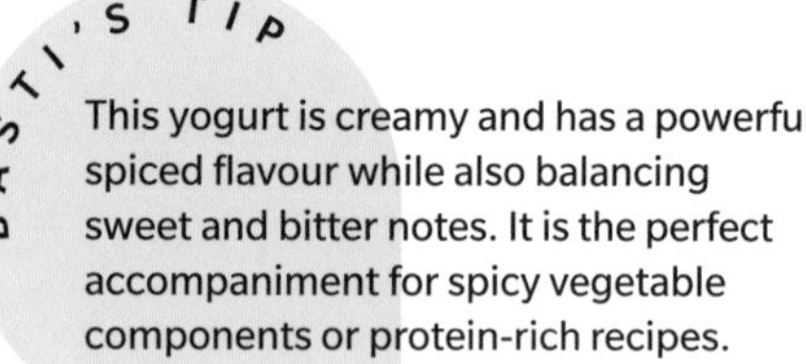

Pear, basil, and walnut topping

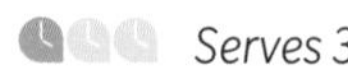

Serves 3

1 large juicy pear, with a bit of bite | 20 basil leaves | 1 small organic lemon | 6 tbsp walnuts, soaked in warm water for 2 hours | 1 tbsp pickled capers | pinch of ground turmeric | ½ tsp freshly ground pepper

Nutritional values per portion: 276 kcal | 13.5g carbohydrate | 21.7g fat | 5.4g protein | 4.4g fibre | 3.1g ALA | 185mg lysine | 43mg calcium | 1mg zinc | 1.3mg iron | 0.1mg B2 | < 0.1mg RE | 3µg iodine | 0.2g salt

Wash, quarter, and core the pear then slice into thin strips. Cut the basil into thin strips. Wash the lemon in hot water and dry it, grate ½ teaspoon of zest and squeeze the juice.

Drain the walnuts in a sieve, rinse under running water, dab dry, and chop roughly. Carefully mix all the topping ingredients in a bowl.

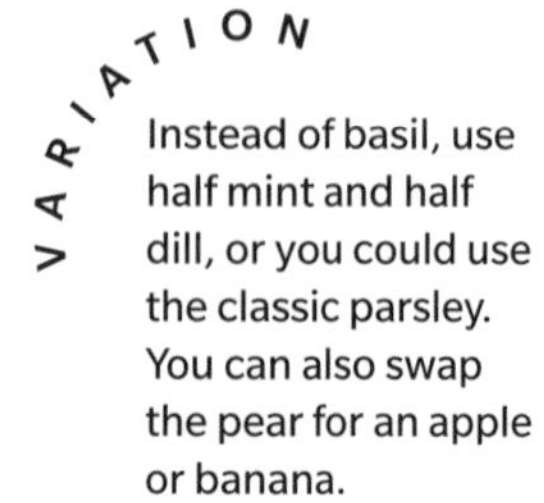

BASTI'S TIP

Soaking the walnuts helps reduce their bitter edge and improve their flavour.

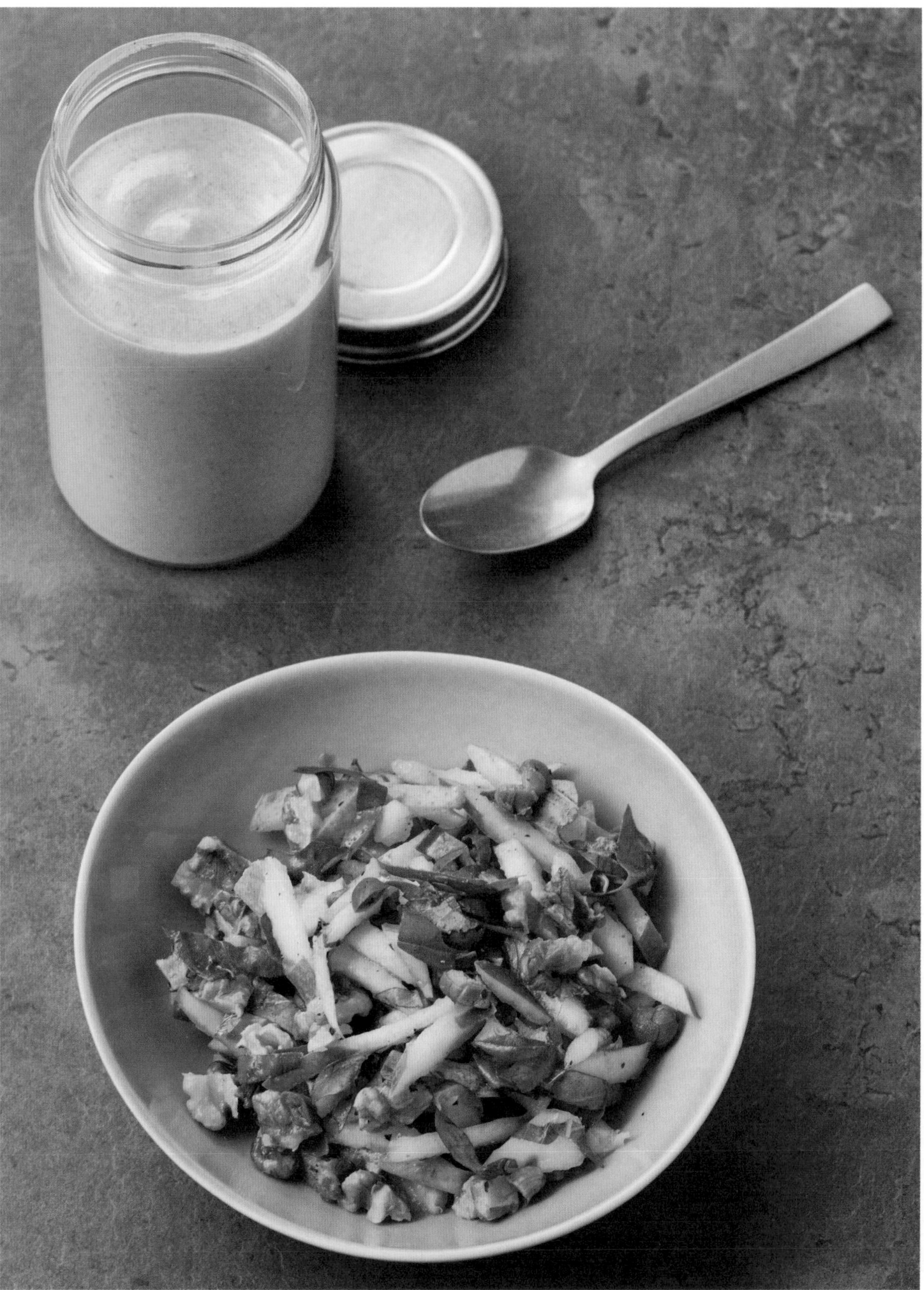

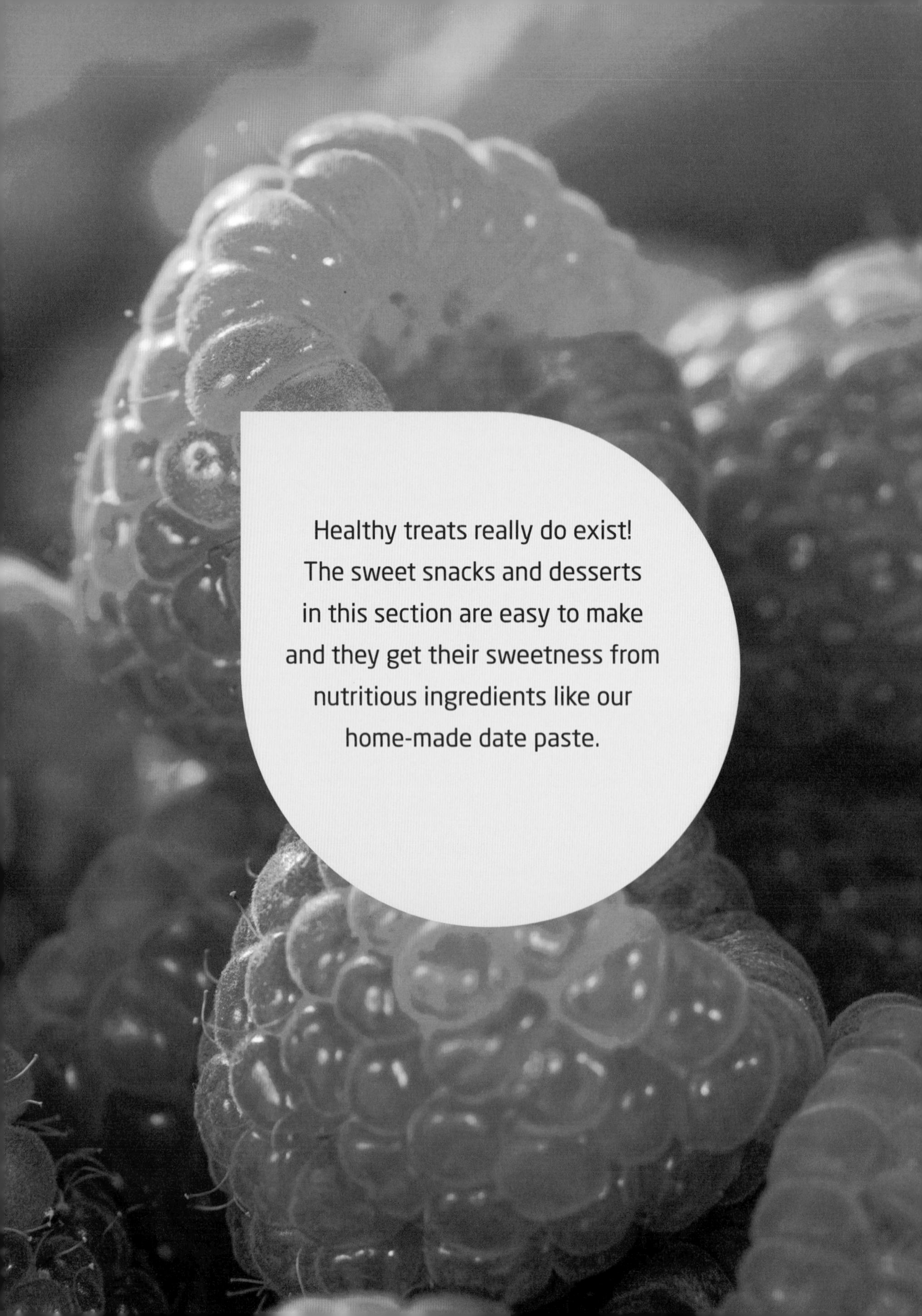

Healthy treats really do exist! The sweet snacks and desserts in this section are easy to make and they get their sweetness from nutritious ingredients like our home-made date paste.

Desserts & sweet treats

Chocolate hazelnut shake with cherry ice cream

Serves 3

Cherry ice cream: 200g (7oz) frozen cherries | 8 Deglet Noor dates, stones removed
Hazelnut shake: 250ml (9fl oz) ice-cold soya milk with calcium | 80g (3oz) Chocolate hazelnut spread (see p.130)
Decoration: 3 cherries | 1 sprig of rosemary

Nutritional values per portion: 242 kcal | 33.3g carbohydrate | 8.7g fat | 6.6g protein | 5.4g fibre | 0.2g ALA | 318mg lysine | 145mg calcium | 0.8mg zinc | 2.7mg iron | 0.1mg B2 | < 0.1mg RE | 10µg iodine | 0.2g salt

Add the frozen cherries and dates to a food processor and purée to create a smooth ice cream using the muddler attachment. Transfer the ice cream to a freezerproof container, seal, and return to the freezer for 30 minutes.

Add the soya milk and chocolate spread to the food processor and mix until you have a nice frothy shake. Get three glasses ready and put two to three little balls of cherry ice cream into each one. Fill the glasses with the shake then decorate with cherries and rosemary.

BASTI'S TIP

If you are making ice cream from frozen fruit, it is important to use a powerful blender and a muddler. The faster you are, the firmer the ice cream will be. If it gets a bit too runny, just spread the ice cream in a 2cm (¾in) thick layer and put it in the freezer for 30 minutes.

VARIATION

If you are short of time and you don't have any hazelnut spread in the fridge, just mix 250g (9oz) of ice-cold soya milk with 1 small ripe banana, a pinch of vanilla powder, and a pinch of salt. This combination also tastes fantastic with the cherry ice cream.

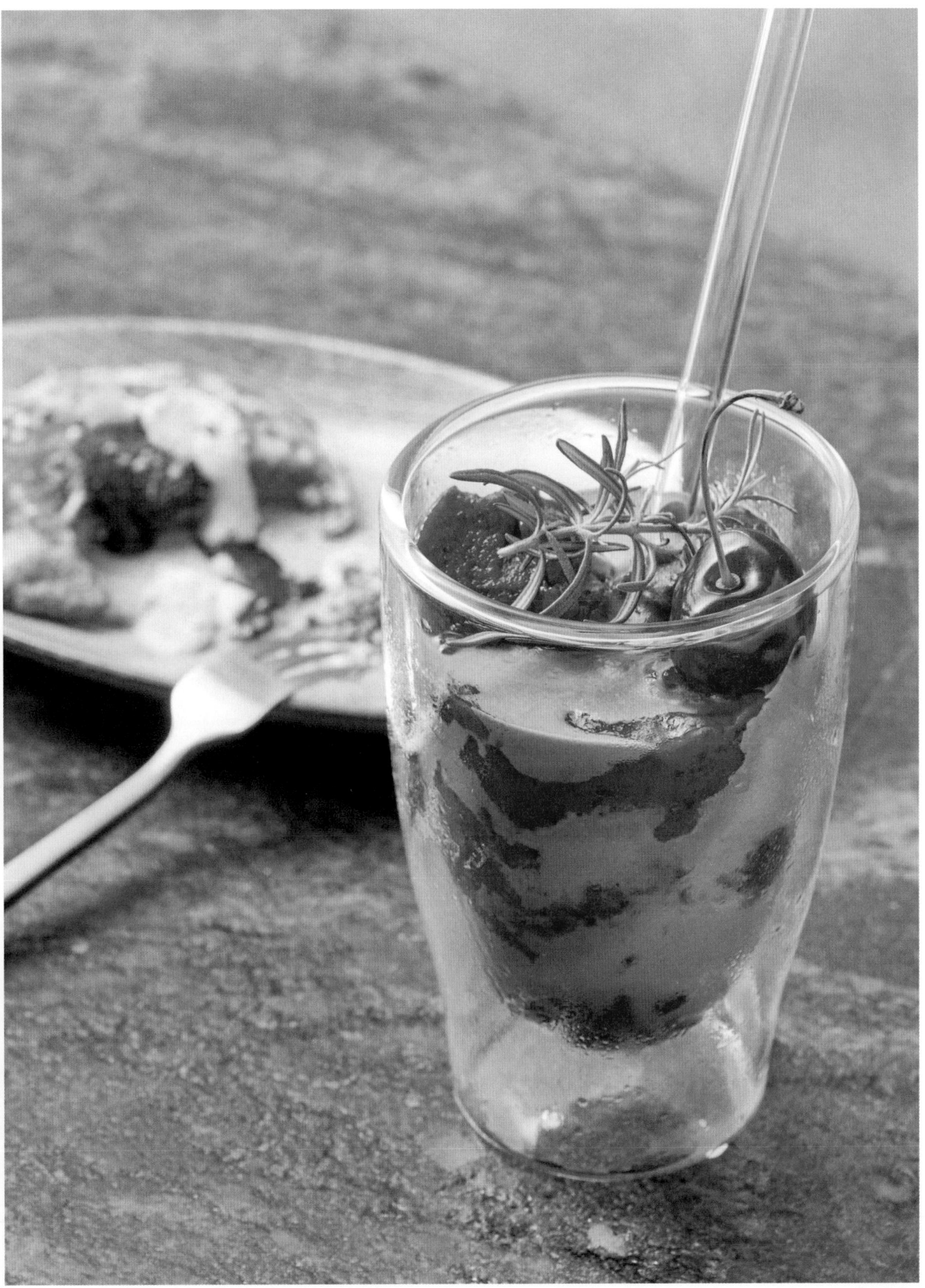

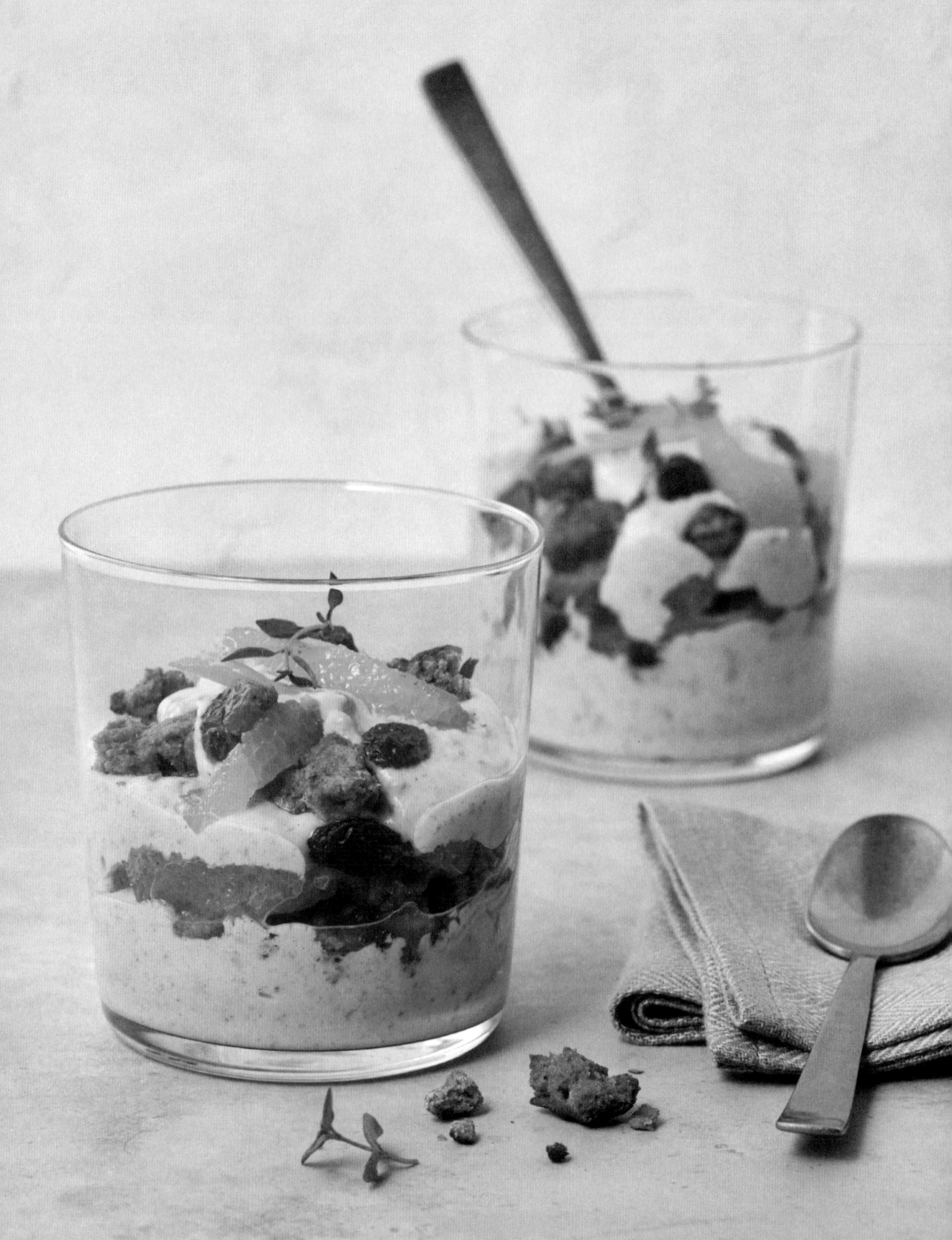

Quark trifle with orange compote and crumble

Serves 3

Cream: 6 Deglet Noor dates, stones removed | 400g (14oz) unsweetened dairy-free quark (such as from Provamel, see tip) | 60g (2oz) white almond nut butter | 2 tsp vanilla powder | 2 tsp organic lemon zest
Orange compote: 4 tbsp raisins | ½ tsp ground cinnamon | 2 organic oranges
Crumble: 50g (1¾oz) wholemeal flour (spelt, wheat, or oat) | 35g (1oz) date paste (see p.97) | 15g (½oz) nut butter (e.g. hazelnut, almond, or peanut) | pinch of salt | 2 tsp olive oil
Decoration: 2 sprigs of thyme

Nutritional values per portion: 545 kcal | 60g carbohydrate | 24g fat | 17.1g protein | 11.3g fibre | 0.4g ALA | 580mg lysine | 387mg calcium | 1.8mg zinc | 3.8mg iron | 0.3mg B2 | < 0.1mg RE | 2µg iodine | 0.5g salt

Put the dates for the cream into a pan with 100ml (3½fl oz) of water along with the raisins and ground cinnamon for the orange compote. Simmer gently until the water has evaporated and the raisins and dates have softened.

Meanwhile, wash the oranges for the compote in hot water, dry them, and use a peeler to remove a 4cm (1½in) long strip of peel. Chop this finely and add to the date and raisin mixture. Segment the flesh of the oranges and squeeze out the juice from the remaining fruit into the date and raisin mixture in the pan.

To make the cream, put the dairy-free quark, almond nut butter, vanilla, and lemon zest into the food processor. Remove the dates from the pan and add to the mixture in the food processor. Process until you have a smooth cream and chill in the fridge for 30 minutes. Add the orange segments to the warm raisin mixture in the pan and leave to infuse without heating.

Preheat the oven to 180°C (160°C fan/350°F/Gas 4). Put all the ingredients for the crumble into a bowl, rub together until you get clumps of around 1cm (½in). Spread these out on a baking tray lined with baking paper and bake for 8–10 minutes in the hot oven (middle shelf) until crisp. Remove from the oven and leave to cool completely.

Get three serving glasses ready. Put 2 tablespoons of the cream mixture into each glass, then add 1 tablespoon of crumble and top with 1 tablespoon of orange compote. Repeat these layers once more. Decorate the trifles with crumble and a couple of thyme leaves.

VARIATION

There are wonderful seasonal options for this dessert: try replacing the oranges in the compote with mango, peach, cherries, or blueberries.

BASTI'S TIP

If you cannot find dairy-free quark or if you are allergic to soya, strain your preferred plant-based yogurt through a clean tea towel placed in a sieve in your fridge for 3–4 hours. This produces a wonderful home-made alternative.

Apple pancakes with yogurt and a blueberry and hemp sauce

Serves 3

Pancakes: 1 large sweet but tangy apple | 1 tsp cider vinegar | 1 tbsp date paste (see p.97) | ½ tsp salt | 150g (5½ oz) wholemeal wheat flour | 25g (1oz) cornflour | 1 tsp bicarbonate of soda (or baking powder) | 1 tsp ground cinnamon | olive oil for cooking
Yogurt: 200g (7oz) plant-based yogurt (soya or coconut) | 1 tbsp grated organic lemon zest | 4 tbsp date paste (see p.97) | 1 tbsp white almond nut butter (optional)
Blueberry and hemp sauce: 200g (7oz) frozen blueberries | 100g (3½oz) banana, peeled | 5 Deglet Noor dates, stoned | 50g (1¾oz) hulled hemp seeds | generous pinch of ground cardamom | pinch of salt
Decoration: 2 tbsp hulled hemp seeds, toasted

Nutritional values per portion: 596 kcal | 79.9g carbohydrate | 20.4g fat | 19.1g protein | 14.9g fibre | 2.5g ALA | 739mg lysine | 101mg calcium | 4.7mg zinc | 5.8mg iron | 0.2mg B2 | < 0.1mg RE | 5μg iodine | 1g salt

First, wash the apple that will be used for the pancakes, remove the core, and slice the fruit into 5mm (¼in) thick discs. Combine the yogurt, lemon zest, date paste, and almond nut butter in a bowl. Put all the ingredients for the blueberry sauce into a food processor with 200ml (7fl oz) of water and purée until smooth.

For the pancakes, add 250ml (9fl oz) of water, the vinegar, date paste, and salt to a bowl and mix. Combine the flour, cornflour, bicarbonate of soda, and cinnamon in a second bowl. Add the vinegar and water mixture, then use a balloon whisk to beat the batter until it has no lumps.

Heat a large non-stick pan over a moderate heat. Brush the pan with a very small amount of oil. Use a small ladle to drop 3–4 dollops of batter into the pan, each measuring roughly 5cm (2in). After about 1–2 minutes, when the pancakes have risen slightly but before the top has dried out, top each one with a slice of apple and press down gently.

Continue cooking the pancakes for 1–2 minutes until the edges are slightly brown, turn carefully and cook for another 2–3 minutes. Transfer the pancakes to a warm plate, and cover with a clean tea towel. Cook the rest of the batter in the same way.

Arrange the pancakes on a plate in overlapping layers. Garnish with a dollop of yogurt and 1–2 tablespoons of the blueberry sauce, then sprinkle with hemp seeds.

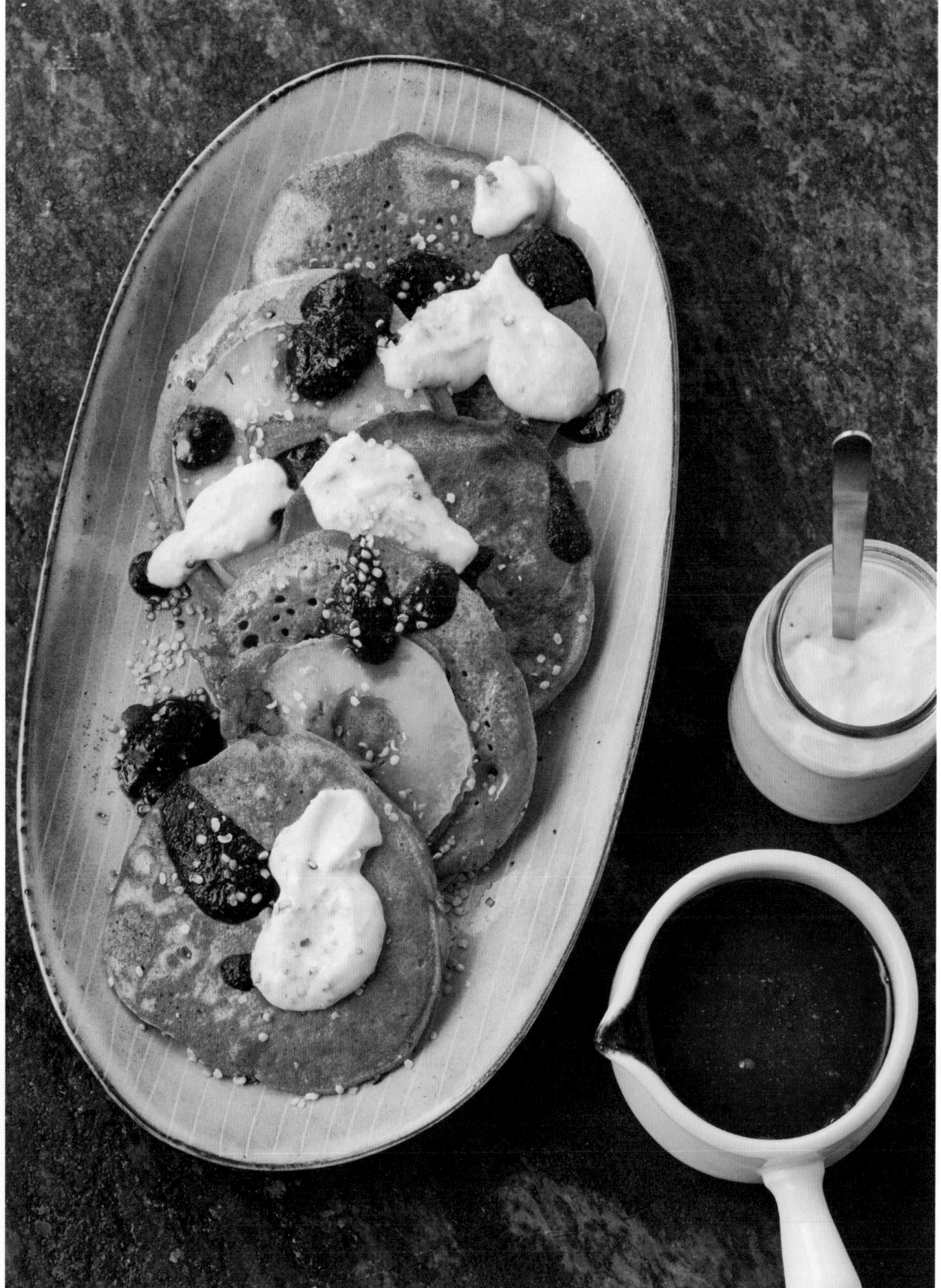

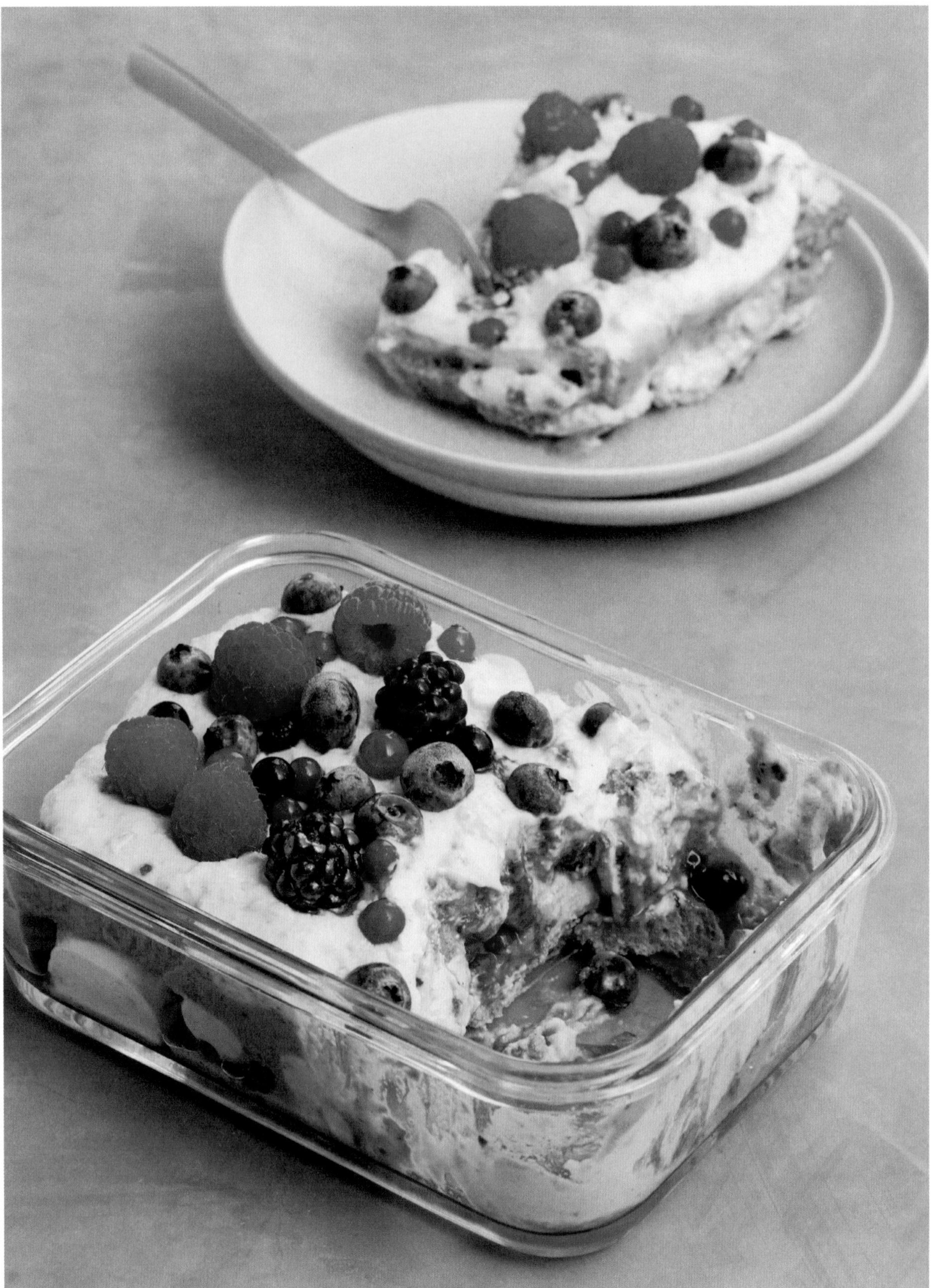

Wholegrain berry tiramisu

Serves 3

Cream: 200g (7oz) unsweetened dairy-free quark (such as Provamel; or see tip p.227) | 60g (2oz) cashews, soaked for 2 hours | 5 Deglet Noor dates, stones removed | 50ml (1¾fl oz) coconut milk | 1 tsp vanilla powder | pinch of salt
Berry sauce: 200ml (7fl oz) soya milk with calcium | 80g (3oz) frozen berries | 3 Deglet Noor dates, stones removed
Also: 8 small slices of wholemeal rusk (or gluten-free rusk) | 100g (3½oz) frozen berries | rectangular dish (about 15 × 15 × 5cm/6 × 6 × 2in)

Nutritional values per portion: 415 kcal | 40.7g carbohydrate | 19.6g fat | 17.4g protein | 10.8g fibre | 0.3g ALA | 760mg lysine | 234mg calcium | 2.7mg zinc | 5.2mg iron | 0.3mg B2 | < 0.1mg RE | 12µg iodine | 0.6g salt

Add all the ingredients for the cream to a powerful food processor and purée until smooth. If you are using a hand-held blender, you will need to soak the dates first or use soft dates. Then transfer the cream to a bowl.

Put the ingredients for the sauce into the food processor (there is no need to wash it), purée until smooth and transfer to a wide bowl. Dip the rusks in the sauce for 20–30 seconds until moistened all the way through. Create a layer of soaked rusks in the dish. If necessary, break the pieces of rusk into appropriate sizes before soaking.

Top the rusks with a layer of half the cream, a couple of spoonfuls of berries, followed by the remaining rusks. Spread the rest of the cream on top. Chill the tiramisu in the fridge for at least 1 hour. Pour over the remaining berry sauce and whole berries before serving.

VARIATION

Instead of making this with berries, you can create a more traditional version using a mixture of 2 small cups of espresso, 1 tbsp of cocoa powder, 3 tbsp of date paste, 1 tbsp of shiro miso, and 250ml (9fl oz) of soya milk with calcium. Soak the rusk in this liquid and sprinkle the tiramisu with cocoa powder.

BASTI'S TIP

It is important to ensure the rusks are moistened all the way through but not falling apart. You may need a bit of practice to get it right.

Peanut butter balls with peach

Serves 3

100g (3½oz) wholemeal rusk (or gluten-free rusk) | 60g (2oz) cooked chickpeas (or white beans, see p.191) | 13 Deglet Noor dates, stones removed | 120g (4oz) crunchy peanut butter | 120ml (4fl oz) soya milk with calcium | pinch of salt | ½ tsp vanilla powder | 4 ripe flat peaches | 3 tbsp cocoa powder

Nutritional values per portion: 625 kcal | 70.6g carbohydrate | 26.2g fat | 25.4g protein | 19.7g fibre | 0.2g ALA | 1135mg lysine | 155mg calcium | 3.9mg zinc | 11mg iron | 0.4mg B2 | < 0.1mg RE | 22µg iodine | 0.5g salt

Break up the rusks in a food processor on a low speed to create crumbs then transfer to a bowl. Add the remaining ingredients apart from the peaches and cocoa powder to the food processor and blend to a smooth, creamy consistency. Add this to the bowl with the rusks and work together by hand to combine. You should end up with a slightly moist, doughy consistency you can mould but is not too dry. Depending on your rusks, you may need slightly more soya milk.

Wash the flat peaches, remove the stones and chop into 2cm (¾in) cubes. Then press 1 tablespoon of dough flat in the palm of your hand, put a cube of peach in the middle and seal the dough around it. Roll the little balls in cocoa powder and enjoy.

VARIATION

You can replace the peach with fresh or dried plums, berries, or other juicy fruit. Or use the mixture to make delicious crunchy cookies by pressing the balls flat on a baking tray and baking at 180°C (160°C fan/350°F/Gas 4) for 10 minutes.

BASTI'S TIP

Put the balls in the freezer for 10 minutes before eating them. You can also keep them for 1–2 days in the fridge in an airtight container, and they make a great portable snack.

Instant date and peanut chocolate snack

Serves 3

6 super-soft, large Medjool dates | 6 tsp crunchy peanut butter | pinch of salt | 6 tsp cocoa powder

Nutritional values per portion: 230 kcal | 23.1g carbohydrate | 11.5g fat | 7.7g protein | 6.4g fibre | 0.1g ALA | 320mg lysine | 40mg calcium | 1.2mg zinc | 4.8mg iron | 0.1mg B2 | < 0.1mg RE | 3µg iodine | 0.3g salt

Slice the dates along one side and remove the stones. Gently fold open the dates, fill each one with 1 teaspoon of peanut butter and sprinkle with salt. Close the dates again and dust with cocoa powder.

BASTI'S TIP

This snack is the perfect solution if you find yourself craving something sweet. The quality of the dates is crucial here. You can get Medjools in any good supermarket, organic store, or speciality Turkish shops. The dates should be large, soft, and have a caramel flavour.

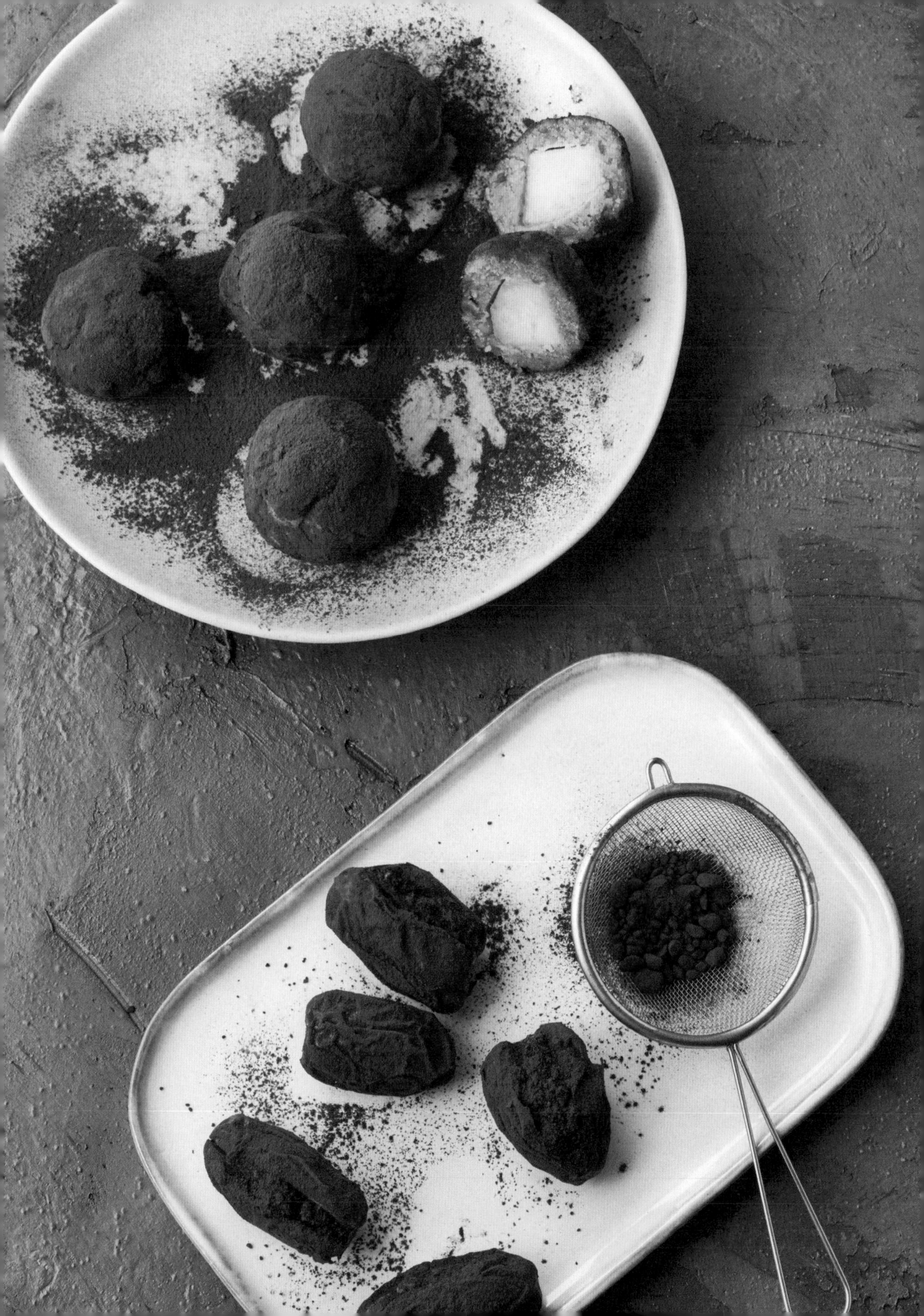

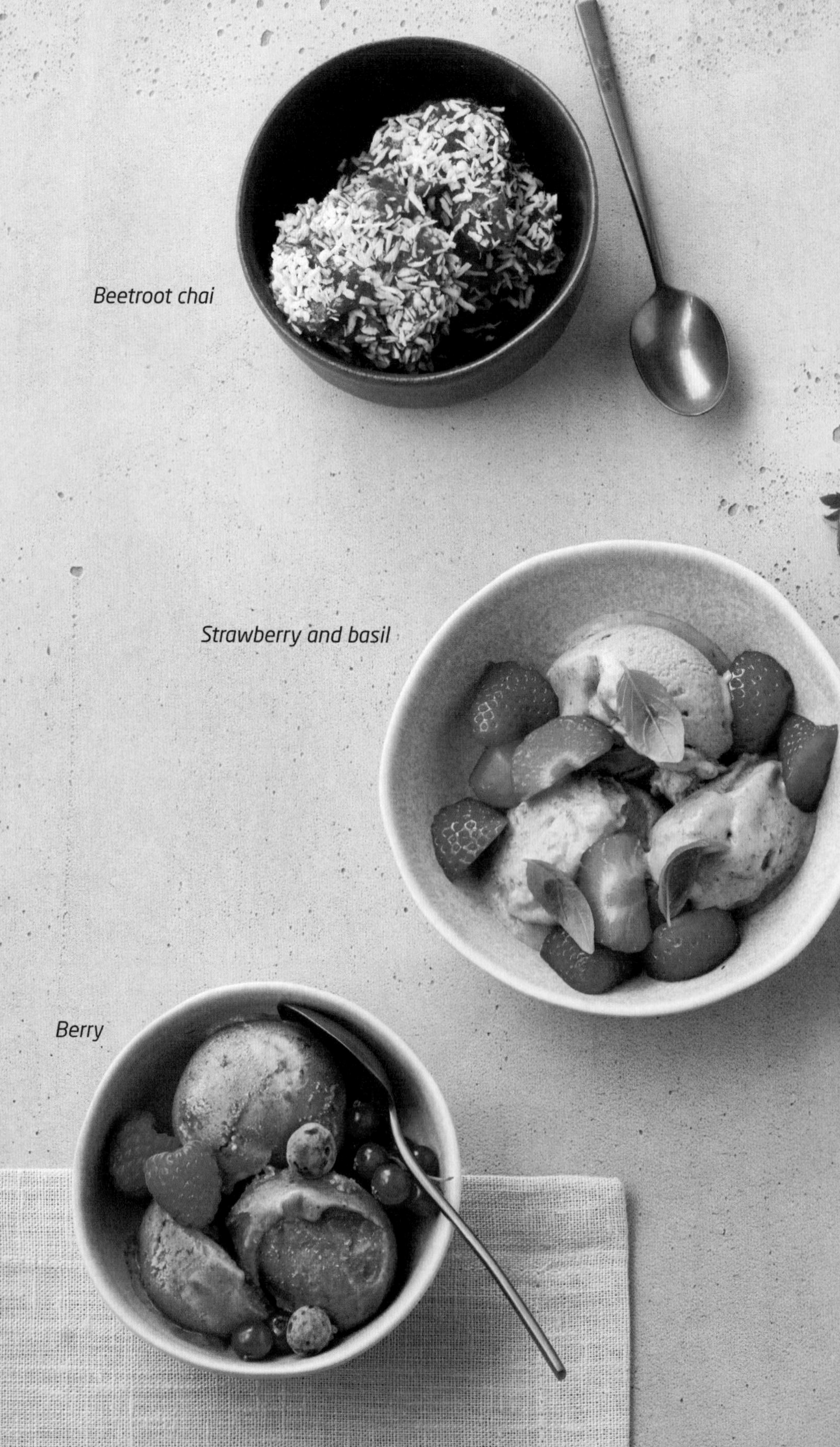

Beetroot chai

Strawberry and basil

Berry

Three varieties of nice cream

Each recipe makes 3 portions

Basic recipe: 250g (9oz) ripe banana (roughly 2 pieces of fruit)

Peel the bananas, slice into 1cm (½in) pieces and put these in the freezer in a sealed container for at least 12 hours.

BASTI'S TIP

I always have 3–4 bananas stored like this in my freezer. That way, I can make some nice cream whenever I fancy.

Beetroot chai: 250g (9oz) frozen banana, sliced (see basic recipe) | 1 tsp ground cinnamon | ½ tsp freshly ground pepper | good pinch of ground cloves | piece of fresh root ginger (3cm/1in), finely chopped | 50ml (1¾fl oz) ice-cold beetroot juice | 5 tbsp desiccated coconut, toasted

Nutritional values per portion: 189 kcal | 18.6g carbohydrate | 10.9g fat | 2.1g protein | 4.5g fibre | < 0.1g ALA | 131mg lysine | 10mg calcium | 0.5mg zinc | 0.9mg iron | 0.1mg B2 | < 0.1mg RE | 2µg iodine | < 0.1g salt

Add all the ingredients except the desiccated coconut to a food processor and blitz until smooth. Scoop balls of ice cream and toss in the coconut before serving.

Strawberry and basil: 250g (9oz) frozen banana, sliced (see basic recipe) | 20g (¾oz) basil + 6 small basil leaves | ½ tsp vanilla powder | 6 strawberries, finely diced

Nutritional values per portion: 93 kcal | 19.9g carbohydrate | 0.4g fat | 1.5g protein | 2.7g fibre | 0.1g ALA | 93mg lysine | 30mg calcium | 0.2mg zinc | 0.9mg iron | 0.1mg B2 | < 0.1mg RE | 3µg iodine | < 0.1g salt

Add all the ingredients except the small basil leaves to a food processor and blitz until smooth. Scoop balls of ice cream and decorate with the strawberries and basil leaves.

Berry: 250g (9oz) frozen banana, in slices (see basic recipe) | 100g (3½oz) frozen berries | good pinch of ground cloves (or ground cinnamon; as preferred) | 4–5 tbsp fresh berries

Nutritional values per portion: 90 kcal | 19.4g carbohydrate | 0.4g fat | 1.2g protein | 3.4g fibre | 0.1g ALA | 70mg lysine | 9mg calcium | 0.2mg zinc | 0.6mg iron | < 0.1mg B2 | < 0.1mg RE | 2µg iodine | <0.1g salt

Add all the ingredients except the fresh berries to a food processor and blitz until smooth. Scoop portions of ice cream and decorate with the fresh berries.

BASTI'S TIP

If you are using a hand-held blender, let the bananas defrost slightly for 3–4 minutes first. A powerful food processor can handle them straight from the freezer.

VARIATION

If you prefer a sweeter or creamier ice cream, add 1 tablespoon of nut butter or date paste (see p.97) to each recipe.

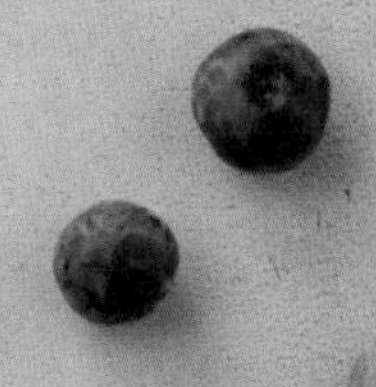

Banana and oat cookies with raisins

Makes 6 cookies or serves 3

2 bananas, peeled (about 200g/7oz) | 20g (¾oz) sesame seeds | 50g (1¾oz) pumpkin seeds | 70g (2½oz) fine oats | 4 tbsp raisins | 1 tbsp organic orange zest

Nutritional values per portion: 336 kcal | 42g carbohydrate | 12.9g fat | 8.7g protein | 6.1g fibre | < 0.1g ALA | 604mg lysine | 78mg calcium | 2.6mg zinc | 3.3mg iron | < 0.1mg B2 | < 0.1mg RE | 3µg iodine | < 0.1g salt

Preheat the oven to 180°C (160°C fan/350°F/Gas 4). Mash the bananas with a fork. Grind the sesame seeds and pumpkin seeds in a food processor to create a flour. Add to a bowl with the other ingredients, combine well by hand and put 6 blobs of cookie mix on a baking tray lined with baking paper.

Shape the blobs so they make roughly 1cm (½in) high mounds and bake the cookies for 15 minutes in the oven (middle shelf). Leave the cookies to cool and enjoy.

BASTI'S TIP

When the cookies come out of the oven, they will be nice and crisp. After a couple of hours, they go soft again. These cookies are the perfect portable snack!

VARIATION

Instead of raisins, you can use other dried fruit or finely chopped dark chocolate (80% cocoa solids).

And you can replace the pumpkin and sesame seeds with any kinds of nuts, seeds, or even coconut flakes.

Carrot cookie dough balls

Serves 3

50g (1¾oz) walnuts | 60g (2oz) carrots | 5 tbsp date paste (see p.97) | 1 tbsp shiro miso | pinch of freshly grated nutmeg | ½ tsp ground cinnamon | ½ tsp freshly ground pepper | 70g (2½oz) fine oats | 50g (1¾oz) desiccated coconut, toasted

Nutritional values per portion: 374 kcal | 28.7g carbohydrate | 24.7g fat | 8.1g protein | 8.6g fibre | 1.7g ALA | 338mg lysine | 42mg calcium | 1.8mg zinc | 2.6mg iron | 0.1mg B2 | 0.3mg RE | 2µg iodine | 0.5g salt

Toast the walnuts in a dry pan over a moderate heat, stirring constantly. Leave the walnuts to cool then grind them in a food processor.

Wash and grate the carrots very finely, add them to a bowl with the date paste, shiro miso, spices, oats, and ground walnuts and knead together. Leave the mixture to rest in the fridge for 20 minutes, then roll little balls from the chilled mix and coat in the toasted desiccated coconut.

BASTI'S TIP

Also nice: Put the balls in the freezer for 10–20 minutes, then eat them ice-cold as a small snack.

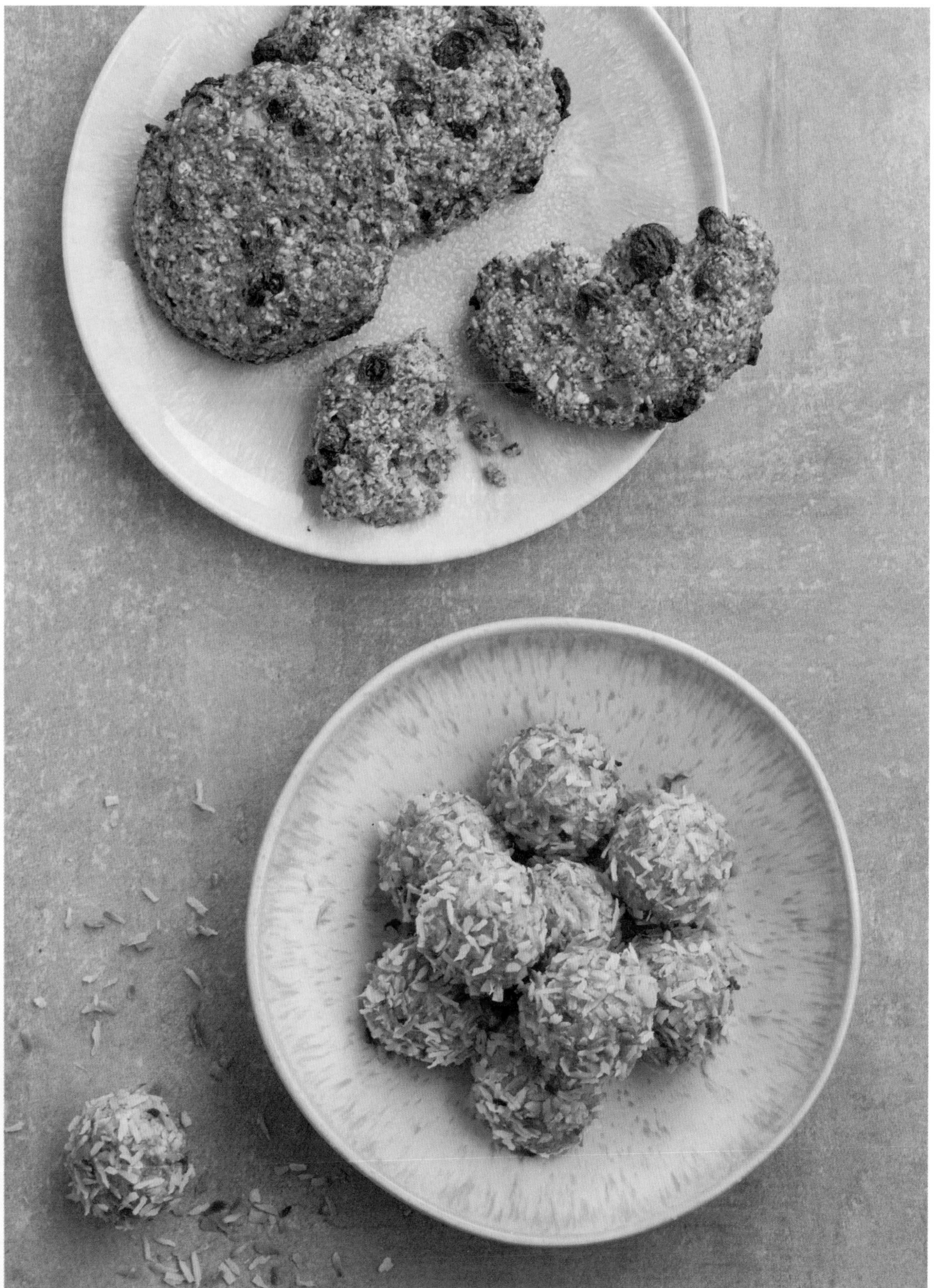

List of references Theory (pp.8–81)

[1] Author's own presentation based on the reasons for a vegan lifestyle following Christian Koeder's *Veganismus – Für die Befreiung der Tiere [Veganism – for the liberation of animals]* (2014).

[2] The Institute for Health Metrics and Evaluation. (2018). Global Health Data Exchange: Germany. Accessed on 1 June 2019. Available at https://bit.ly/2HWqg9w

[3] The Institute for Health Metrics and Evaluation. (2018). Global Health Data Exchange: Switzerland. Accessed on 1 June 2019. Available at https://bit.ly/2Ei7mKk

[4] The Institute for Health Metrics and Evaluation. (2018). Global Health Data Exchange: Austria. Accessed on 1 June 2019. Available at https://bit.ly/2VLXfrK

[5] GBD 2017 Diet Collaborators. (2019). Health effects of dietary risks in 195 countries, 1990–2017: a systematic analysis for the Global Burden of Disease Study 2017. Lancet, 0140-6736(19), 30041–30048.

[6] World Cancer Research Fund & American Institute for Cancer Research. (2007). Food, Nutrition, Physical Activity and the Prevention of Cancer: A Global Perspective. Washington DC: AICR.

[7] American Heart Association. (2017). Why Should I Limit Sodium? Accessed on 1 June 2019. Available at https://bit.ly/2JoZlas

[8] German Nutrition Society (Deutsche Gesellschaft für Ernährung). (2016). *Ausgewählte Fragen und Antworten zu Speisesalz. [Selected questions and answers on table salt]* Accessed on 1 June 2019. Available at https://bit.ly/2Hr8ayj

[9] GBD 2017 Diet Collaborators. (2019). Health effects of dietary risks in 195 countries, 1990–2017: a systematic analysis for the Global Burden of Disease Study 2017. Lancet, 0140-6736(19), 30041–30048.

[10] German Nutrition Society (Deutsche Gesellschaft für Ernährung). (2017). *Vollwertig essen und trinken nach den 10 Regeln der DGE [Healthy eating and drinking following the German Nutrition Society's 10 rules]* (10th edition). Accessed on 1 June 2019. Available at https://bit.ly/2nZ7SSo

[11] German Nutrition Society (Deutsche Gesellschaft für Ernährung). (no date). *Vollwertig essen und trinken nach den 10 Regeln der DGE: [Healthy eating and drinking following the German Nutrition Society's 10 rules]* 1. *Lebensmittelvielfalt genießen – Nachhaltigkeit.* [Enjoy food diversity – sustainability] Accessed on 1 June 2019. Available at https://bit.ly/1BGSSy0

[12] Lenihan-Geels, G., Bishop, K. S. & Ferguson, L. R. (2013). Alternative Sources of Omega-3 Fats: Can We Find a Sustainable Substitute for Fish? Nutrients, 5(4), 1301–1315.

[13] Carlson, D. L. & Hites, R. A. (2005). Polychlorinated biphenyls in salmon and salmon feed: global differences and bioaccumulation. Environ Sci Technol, 39(19), 7389–7395.

[14] Rittenau, N. (2018). *Vegan-Klischee ade! [Goodbye Vegan Cliché!] Wissenschaftliche Antworten auf kritische Fragen zu veganer Ernährung [Scientific answers to critical questions about the vegan diet]* (5th edition). Mainz: Ventil.

[15] Hendel, B. (2016). *Das Magnesium Buch. [The Magnesium Book]* Kirchzarten, near Freiburg: VAK Verlags GmbH, 291–298.

[16] Wang, M. Yu, M. Fang, L. & Hu, R.Y. (2015). Association between sugar-sweetened beverages and type 2 diabetes: A meta-analysis. J Diabetes Investig, 6(3), 360–366.

[17] Zong, G., Gao, A., Hu, F.B. & Sun, Q. (2016). Whole Grain Intake and Mortality from All Causes, Cardiovascular Disease, and Cancer: A Meta-Analysis of Prospective Cohort Studies. Circulation, 133(24), 2370–2380.

[18] Wang, X., Ouyang, Y., Liu, J., Zhu, M., Zhao, G., Bao, W. & Hu, F.B. (2014). Fruit and vegetable consumption and mortality from all causes, cardiovascular disease, and cancer: systematic review and dose-response meta-analysis of prospective cohort studies. *BMJ*, 4490.

[19] Chen, G.C. Zhang, R., Martínez-González, M.A., Zhang, Z.L., Bonaccio, M., van Dam, R.M. & Qi, L.Q. (2017). Nut consumption in relation to all-cause and cause-specific mortality: a meta-analysis 18 prospective studies. Food Funct, 8(11), 3893–3905.

[20] Li, H., Li, J., Shen, Y., Wang, J. & Zhou, D. (2017). Legume Consumption and All-Cause and Cardiovascular Disease Mortality. Biomed Res Int, 8450618.

[21] Larsson, S.C. & Orsini, N. (2014). Red meat and processed meat consumption and all-cause mortality: a meta-analysis. Am J Epidemiol, 179(3), 282–289.

[22] Stehle, P., Oberritter, H., Büning-Fesel, M. & Heseker, H. (2005). *Grafische Umsetzung von Ernährungsrichtlinien – traditionelle und neue Ansätze. [Graphic implementation of nutritional guidelines – traditional and new approaches] Ernährungs-Umschau,* [Nutrition Review] 52(4), 128–135.

[23] Minister of Health. (2019). Canada's Food Guide – Eat well. Live well. Accessed on 1 June 2019. Available at https://bit.ly/2S9e2m5

[24] U.S. Department of Health and Human Services and U.S. Department of Agriculture. (2015). 2015–2020 Dietary Guidelines for Americans (8th Edt.). Accessed on 1 June 2019. Available at https://bit.ly/21N65zL

[25] World Health Organization. (2015). Healthy Diet – Fact Sheet N°394. Accessed on 01 June 2018. Available at http://bit.ly/2Fxuxzn

[26] Harvard T.H. Chan – School of Public Health. (2011). Healthy Eating Plate. Accessed on 18 May 2019. Available at https://bit.ly/1YSW4OJ

[27] Skerrett, P. J. & Willett, W. C. (2010). Essentials of Healthy Eating: A Guide. J Midwifery Womens Health, 55(6), 492–501.

[28] Oyebode, O., Gordon-Dseagu, V., Walker, A. & Mindell, J. S. (2014). Fruit and vegetable consumption and all-cause, cancer and CVD mortality: analysis of Health Survey for England data. J Epidemiol Community Health, 68(9), 856–862.

[29] Nguyen, B., Bauman, A., Gale, J., Banks, E., Kritharides, L. & Ding, D. (2016). Fruit and vegetable consumption and all-cause mortality: evidence from a large Australian cohort study. Int J Behav Nutr Phys Act, 13, 9.

[30] Boeing, H., Bechthold, A., Bub, A., Ellinger, S., Haller, D., Kroke, A. et al. (2012). German Nutrition Society (Deutsche Gesellschaft für Ernährung): *Stellungnahme – Gemüse und Obst in der Prävention ausgewählter chronischer Krankheiten. [Position paper – vegetables and fruit in the prevention of specific chronic illnesses]* Accessed on 01 June 2018. Available at https://bit.ly/2H8GzAf

[31] Boeing, H., Bechthold, A., Bub, A., Ellinger, S., Haller, D., Kroke, A. et al. (2012). German Nutrition Society (Deutsche Gesellschaft für Ernährung): *Stellungnahme – Gemüse und Obst in der Prävention ausgewählter chronischer Krankheiten. [Position paper – vegetables and fruit in the prevention of specific chronic illnesses]* Accessed on 01 June 2018. Available at https://bit.ly/2H8GzAf

[32] Boivin, D., Lamy, S., Lord-Dufour, S., Jackson, J., Beaulieu, E., Côté, M., Moghrabi, A., Barrette, S., Gingras, D. & Beliveau, R. (2009). Antiproliferative and antioxidant activities of common vegetables: A comparative study. Food Chem., 112(2), 374–380.

[33] Boivin, D., Lamy, S., Lord-Dufour, S., Jackson, J., Beaulieu, E., Côté, M., Moghrabi, A., Barrette, S., Gingras, D. & Beliveau, R. (2009). Antiproliferative and antioxidant activities of common vegetables: A comparative study. Food Chem., 112(2), 374–380.

[34] Meng, H., Hu, W., Chen, Z. & Shen, Y. (2014). Fruit and vegetable intake and prostate cancer risk: a meta-analysis. Asia Pac J Clin Oncol, 10(2), 133–140.

[35] Liu, B., Mao, Q., Cao, M. & Xie, L. (2012). Cruciferous vegetables intake and risk of prostate cancer: a meta-analysis. Int J Urol, 19(2), 134–141.

[36] Nicastro, H. L., Ross, S. A. & Milner, J. A. (2015). Garlic and onions: Their cancer prevention properties. Cancer Prev Res (Phila), 8(3), 181–189.

[37] Wu, Q. J., Yang, Y. Wang, J., Han, L. H. & Xiang, Y. B. (2013). Cruciferous vegetable consumption and gastric cancer risk: a meta-analysis of epidemiological studies. Cancer Sci, 104(8), 1067–1073.

[38] Turati, F., Pelucchi, C., Guercio, V., La Vecchia, C. & Galeone, C. (2015). Allium vegetable intake and gastric cancer: a case-control study and meta-analysis. Mol Nutr Food Res, 59(1), 171–179.

[39] Wu, Q. J., Yang, Y., Vogtmann, E., Wang, J., Han, L. H., Li, H. L. & Xiang, Y. B. (2013). Cruciferous vegetables intake and the risk of colorectal cancer: a meta-analysis of observational studies. Ann Oncol, 24(4), 1079–1087.

[40] Boivin, D., Lamy, S., Lord-Dufour, S., Jackson, J., Beaulieu, E., Côté, M. et al. (2009). Antiproliferative and antioxidant activities of common vegetables: A comparative study. Food Chem, 112(2), 374–380.

[41] Zhou, X. F., Ding, Z. S. & Liu, N. B. (2013). Allium vegetables and risk of prostate cancer: evidence from 132.192 subjects. Asian Pac J Cancer Prev, 14(7), 4131–4134.

[42] Boivin, D., Lamy, S., Lord-Dufour, S., Jackson, J., Beaulieu, E., Côté, M. et al. (2009). Antiproliferative and antioxidant activities of common vegetables: A comparative study. Food Chem, 112(2), 374–380.

[43] Bognar, A. (1995). *Vitaminverluste bei der Lagerung und Zubereitung von Lebensmitteln.* [Loss of vitamins when storing and preparing foods] Ernährung/Nutrition, 19(11), 551–554.

[44] Koerber, K., Männle, T. & Leitzmann, C. (2012). *Vollwert-Ernährung – Konzeption einer zeitgemäßen und nachhaltigen Ernährung [Wholesome nutrition – devising a contemporary and sustainable diet]* (11th edition) Stuttgart: Karl F. Hauf Verlag, 245.

[45] Koerber, K., Männle, T. & Leitzmann, C. (2012). *Vollwert-Ernährung – Konzeption einer zeitgemäßen und nachhaltigen Ernährung [Wholesome*

nutrition – devising a contemporary and sustainable diet] (11th edition). Stuttgart: Karl F. Haug Verlag, 239.
[46] Hahn, A., Ströhle, A. & Wolters, M. (2016). *Ernährung – Physiologische Grundlagen, Prävention, Therapie* [*Nutrition – physiological principles, prevention, therapy*] (3rd edition). Stuttgart: Wissenschaftliche Verlagsgesellschaft Stuttgart, 472.
[47] Mercader, J. (2009). Mozambican grass seed consumption during the Middle Stone Age. *Science*, 326(5960), 1680–1683.
[48] The Oldways Whole Grains Council. (2017). Summary of Recent Research on Whole Grains and Health (2017 edt.). Accessed on 1 June 2019. Available at http://bit.ly/2r1rFHC
[49] Aune, D., Keum, N., Giovannucci, E., Fadnes, L. T., Boffetta, P., Greenwood, D. C., Tonstad, S., Vatten, L. J., Riboli, E. & Norat, T. (2016). Whole grain consumption and risk of cardiovascular disease, cancer, and all cause and cause specific mortality: systematic review and dose-response meta-analysis of prospective studies. *BMJ*, 353, i2716.
[50] Davis, B. & Vesanto, M. (2014). *Becoming Vegan – The comprehensive Edition*. Tennessee: Book Publishing Company, 170.
[51] Klose, C. & Arendt, E. K. (2012). Proteins in oats; their synthesis and changes during germination: a review. Crit Rev Food Sci Nutr, 52(7), 629–39.
[52] Chavan, J. K. & Kadam, S. S. (1989). Nutritional improvement of cereals by sprouting. Crit Rev Food Sci Nutr, 28(5), 401–437.
[53] U.S. Department of Agriculture, Agricultural Research Service. (2010). USDA Database for the Oxygen Radical Absorbance Capacity (ORAC) of Selected Foods, Release 2. Accessed on 10 May 2019. Available at https://bit.ly/30fkGZe
[54] Caracuta, V., Vardi, J., Paz, Y. & Boaretto, E. (2017). Farming legumes in the pre-pottery Neolithic: New discoveries from the site of Ahihud (Israel). PLoS One, 12(5), e0177859.
[55] Shurtleff, W. & Aoyagi, A. (1979). *The Book of Tofu: Protein Source of the Future – Now!* New York: Ballantine Books.
[56] Shurtleff, W. & Aoyagi, A. (1979). *The Book of Tempeh – A Super Soyfood from Indonesia*. New York: Harper & Row.
[57] Souci, S. W., Fachmann, W. & Kraut H. (2016). *Die Zusammensetzung der Lebensmittel – Nährwerttabellen* [*The composition of food – nutritional tables*] (8th edition). Stuttgart: Wissenschaftliche Verlagsgesellschaft.
[58] Deshpande, S. S. (1992). Food legumes in human nutrition: a personal perspective. Crit Rev Food Sci Nutr, 32(4), 333–363.
[59] Marventano, S., Izquierdo-Pulido, M., Sánchez-González, C., Godosm, J., Speciani, A., Galvano, F. & Grosso, G. (2017). Legume consumption and CVD risk: a systematic review and meta-analysis. Public Health Nutr, 20(2), 245-254.
[60] Li, J. & Mao, Q. (2017). Legume intake and risk of prostate cancer: a meta-analysis of prospective cohort studies. Oncotarget, 8(27), 44776–44784.
[61] Zhu, B., Sun, Y., Qi, L., Zhong, R. & Miaoa, X. (2015). Dietary legume consumption reduces risk of colorectal cancer: evidence from a meta-analysis of cohort studies. Sci Rep, 5, 8797.
[62] U.S. Department of Agriculture, Agricultural Research Service. (2010). USDA Database for the Oxygen Radical Absorbance Capacity (ORAC) of Selected Foods, Release 2. Accessed on 10 May 2019. Available at https://bit.ly/30fkGZe
[63] Zanovec, M., O'Neil, C. E. & Nicklas, T. A. (2011). Comparison of Nutrient Density and Nutrient-to-Cost between Cooked and Canned Beans. Food and Nutrition Sciences, 2, 66–73.
[64] Duyff, R. L., Mount, J. R. & Jones, J. B. (2011). Sodium Reduction in Canned Beans After Draining. Journal of Culinary Science & Technology Rinsing. 9(2), 106–112.
[65] Cao, G., Alessio, H.M. & Cutler, R.G. (1993). Oxygen-radical absorbance capacity assay for antioxidants. Free Radic Biol Med, 14(3), 303–311.
[66] Davey, G. K., Spencer, E. A., Appleby, P. N., Allen, N. E., Knox, K. H. & Key, T. J. (2003). EPIC-Oxford: lifestyle characteristics and nutrient intakes in a cohort of 33 883 meat-eaters and 31 546 non meat-eaters in the UK. Public Health Nutr, 6(3), 259–269.
[67] Young, V. R. & Pellett, P. L. (1994). Plant proteins in relation to human protein and amino acid nutrition. Am J Clin Nutr, 59 (5), 1203–1212.
[68] Neumeister, U. (2016). Veggiewahn – Eine Aufarbeitung der Irrtümer und Missverständnisse des Vegetarismus. [Veggie mania – a reappraisal of vegetarian mistakes and misunderstandings] Linz: Freya, 123.
[69] Hoffman, J. R. & Falvo, M. J. (2004). Protein – Which is Best? J Sports Sci Med, 3(3), 118–130.
[70] Avilés-Gaxiola, S., Chuck-Hernández, C. & Serna Saldívar, S. O. (2018). Inactivation Methods of Trypsin Inhibitor in Legumes: A Review. Concise Reviews & Hypotheses in Food Science. J Food Sci, 83(1), 17–29.
[71] Thompson, L. U., Rea, R. L. & Jenkins, D. J.A. (1983). Effect of Heat Processing on Hemagglutinin Activity in Red Kidney Beans. J Food Sci, 48(1), 235–236.
[72] Schlemmer, U., Frølich, W., Prieto, R. M. & Grases, F. (2009). Phytate in foods and significance for humans: food sources, intake, processing, bioavailability, protective role and analysis. Mol Nutr Food Res, 53(2), 330–375.
[73] Winham, D. M. & Hutchins, A. M. (2011). Perceptions of flatulence from bean consumption among adults in 3 feeding studies. Nutr J, 10, 128.
[74] Jood, S., Mehta, U., Singh, R. & Bhat, C. M. (1985). Effect of processing on flatus-producing factors in legumes. J Agric Food Chem, 33(2), 268–271.
[75] Larijani, B., Esfahani, M. M., Moghimi, M., Ardakani, M. R.S., Keshavarz, M., Kordafshari, G., Nazem, E., Ranjbar, S. H., Kenari, H. M. & Zargaran, A. (2016). Prevention and Treatment of Flatulence From a Traditional Persian Medicine Perspective. Iran Red Crescent Med J, 18(4), e23664.
[76] Ibrahim, S. S., Habiba, R. A., Shatta, A. A. & Embaby, H. E. (2002). Effect of soaking, germination, cooking and fermentation on antinutritional factors in cowpeas. Nahrung, 46(2), 92–95.
[77] U.S. Department of Agriculture, Agricultural Research Service. (2010). USDA Database for the Oxygen Radical Absorbance Capacity (ORAC) of Selected Foods, Release 2. Accessed on 10 May 2019. Available at https://bit.ly/30fkGZe
[78] Gardener, H., Moon, Y.P., Rundek, T., Elkind, M.S. & Sacco, R.L. (2018). Diet Soda and Sugar-Sweetened Soda Consumption in Relation to Incident Diabetes in the Northern Manhattan Study. Curr Dev Nutr, 2(5), nzy008.
[79] Muraki, I., Imamura, F., Manson, J. E., Hu, F. B., Willett, W. C., van Dam, R. M. & Sun, Q. (2013). Fruit consumption and risk of type 2 diabetes: results from three prospective longitudinal cohort studies. BMJ, 347, 5001.
[80] Feig, D.I. (2010). Sugar-sweetened beverages and hypertension. Future Cardiol, 6(6), 773–776.
[81] Muraki, I., Imamura, F., Manson, J. E., Hu, F. B., Willett, W. C., van Dam, R. M. & Sun, Q. (2013). Fruit consumption and risk of type 2 diabetes: results from three prospective longitudinal cohort studies. BMJ, 347, 5001.
[82] Borgi, L., Muraki, I., Satija, A., Willett, W.C., Rimm, E.B. & Forman, J.P. (2016). Fruit and vegetable consumption and the incidence of Hypertension in three prospective cohort studies. Hypertension, 67(2), 288–293.
[83] Gan, Y., Tong, X., Li, L., Cao, S., Yin, X., Gao, C. et al. (2015). Consumption of fruit and vegetable and risk of coronary heart disease: a meta-analysis of prospective cohort studies. Int J Cardiol, 183, 129–137.
[84] Hu, D., Huang, J., Wang, Y., Zhang, D., Qu, Y. (2014). Fruits and vegetables consumption and risk of stroke: a meta-analysis of prospective cohort studies. Stroke, 45(6), 1613–1619.
[85] Wang, Q., Chen, Y., Wang, X., Gong, G., Li, G. & Li, C. (2014). Consumption of fruit, but not vegetables, may reduce risk of gastric cancer: results from a meta-analysis of cohort studies. Eur J Cancer, 50(8), 1498–1509.
[86] Bertoia, M. L., Mukamal, K. J., Cahill, L. E., Hou, T., Ludwig, D. S., Mozaffarian, D. et al. (2015). Changes in Intake of Fruits and Vegetables and Weight Change in United States Men and Women Followed for Up to 24 Years: Analysis from Three Prospective Cohort Studies. PLoS Med, 12(9), e1001878.
[87] Petta, S., Marchesini, G., Caracausi, L., Macaluso, F. S., Camm., C, Ciminnisi, S. et al. (2013). Industrial, not fruit fructose intake is associated with the severity of liver fibrosis in genotype 1 chronic hepatitis C patients. J Hepatol, 59(6), 1169–1176.
[88] U.S. Department of Agriculture, Agricultural Research Service. (2010). USDA Database for the Oxygen Radical Absorbance Capacity (ORAC) of Selected Foods, Release 2. Accessed on 10 May 2019. Available at https://bit.ly/30fkGZe
[89] Bonwick, G. & Birch, C. S. (2013). Antioxidants in Fresh and Frozen Fruit and Vegetables: Impact Study of Varying Storage Conditions. Accessed on 01 June 2019. Available at https://bit.ly/2JGcADI
[90] Bouzari, A., Holstege, D. & Barrett, D. M. (2015). Vitamin retention in eight fruits and vegetables: a comparison of refrigerated and frozen storage. J Agric Food Chem, 63(3), 957–962.
[91] Vogelreuter, A. (2012). *Nahrungsmittelunverträglichkeiten: Lactose – Fructose – Histamin – Gluten.* [*Food intolerances: lactose – fructose – histamine – gluten*] Stuttgart: Wissenschaftliche Verlagsgesellschaft Stuttgart.
[92] Elmadfa, I., Aign, W., Muskat, E. & Fritzsche, D. (2017). *Die große GU Nährwert-Kalorien-Tabelle.* [*The big GU nutritional value – calories table*] München: Gräfe und Unzer Verlag. 118.
[93] Vogelreuter, A. (2012). *Nahrungsmittelunverträglichkeiten: Lactose – Fructose – Histamin – Gluten.* [*Food intolerances: lactose – fructose – histamine – gluten*] Stuttgart: Wissenschaftliche Verlagsgesellschaft Stuttgart.
[94] Schäfer, K., Reese, I., Ballmer-Weber, B. K., Beyer, K., Erdmann, S., Fuchs, T. et al. (2010). *Stellungnahme der AG Nahrungsmittelallergie in der Deutschen*

Gesellschaft für Allergologie und klinische Immunologie (DGAKI) – Fruktosemalabsorption. [Position paper by the food allergy working group at the German Society for Allergology and Clinical Immunology (DGAKI) – Fructose malabsorption] Allergo J, 19, 66–69.

[95] Fujisawa, T., Mulligan, K., Wada, L., Schumacher, L., Riby, J. & Kretchmer, N. (1993). The effect of exercise absorption. Am J Clin Nutr, 58(1), 75–79.

[96] Ferraris, R. P. (2001). Dietary and developmental regulation of intestinal sugar transport. Biochem J, 360(Pt 2), 265–276.

[97] Whitney, E. N. & Rolfes, S. R. (2018). *Understanding Nutrition*. Boston: Cengage Learning, 78.

[98] U.S. Department of Agriculture, Agricultural Research Service. (2010). USDA Database for the Oxygen Radical Absorbance Capacity (ORAC) of Selected Foods, Release 2. Accessed on 10 May 2019. Available at https://bit.ly/30fkGZe

[99] Eaton, S. B. & Konner, M. (1985). Paleolithic nutrition. A consideration of its nature and current implications. N Engl J Med, 312(5), 283–289.

[100] Sabat., J., Ros, E. & Salas-Salvadó., J. (2006). Nuts: nutrition and health outcomes. Br J Nutr, 96(2), 1–2.

[101] Jackson, C. L. & Hu, F. B. (2014). Long-term associations of nut consumption with body weight and obesity. Am J Clin Nutr, 100(1), 408–411.

[102] Brennan, A. M., Sweeney, L. L., Liu, X. & Mantzoros, C. S. (2010). Walnut consumption increases satiation but has no effect on insulin resistance or the metabolic profile over a 4-day period. Obesity (Silver Spring), 18(6), 1176–1182.

[103] Mattes, R. D. & Dreher, M. L. (2010). Nuts and healthy body weight maintenance mechanisms. Asia Pac J Clin Nutr, 19(1), 137–141.

[104] U.S. Department of Agriculture, Agricultural Research Service. (2010). USDA Database for the Oxygen Radical Absorbance Capacity (ORAC) of Selected Foods, Release 2. Accessed on 10 May 2019. Available at https://bit.ly/30fkGZe

[105] Ros, E. & Mataix, J. (2006). Fatty acid composition of nuts – implications for cardiovascular health. Br J Nutr. 96(2), 29–35.

[106] Kajla, P., Sharma, A. & Sood, D. R. (2015). Flaxseed – a potential functional food source. J Food Sci Technol, 52(4), 1857–1871.

[107] Rodriguez-Leyva, D., Weighell, W., Edel, A. L., LaVallee, R., Dibrov, E., Pinneker, R. et al. (2013). Potent antihypertensive action of dietary flaxseed in hypertensive patients. Hypertension, 62(6), 1081–1089.

[108] McCann, S. E., Thompson, L. U., Nie, J., Dorn, J., Trevisan, M. & Shields, P. G. (2010). Dietary lignan intakes in relation to survival among women with breast cancer: the Western New York Exposures and Breast Cancer (WEB) Study. Breast Cancer Res Treat, 122(1), 229–235.

[109] Demark-Wahnefried, W., Polascik, T. J., George, S. L., Switzer, B. R., Madden, J. F., Ruffin, M. T. et al. (2008). Flaxseed Supplementation (not Dietary Fat Restriction) Reduces Prostate Cancer Proliferation Rates in Men Presurgery. Cancer Epidemiol Biomarkers Prev, 17(12), 3577–3587.

[110] Malcolmson, L. J., Przybylski, R. & Daun, J. K. (2000). Storage stability of milled flaxseed. Journal of the American Oil Chemists' Society, 77(3), 235–238.

[111] Greger, M. (2016). How not to die – *Entdecken Sie Nahrungsmittel, die Ihr Leben verlängern und bewiesenermaßen Krankheiten vorbeugen und heilen*. *[How not to die – discover the foods scientifically proven to prevent and reverse disease]* Kandern: Unimedica, 313.

[112] Chen, Z. Y., Ratnayake, W. M.N. & Cunnane, S. C. (1994). Oxidative stability of flaxseed lipids during baking. J Am Oil Chem Soc, 71(6), 629–632.

[113] Hyvärinen, H. K., Pihlava, J. M., Hiidenhovi, J. A., Hietaniemi, V., Korhonen, H. J. & Ryhänen, E. L. (2006). Effect of processing and storage on the stability of flaxseed lignin added to bakery products. J Agric Food Chem, 54(1), 48–53.

[114] Hyvärinen, H. K., Pihlava, J. M., Hiidenhovi, J. A., Hietaniemi, V., Korhonen, H. J. & Ryhänen, E. L. (2006). Effect of processing and storage on the stability of flaxseed lignin added to bakery products. J Agric Food Chem, 54(1), 48–53.

[115] Guasch-Ferré, M., Bulló, M., Martínez-González, M. Á., Ros, E., Corella, D., Estruch, R. et al. (2013). Frequency of nut consumption and mortality risk in the PREDIMED nutrition intervention trial. BMC Med, 11, 164.

[116] Albert, C. M., Gaziano, J. M., Willett, W. C. & Manson, J. E. (2002). Nut consumption and decreased risk of sudden cardiac death in the Physicians' Health Study. Arch Intern Med, 162(12), 1382–1387.

[117] US Food and Drug Administration. (2003). Qualified Health Claims: Letter of Enforcement Discretion – Nuts and Coronary Heart Disease (Docket No 02P-0505). Accessed on 01 June 2018. Available at https://bit.ly/2pl6Blu

[118] German Nutrition Society (Deutsche Gesellschaft für Ernährung). (2016). 13. DGE-Ernährungsbericht. [13th DGE nutrition report] Bonn: DGE.

[119] Taylor, H., Webster, K., Gray, A. R., Tey, S. L., Chisholm, A., Bailey, K. et al. (2018). The effects of 'activating' almonds on consumer acceptance and gastrointestinal tolerance. Eur J Nutr, 57(8), 2771–2783.

[120] Kumari, S.V. (2017). The Effect of Soaking Almonds and Hazelnuts on Phytate and Mineral Concentrations. Accessed on 01 June 2019. Available at https://bit.ly/2EBXWtd

[121] Klich, M. A. (2007). *Aspergillus flavus*: the major producer of aflatoxin. Mol Plant Pathol, 8(6), 713–722.

[122] Ramesh, J., Sarathchandra, G. & Sureshkumar, V. (2013). Survey of market samples of food grains and grain flour for Aflatoxin B1 contamination. Int J Curr Microbiol App Sci, 2(5), 184–188.

[123] Kumar, P., Mahato, D. K., Kamle, M., Mohanta, T. K. & Kang, S. G. (2016). Aflatoxins: A Global Concern for Food Safety, Human Health and Their Management. Front Microbiol, 7, 2170.

[124] Brunke, H., Alston, J. M., Gray, R. S. & Sumner, D. A. (2004). Industry-mandated testing to improve food safety: the new US marketing order for pistachios. Agrarwirtschaft, 53(8), 334–343.

[125] *Bayerisches Landesamt für Gesundheit und Lebensmittelsicherheit*. [Bavarian Health and Food Safety Authority] (2014). *Untersuchung von Erdnusscreme und Erdnussbutter auf Aflatoxine – Untersuchungsergebnisse* 2014. *[Investigating peanut butter for aflatoxins – research results 2014]* Accessed on 01 June 2018. Available at https://bit.ly/2uqK3eA

[126] *Stiftung Warentest*. [German consumer organization] (2017). *Nüsse – Wie viel Schadstoffe stecken in Haselnüssen und Walnüssen? [Nuts – how many toxins are contained in hazelnuts and walnuts?]* Test, 11, 10–14.

[127] Jubert, C., Mata, J., Bench, G., Dashwood, R., Pereira, C., Tracewell, W. et al. (2009). Effects of chlorophyll and chlorophyllin on low-dose aflatoxin B1 pharmacokinetics in human volunteers. Cancer Prev Res (Phila). 2(12), 1015–1022.

[128] *Stiftung Warentest*. [German consumer organization] (2017). *Besser ganze Kerne kaufen. [Buying better whole seeds]* Test, 11, 10–14.

[129] Rimbach, G., Nagursky, J. & Erbersdobler, H.F. (2015). *Lebensmittel – Warenkunde für Einsteiger [Food – product expertise for beginners]* (2nd edition). Berlin: Springer Verlag, 171.

[130] Von Braunsweig, R. (2018). *Pflanzenöle – über 50 starke Helfer für Genuss und Hautpflege [Plant oils – over 50 powerful assistants for enjoyment and skin care]* (6th edition). Wiggensbach: Stadelmann Verlag, 52.

[131] Pohl, S. (2018). *Das Ölbuch – Pflanzenöle kompakt erklärt [The oil book – a compact guide to plant oils]* (5th edition). Wiggensbach: Stadelmann Verlag, 23.

[132] Pohl, S. (2018). *Das Ölbuch – Pflanzenöle kompakt erklärt [The oil book – a compact guide to plant oils]* (5th edition). Wiggensbach: Stadelmann Verlag, 61.

[133] Lawson, H. (1995). *Food Oils and Fats – Technology, Utilization and Nutrition*. New York: Chapman & Hall, 7f.

[134] Fiebig, H.J., Matthäus, B. & Schiekiera, K. (2016). *Warenkunde Öl. [Product expertise: oil]* Berlin: Stiftung Warentest, 27f.

[135] Matthäus, B. (2014). *Fette und Öle: Grundlagenwissen und praktische Verwendung. [Fats and oils: basic knowledge and practical use]* Ernährungs Umschau, 3, 162–170.

[136] Fiebig, H.J., Matthäus, B. & Schiekiera, K. (2016). *Warenkunde Öl. [Product expertise: oil]* Berlin: Stiftung Warentest, 62f.

[137] Krist, S., Buchbauer, G. & Klausberger, C. (2008). *Lexikon der pflanzlichen Fette und Öle. [Dictionary of plant-based fats and oils]* Vienna: Springer, 5f.

[138] Fiebig, H.J., Matthäus, B. & Schiekiera, K. (2016). *Warenkunde Öl. [Product expertise: oil]* Berlin: Stiftung Warentest, 42.

[139] Rimbach, G., Nagursky, J. & Erbersdobler, H.F. (2015). *Lebensmittel – Warenkunde für Einsteiger [Food – product expertise for beginners]* (2nd edition). Berlin: Springer Verlag, 179–184.

[140] Pohl, S. (2018). *Das Ölbuch – Pflanzenöle kompakt erklärt [The oil book – a compact guide to plant oils]* (5th edition). Wiggensbach: Stadelmann Verlag, 60.

[141] Fiebig, H.J., Matthäus, B. & Schiekiera, K. (2016). *Warenkunde Öl. [Product expertise: oil]* Berlin: Stiftung Warentest, 79.

[142] Fiebig, H.J., Matthäus, B. & Schiekiera, K. (2016). *Warenkunde Öl. [Product expertise: oil]* Berlin: Stiftung Warentest, 31.

[143] Pohl, S. (2018). *Das Ölbuch – Pflanzenöle kompakt erklärt [The oil book – a compact guide to plant oils]* (5th edition). Wiggensbach: Stadelmann Verlag, 61.

[144] Fiebig, H.J., Matthäus, B. & Schiekiera, K. (2016). *Warenkunde Öl. [Product expertise: oil]* Berlin: Stiftung Warentest, 82.

[145] De Alzaa, F., Guillaume, C. & Ravetti, L. (2018). Evaluation of Chemical and Physical Changes in Different Commercial Oils during Heating. Acta Scientific, 2(6), 2–11.

[146] Marcus, J.B. (2013). *Culinary Nutrition – The Science and Practice of Healthy Cooking*. Waltham: Academic Press, 61.

[147] The Vegetarian Health Institute. (2012). Smoke Point of Oils. Accessed on 01 June 2019. Available at https://bit.ly/2yGD2qQ

[148] The Culinary Institute of America. (2011). *The Professional Chef.* New Jersey: Wiley, 232f.

[149] Fiebig, H.J., Matthäus, B. & Schiekiera, K. (2016). *Warenkunde Öl. [Product expertise: oil]* Berlin: Stiftung Warentest, 32.

[150] Fiebig, H.J., Matthäus, B. & Schiekiera, K. (2016). *Warenkunde Öl. [Product expertise: oil]* Berlin: Stiftung Warentest, 70.

[151] Clodoveo, M.L., Camposeo, S., De Gennaro, B., Pascuzzi, S. & Roselli, L. (2014). In the ancient world, virgin olive oil was called 'liquid gold' by Homer and 'the great healer' by Hippocrates. Why has this mythic image been forgotten? Food Research International, 62, 1062–1068.

[152] Casal, S., Malheiro, R., Sendas, A., Oliveira, B.P. & Pereira, J.A. (2010). Olive oil stability under deep-frying conditions. Food Chem Toxicol, 48(10), 2972–2979.

[153] Chiou, A. & Kalogeropoulos, N. (2017). Virgin Olive Oil as Frying Oil. Compr Rev Food Sci Food Saf, 16(4), 632–646.

[154] Allouche, Y., Jiménez, A., Gaforio, J.J., Uceda, M. & Beltrán, G. (2007). How heating affects extra virgin olive oil quality indexes and chemical composition. J Agric Food Chem, 55(23), 964–69654.

[155] Sacchi, R., Paduano, A., Savarese, M., Vitaglione, P. & Fogliano, V. (2014). Extra virgin olive oil: from composition to 'molecular gastronomy' Cancer Treat Res, 159, 325–338.

[156] Warner K. 2009. Flavor changes during frying. In: Sahin, S., Sumnu, S. G. editors. *Advances in deep-fat frying of foods.* Boca Raton: CRC Press, 201–213.

[157] Lawson, H. (1995). *Food Oils and Fats – Technology, Utilization and Nutrition.* New York: Chapman & Hall, 213.

[158] Clarke, R., Frost, C., Collins, R., Appleby, P. & Peto, R. (1997). Dietary lipids and blood cholesterol: quantitative meta-analysis of metabolic ward studies. BMJ, 314(7074), 112–117.

[159] Guasch-Ferré, M., Hu, F.B., Martínez-González, M.A., Fitó, M., Bulló, M., Estruch, R. et al. (2014). Olive oil intake and risk of cardiovascular disease and mortality in the PREDIMED Study. BMC Med, 12, 78.

[160] Azambuja, P., de Souza, L., Marcadenti, A. & Portal, V.L. (2017). Effects of Olive Oil Phenolic Compounds on Inflammation in the Prevention and Treatment of Coronary Artery Disease. Nutrients, 9(10), 1087.

[161] George, E.S., Marshall, S., Mayr, H.L., Trakman, G.L., Tatucu-Babet, O.A., Lassemillante, A.M. (2018). The effect of high-polyphenol extra virgin olive oil on cardiovascular risk factors: A systematic review and meta-analysis. Crit Rev Food Sci Nutr, 1–24.

[162] Omar, S.H. (2010). Oleuropein in Olive and its Pharmacological Effects. Sci Pharm, 78(2), 133–154.

[163] Pang, K.L. & Chin, K.Y. (2018). The Biological Activities of Oleocanthal from a Molecular Perspective. Nutrients, 10(5), 570.

[164] Ramírez-Anaya, J.P., Samaniego-Sánchez, C., Castañeda-Saucedo, M.C., Villalón-Mir, M. & de la Serrana, H.L. (2015). Phenols and the antioxidant capacity of Mediterranean vegetables prepared with extra virgin olive oil using different domestic cooking techniques. Food Chem, 188, 430–438.

[165] Carnevale, R., Silvestri, R., Loffredo, L., Novo, M., Cammisotto, V., Castellani, V. et al. (2018). Oleuropein, a component of extra virgin olive oil, lowers postprandial glycaemia in healthy subjects. Br J Clin Pharmacol, 84(7), 1566–1574.

[166] Soriguer, F., Esteva, I., Rojo-Martinez, G., Ruiz de Adana, M.S., Dobarganes, M.C., García-Almeida, J.M. et al. (2004). Oleic acid from cooking oils is associated with lower insulin resistance in the general population (Pizarra study). Eur J Endocrinol, 150(1), 33–39.

[167] Bültjer, U. (2015). *Lexikon der Kräuter und Gewürze. [Dictionary of herbs and spices]* Munich: Bassermann Verlag, 240.

[168] Budak, N.H., Aykin, E., Seydim, A.C., Greene, A.K. & Guzel-Seydim, Z.B. (2014). Functional Properties of Vinegar. J Food Sci, 79(5), 757–764.

[169] Bültjer, U. (2015). *Lexikon der Kräuter und Gewürze. [Dictionary of herbs and spices]* Munich: Bassermann Verlag, 241.

[170] Johnston, C.S., Quagliano, S. & White, S. (2013). Vinegar ingestion at mealtime reduced fasting blood glucose concentrations in healthy adults at risk for type 2 diabetes. J Funct Foods, 5(4), 2007–2011.

[171] Budak, N.H., Aykin, E., Seydim, A.C., Greene, A.K. & Guzel-Seydim, Z.B. (2014). Functional Properties of Vinegar. J Food Sci, 79(5), 757–764.

[172] Mitrou, P., Petsiou, E., Papakonstantinou, E., Maratou, E., Lambadiari, V., Dimitriadis, P. et al. (2015). Vinegar Consumption Increases Insulin-Stimulated Glucose Uptake by the Forearm Muscle in Humans with Type 2 Diabetes. J Diabetes Res, 2015, 175204.

[173] Liatis, S., Grammatikou, S., Poulia, K.A., Perrea, D., Makrilakis, K., Diakoumopoulou, E. & Katsilambros, N. (2010). Vinegar reduces postprandial hyperglycaemia in patients with type II diabetes when added to a high, but not to a low, glycaemic index meal. Eur J Clin Nutr, 64(7), 727–732.

[174] Mitrou, P., Petsiou, E., Papakonstantinou, E., Maratou, E, Lambadiari, V., Dimitriadis, P. et al. (2015). The role of acetic acid on glucose uptake and blood flow rates in the skeletal muscle in humans with impaired glucose tolerance. Eur J Clin Nutr, 69(6), 734–739.

[175] Mitrou, P., Petsiou, E., Papakonstantinou, E., Maratou, E., Lambadiari, V., Dimitriadis, P. et al. (2015). Vinegar Consumption Increases Insulin-Stimulated Glucose Uptake by the Forearm Muscle in Humans with Type 2 Diabetes. J Diabetes Res, 2015, 175204.

[176] Johnston, C.S. & Buller, A.J. (2005). Vinegar and peanut products as complementary foods to reduce postprandial glycemia. J Am Diet Assoc, 105(12), 1939–1942.

[177] Sugiyama, M., Tang, A.C., Wakaki, Y. & Koyama, W. (2003). Glycemic index of single and mixed meal foods among common Japanese foods with white rice as a reference food. Eur J Clin Nutr, 57(6), 743–752.

[178] Ostman, E.M., Liljeberg Elmstahl, H.G. & Bjorck, I.M. (2001). Inconsistency between glycemic and insulinemic responses to regular and fermented milk products. Am J Clin Nutr, 74, 96–100.

[179] Leeman, M., Ostman, E. & Björck. I. (2005). Vinegar dressing and cold storage of potatoes lowers postprandial glycaemic and insulinaemic responses in healthy subjects. Eur J Clin Nutr, 59(11), 1266–1271.

[180] Johnston, C.S., Quagliano, S. & White, S. (2013). Vinegar ingestion at mealtime reduced fasting blood glucose concentrations in healthy adults at risk for type 2 diabetes. J Funct Foods, 5(4), 2007–2011.

[181] Sherwani, S.I., Khan, H.A., Ekhzaimy, A., Masood, A. & Sakharkar, M.K. (2016). Significance of HbA1c Test in Diagnosis and Prognosis of Diabetic Patients. Biomark Insights, 11, 95–104.

[182] Johnston, C.S., White, A.M. & Kent, S.M. (2009). Preliminary evidence that regular vinegar ingestion favorably influences hemoglobin A1c values in individuals with type 2 diabetes mellitus. Diabetes Res Clin Pract, 84(2), e15–17.

[183] Ostman, E., Granfeldt, Y., Persson, L. & Björck, I. (2005). Vinegar supplementation lowers glucose and insulin responses and increases satiety after a bread meal in healthy subjects. Eur J Clin Nutr, 59(9), 983–938.

[184] Beheshti, Z., Chan, Y.H., Nia, H.S., Hajihosseini, F., Nazari, R., Shaabani, M. & Omran, M.T. (2012). Influence of apple cider vinegar on blood lipids. Life Science Journal, 9(4), 2431–2440.

[185] Johnston, C.S., Steplewska, I., Long, C.A., Harris, L.N., Ryals, R.H. (2010). Examination of the antiglycemic properties of vinegar in healthy adults. Ann Nutr Metab, 56(1), 74–79.

[186] Kondo, T., Kishi, M., Fushimi, T., Ugajin, S. & Kaga, T. (2009). Vinegar intake reduces body weight, body fat mass, and serum triglyceride levels in obese Japanese subjects. Biosci Biotechnol Biochem, 73(8), 1837–1843.

[187] Kondo, T., Kishi, M., Fushimi, T., Ugajin, S. & Kaga, T. (2009). Vinegar intake reduces body weight, body fat mass, and serum triglyceride levels in obese Japanese subjects. Biosci Biotechnol Biochem, 73(8), 1837–1843.

[188] Benmeir, P., Lusthaus, S., Weinberg, A., Neuman, A. & Eldad, A. (1994). Facial chemical burn. Burns, 20(3), 282.

[189] Takano-Lee, M., Edman, J.D., Mullens, B.A. & Clark, J.M. (2004). Home remedies to control head lice: assessment of home remedies to control the human head louse, *Pediculus humanus capitis* (Anoplura: Pediculidae). J Pediatr Nurs, 19(6), 393–398.

[190] Zheng, L.W., Li, D., Lu, J.Z., Hu, W., Chen, D. & Zhou, X.D. (2014). Effects of vinegar on tooth bleaching and dental hard tissues in vitro. Sichuan Da Xue Xue Bao Yi Xue Ban, 45(6), 933–936.

[191] Willershausen, I., Weyer, V., Schulte, D., Lampe, F., Buhre, S. & Willershausen, B. (2014). In vitro study on dental erosion caused by different vinegar varieties using an electron microprobe. Clin Lab, 60(5), 783–790.

[192] Gambon, D.L., Brand, H.S. & Veerman, E.C. (2012). Unhealthy weight loss. Erosion by apple cider vinegar. Ned Tijdschr Tandheelkd, 119(12), 589–591.

[193] Bültjer, U. (2015). *Lexikon der Kräuter und Gewürze. [Dictionary of herbs and spices]* Munich: Bassermann Verlag, 241.

[194] Bültjer, U. (2015). *Lexikon der Kräuter und Gewürze. [Dictionary of herbs and spices]* Munich: Bassermann Verlag, 241.

[195] U.S. Department of Agriculture, Agricultural Research Service. (2010). USDA Database for the Oxygen Radical Absorbance Capacity (ORAC) of Selected Foods, Release 2. Accessed on 10 May 2019. Available at https://bit.ly/30fkGZe

[196] Bültjer, U. (2015). *Lexikon der Kräuter und Gewürze. [Dictionary of herbs and spices]* Munich: Bassermann Verlag, 8.

[197] Teuscher, E. (2018). *Gewürze und Küchenkräuter – Gewinnung, Inhaltsstoffe, Wirkungen [Spices and kitchen herbs – extraction, constituents, effects]* (2nd edition). Stuttgart: Wissenschaftliche Verlagsgesellschaft, 56.

[198] U.S. Department of Agriculture, Agricultural Research Service. (2010). USDA Database for the Oxygen Radical Absorbance Capacity (ORAC) of

Selected Foods, Release 2. Accessed on 10 May 2019. Available at https://bit.ly/30fkGZe
[199] Rimbach, G., Nagursky, J. & Erbersdobler, H.F. (2015). *Lebensmittel – Warenkunde für Einsteiger* [*Food – product expertise for beginners*] (2nd edition). Berlin: Springer Verlag.
[200] Teuscher, E. (2018). *Gewürze und Küchenkräuter – Gewinnung, Inhaltsstoffe, Wirkungen* [*Spices and kitchen herbs – extraction, constituents, effects*] (2nd edition). Stuttgart: Wissenschaftliche Verlagsgesellschaft. 261–282.
[201] Von Koerber, K., Männle, T. & Leitzmann, C. (2012). *Vollwert-Ernährung – Konzeption einer zeitgemäßen und nachhaltigen Ernährung* [*Wholesome nutrition – devising a contemporary and sustainable diet*] (11th edition). Stuttgart: Karl F. Haug Verlag, 327–335.
[202] Bültjer, U. (2015). *Lexikon der Kräuter und Gewürze.* [*Dictionary of herbs and spices*] Munich: Bassermann Verlag.
[203] Bendel, L. (2018). *Kräuter & Gewürze – Das große Lexikon.* [*Herbs & spices – the big dictionary*] Cologne: Anaconda.
[204] Maghbooli, M., Golipour, F., Moghimi Esfandabadi, A. & Yousefi, M. (2014). Comparison between the efficacy of ginger and sumatriptan in the ablative treatment of the common migraine. Phytother Res, 28(3), 412–415.
[205] Kashefi, F., Khajehei, M., Tabatabaeichehr, M., Alavinia, M. & Asili, J. (2014). Comparison of the effect of ginger and zinc sulfate on primary dysmenorrhea: a placebo-controlled randomized trial. Pain Manag Nurs, 15(4), 826–833.
[206] Palatty, P.L., Haniadka, R., Valder, B., Arora, R. & Baliga, M.S. (2013). Ginger in the prevention of nausea and vomiting: a review. Crit Rev Food Sci Nutr, 53(7), 659–669.
[207] Mnif, S. & Aifa, S. (2015). Cumin (*Cuminum cyminum L.*) from traditional uses to potential biomedical applications. Chem Biodivers, 12(5), 733–742.
[208] Zare, R., Heshmati, F., Fallahzadeh, H. & Nadjarzadeh, A. (2014). Effect of cumin powder on body composition and lipid profile in overweight and obese women. Complement Ther Clin Pract, 20(4), 297–301.
[209] Gupta, S.C., Patchva, S. & Aggarwal, B.B. (2013). Therapeutic Roles of Curcumin: Lessons Learned from Clinical Trials. AAPS J, 15(1), 195–218.
[210] Siruguri, V. & Bhat, R.V. (2015). Assessing intake of spices by pattern of spice use, frequency of consumption and portion size of spices consumed from routinely prepared dishes in southern India. Nutr J, 14, 7.
[211] Stohs, S.J., Chen, O., Ray, S.D., Ji, J., Bucci, L.R. & Preuss, H.G. (2020). Highly Bioavailable Forms of Curcumin and Promising Avenues for Curcumin-Based Research and Application: A Review. Molecules, 25(6), 1397.
[212] Shoba, G., Joy, D., Joseph, T., Majeed, M., Rajendran, R. & Srinivas, P.S. (1998). Influence of piperine on the pharmacokinetics of curcumin in animals and human volunteers. Planta Med, 64(4), 353–356.
[213] Hewlings, S.J. & Kalman, D.S. (2017). Curcumin: A Review of Its [*sic*] Effects on Human Health. Foods, 6(10), 92.
[214] Periasamy, G., Karim, A., Gibrelibanos, M., Gebremedhin, G., Preedy, V. R., Hrsg: Gilani, A. (2016). Nutmeg (*Myristica fragrans* Houtt.) Oils. In: *Essential Oils in Food Preservation, Flavor and Safety*. London Academic Press, 607–616.
[215] Idle, J.R. (2005). Christmas gingerbread (Lebkuchen) and Christmas cheer – review of the potential role of mood elevating amphetamine-like compounds formed in vivo and in furno. Prague Med Rep, 106(1), 27–38.
[216] Scholefield, J.H. (1986). Nutmeg – an unusual overdose. Arch Emerg Med, 3(2), 154–155.
[217] Williams, E.Y. & West, F. (1968). The use of nutmeg as a psychotrpic [sic] drug. Report of two cases. J Natl Med Assoc, 60(4), 289–290.
[218] Rimbach, G., Nagursky, J. & Erbersdobler, H.F. (2015). *Lebensmittel – Warenkunde für Einsteiger* [*Food – product expertise for beginners*] (2nd edition). Berlin: Springer Verlag, 265.
[219] U.S. Department of Agriculture, Agricultural Research Service. (2010). USDA Database for the Oxygen Radical Absorbance Capacity (ORAC) of Selected Foods, Release 2. Accessed on 10 May 2019. Available at https://bit.ly/30fkGZe
[220] Teuscher, E. (2018). *Gewürze und Küchenkräuter – Gewinnung, Inhaltsstoffe, Wirkungen* [*Spices and kitchen herbs – extraction, constituents, effects*] (2nd edition). Stuttgart: Wissenschaftliche Verlagsgesellschaft, 177–179.
[221] Cortés-Rojas, D.F., Fernandes de Souza, C.R. & Oliveira, W.P. (2014). Clove (*Syzygium aromaticum*): a precious spice. Asian Pac J Trop Biomed, 4(2), 90–96.
[222] Rimbach, G., Nagursky, J. & Erbersdobler, H.F. (2015). *Lebensmittel – Warenkunde für Einsteiger* [*Food – product expertise for beginners*] (2nd edition). Berlin: Springer Verlag, 273.
[223] *Umweltbundesamt*. [German Environment Agency] (2016). *Polyzyklische Aromatische Kohlenwas- serstoffe Umweltschädlich! Giftig! Unvermeidbar?* [*Polycyclic aromatic hydrocarbons: Environmentally unfriendly! Toxic! Unavoidable?*] Accessed on 01 June 2019. Available at https://bit.ly/2F1A2JQ
[224] Tormo, M.A., Campillo, J.E., Viña, J., Gómez-Encinas, J., Borrás, C., Torres, M.D. & Campillo, C. (2013). The mechanism of the antioxidant effect of smoked paprika from La Vera, Spain. CyTa, 11(2), 114–118.
[225] Gomaa, E.A., Gray, J.I., Rabie, S., Lopez-Bote, C. & Booren, A.M. (1993). Polycyclic aromatic hydrocarbons in smoked food products and commercial liquid smoke flavourings. Food Addit Contam, 10(5), 503–521.
[226] Sanati, S., Razavi, B.M. & Hosseinzadeh, H. (2018). A review of the effects of *Capsicum annuum L.* and its constituent, capsaicin, in metabolic syndrome. Iran J Basic Med Sci, 21(5), 439–448.
[227] Srinivasan, K. (2016). Biological Activities of Red Pepper (*Capsicum annuum*) and Its Pungent Principle Capsaicin: A Review. Crit Rev Food Sci Nutr, 56(9), 1488-1500.
[228] Butt, M.S., Pasha, I., Sultan, M.T., Randhawa, M.A., Saeed, F. & Ahmed, W. (2013). Black pepper and health claims: a comprehensive treatise. Crit Rev Food Sci Nutr, 53(9), 875–886.
[229] Bezerra, D.P., Nascimento Soares, A.K. & Pergentino de Sousa, D. (2016). Overview of the Role of Vanillin on Redox Status and Cancer Development. Oxid Med Cell Longev, 2016, 9734816.
[230] Fotland, T.Ø., Paulsen, J.E., Sanner, T., Alexander, J. & Husøy, T. (2012). Risk assessment of coumarin using the bench mark dose (BMD) approach: children in Norway which regularly eat oatmeal porridge with cinnamon may exceed the TDI for coumarin with several folds. Food Chem Toxicol, 50(3–4), 903–912.
[231] Shen, Y., Jia, L.N., Honma, N., Hosono, T., Ariga,T. & Seki, T. (2012). Beneficial Effects of Cinnamon on the Metabolic Syndrome, Inflammation, and Pain, and Mechanisms Underlying These Effects – A Review. J Tradit Complement Med, 2(1), 27–32.
[232] Rimbach, G., Nagursky, J. & Erbersdobler, H.F. (2015). *Lebensmittel – Warenkunde für Einsteiger* [*Food – product expertise for beginners*] (2nd edition). Berlin: Springer Verlag.
[233] Teuscher, E. (2018). *Gewürze und Küchenkräuter – Gewinnung, Inhaltsstoffe, Wirkungen* [*Spices and kitchen herbs – extraction, constituents, effects*] (2nd edition). Stuttgart: Wissenschaftliche Verlagsgesellschaft. 261–282.
[234] Von Koerber, K., Männle, T. & Leitzmann, C. (2012). *Vollwert-Ernährung – Konzeption einer zeitgemäßen und nachhaltigen Ernährung* [*Wholesome nutrition – devising a contemporary and sustainable diet*] (11th edition). Stuttgart: Karl F. Haug Verlag, 327–335.
[235] Bültjer, U. (2015). *Lexikon der Kräuter und Gewürze.* [*Dictionary of herbs and spices*] Munich: Bassermann Verlag.
[236] Bendel, L. (2018). *Kräuter & Gewürze – Das große Lexikon.* [*Herbs & spices – the big dictionary*] Cologne: Anaconda.
[237] Beauchamp, G.K. (2016). Why do we like sweet taste: A bitter tale? Physiol Behav, 164(Pt B), 432–437.
[238] Drewnowski, A., Mennella, J.A., Johnson, S.L. & Bellisle, F. (2012). Sweetness and Food Preference. J Nutr, 142(6), 1142–1148.
[239] Murray, R.D. (2017). Savoring Sweet: Sugars in Infant and Toddler Feeding. Ann Nutr Metab, 70(3), 38–46.
[240] Rimbach, G., Nagursky, J. & Erbersdobler, H.F. (2015). *Lebensmittel – Warenkunde für Einsteiger* [*Food – product expertise for beginners*] (2nd edition). Berlin: Springer Verlag, 238.
[241] Von Koerber, K., Männle, T. & Leitzmann, C. (2012). *Vollwert-Ernährung – Konzeption einer zeitgemäßen und nachhaltigen Ernährung* [*Wholesome nutrition – devising a contemporary and sustainable diet*] (11th edition). Stuttgart: Karl F. Haug Verlag, 339.
[242] Statista. [German market research company] (2019). Pro-Kopf-Konsum von Zucker in Deutschland in den Jahren 1950/51 bis 2015/16 (in Kilogramm Weißzuckerwert). [Per capita consumption of sugar in Germany in the years 1950/51 to 2015/16 (expressed as kilograms white sugar)] Accessed on 01 June 2019. Available at https://bit.ly/2dpjClv
[243] Harvard Health Letter. (2011). Abundance of fructose not good for the liver, heart. Accessed on 01 June 2019. Available at http://bit.ly/2AiZdka
[244] Rimbach, G., Nagursky, J. & Erbersdobler, H.F. (2015). *Lebensmittel – Warenkunde für Einsteiger* [*Food – product expertise for beginners*] (2nd edition). Berlin: Springer Verlag, 259.
[245] Moeller, S.M., Fryhofer, S.A., Osbahr, A.J. & Robinowitz, C.B. (2009). The effects of high fructose syrup. J Am Coll Nutr, 28(6), 619–626.
[246] Rimbach, G., Nagursky, J. & Erbersdobler, H.F. (2015). *Lebensmittel – Warenkunde für Einsteiger* [*Food – product expertise for beginners*] (2nd edition). Berlin: Springer Verlag, 258.
[247] Lustig, R.H., Schmidt, L.A. & Brindis, C.D. (2012). Public health: The toxic truth about sugar. Nature, 482(7383), 27–29.
[248] Radulian, G., Rusu, E., Dragomir, A. & Posea, M. (2009). Metabolic effects of low glycaemic index diets. Nutr J, 8, 5.
[249] Yan, L.J. (2014). Pathogenesis of Chronic Hyperglycemia: From Reductive Stress to Oxidative Stress. J Diabetes Res, 2014, 137919.

[250] Bhupathiraju, S.N., Tobias, D.K., Malik, V.S., Pan, A., Hruby, A., Manson, J.E. et al. (2014). Glycemic index, glycemic load, and risk of type 2 diabetes: results from 3 large US cohorts and an updated meta-analysis. Am J Clin Nutr, 100(1), 218–232.

[251] Greenwood, D.C., Threapleton, D.E., Evans, C.E., Cleghorn, C.L., Nykjaer, C., Woodhead, C. & Burley, V.J. (2013). Glycemic Index, Glycemic Load, Carbohydrates, and Type 2 Diabetes: Systematic review and dose–response meta-analysis of prospective studies. Diabetes Care, 36(12), 4166–4171.

[252] Livesey, G. & Livesey, H. (2019). Coronary Heart Disease and Dietary Carbohydrate, Glycemic Index, and Glycemic Load: Dose-Response Meta-analyses of Prospective Cohort Studies. Mayo Clin Proc Innov Qual Outcomes, 3(1), 52–69.

[253] Ma, X.Y., Liu, J.P. & Song, Z.Y. (2012). Glycemic load, glycemic index and risk of cardiovascular diseases: meta-analyses of prospective studies. Atherosclerosis, 223(2), 491–496.

[254] Petta, S., Marchesini, G., Caracausi, L., Macaluso, F. S., Cammà, C., et al. (2013). Industrial, not fruit fructose intake is associated with the severity of liver fibrosis in genotype 1 chronic hepatitis C patients. J Hepatol, 59(6), 1169–1176.

[255] Jensen, T., Abdelmalek, M.F., Sullivan, S., Nadeau, K.J., Green, M. & Roncal, C. (2018). Fructose and Sugar: A Major Mediator of Nonalcoholic Fatty Liver Disease. J Hepatol, 68(5), 1063–1075.

[256] Kelishadi, R., Mansourian, M., Heidari-Beni, M. (2014). Association of fructose consumption and components of metabolic syndrome in human studies: a systematic review and meta-analysis. Nutrition, 30(5), 503–510.

[257] Deutsche Adipositas-Gesellschaft e.V. (DAG) [German Obesity Society], Deutsche Diabetes Gesellschaft e.V. (DDG) [German Diabetes Society] & Deutsche Gesellschaft für Ernährung e.V. (DGE) [German Nutrition Society]. (2018). *Konsensuspapier – Quantitative Empfehlung zur Zuckerzufuhr in Deutschland. [Consensus paper – quantitative recommendation on sugar consumption in Germany]* Accessed on 01 June 2019. Available at https://bit.ly/2spdeLm

[258] *Statista.* [German market research company] (2019). *Pro-Kopf-Konsum von Zucker in Deutschland in den Jahren 1950/51 bis 2015/16 (in Kilogramm Weißzuckerwert). [Per capita consumption of sugar in Germany in the years 1950/51 to 2015/16 (expressed as kilograms white sugar)]* Accessed on 01 June 2019. Available at https://bit.ly/2dpjClv

[259] Erickson, J. & Slavin, J. (2015). Total, added, and free sugar: Are restrictive guidelines science-based or achievable? Nutrients, 7, 2866–2878.

[260] Von Koerber, K., Männle, T. & Leitzmann, C. (2012). *Vollwert-Ernährung – Konzeption einer zeitgemäßen und nachhaltigen Ernährung [Wholesome nutrition – devising a contemporary and sustainable diet]* (11th edition). Stuttgart: Karl F. Haug Verlag, 340.

[261] Wise, P.M., Nattress, L., Flammer, L.J., Beauchamp, G.K. (2015). Reduced dietary intake of simple sugars alters perceived sweet taste intensity but not perceived pleasantness. Am J Clin Nutr, 103(1), 50–60.

[262] Wong, A., Young, D.A., Emmanouil, D.E., Wong, L.M., Waters, A.R. & Booth, M.T. (2013). Raisins and oral health. J Food Sci, 78(1), A26–29.

[263] Sadler, M.J. (2016). Dried fruit and dental health. Int J Food Sci Nutr, 67(8), 944-959.

[264] *Rapunzel Naturkost.* [Food manufacturer] (no date). *Natürlich süßen – mit alternativen Süßungsmitteln und Rohrzucker.* [Natural sweeteners – using alternative sweeteners and cane sugar] Accessed on 01 June 2019. Available at https://bit.ly/2XvyTn2

[265] Phillips, K.M., Carlsen, M.H. & Blomhoff, R. (2009). Total antioxidant content of alternatives to refined sugar. J Am Diet Assoc, 109(1), 64–71.

[266] Goossens, J. & Roè, H. (1994) Erythritol: A new bulk sweetener. International Food Ingredients, 1(2), 27–33.

[267] Ishikawa, M., Miyashita, M., Kawashima, Y., Nakamura, T., Saitou, N. & Modderman, J. (1996). Effects of oral administration of erythritol on patients with diabetes. Regul Toxicol Pharmacol, 24(2), 303–308.

[268] Mäkinen, K.K. (2016). Gastrointestinal Disturbances Associated with the Consumption of Sugar Alcohols with Special Consideration of Xylitol: Scientific Review and Instructions for Dentists and Other Health-Care Professionals. Int J Dent, 2016, 5967907.

[269] Munro, I.C., Berndt, W.O., Borzelleca, J.F., Flamm, G., Lynch, B.S., Kennepohl, E. et al. (1998). Erythritol: an interpretive summary of biochemical, metabolic, toxicological and clinical data. Food Chem Toxicol, 36(12), 1139–1174.

[270] Bohacek, H. (2018). *E-NUMMERN LISTE: Die Zusatzstoffe in unseren Nahrungsmitteln. [E-NUMBERS LIST: the additives in our foods]* Accessed on 01 June 2019. Available at https://bit.ly/2NCqmdl

[271] Falony, G., Honkala, S., Runnel, R., Olak, J., Nõmmela, R., Russak, S. et al. (2016). Long-Term Effect of Erythritol on Dental Caries Development during Childhood: A Posttreatment Survival Analysis. Caries Res, 50(6), 579–588.

[272] den Hartog, G.J., Boots, A.W., Adam-Perrot, A., Brouns, F., Verkooijen, I.W., Weseler, A.R. et al. (2010). Erythritol is a sweet antioxidant. Nutrition, 26(4), 449–458.

[273] Bernt, W.O., Borzelleca, J.F., Flamm, G. & Munro, I.C. (1996). Erythritol: a review of biological and toxicological studies. Regul Toxicol Pharmacol, 24(2), 191–197.

[274] Arrigoni, E., Brouns, F. & Amadò, R. (2005). Human gut microbiota does not ferment erythritol. Br J Nutr, 94(5), 643–646.

[275] Greenhill, C. (2014). Gut microbiota: not so sweet – artificial sweeteners can cause glucose intolerance by affecting the gut microbiota. Nat Rev Endocrinol, 10(11), 637.

[276] Suez, J., Korem, T., Zeevi, D., Zilberman-Schapira, G., Thaiss, C.A., Maza, O. et al. (2014). Artificial sweeteners induce glucose intolerance by altering the gut microbiota. Nature, 514(7521), 181–186.

[277] Frankenfeld, C.L., Sikaroodi, M., Lamb, E., Shoemaker, S. & Gillevet, P.M. (2015). High-intensity sweetener consumption and gut microbiome content and predicted gene function in a cross-sectional study of adults in the United States. Ann Epidemiol, 25(10), 736–742.

[278] Ciappuccini, R., Ansemant, T., Maillefert, J.F., Tavernier, C. & Ornetti, P. (2010). Aspartame-induced fibromyalgia, an unusual but curable cause of chronic pain. Clin Exp Rheumatol, 28(63), 131–133.

[279] Jacob, S.E. & Stechschulte, S. (2008). Formaldehyde, aspartame, and migraines: a possible connection. Dermatitis, 19(3), E10–1.

[280] Roberts, H.J. (2008). Overlooked aspartame-induced hypertension. South Med J, 101(9), 969.

[281] Lindseth, G.N., Coolahan, S.E., Petros, T.V. & Lindseth, P.D. (2014). Neurobehavioral effects of aspartame consumption. Res Nurs Health, 37(3), 185–193.

[282] Pretorius, E. (2012). GUT bacteria and aspartame: why are we surprised? Eur J Clin Nutr, 66(8), 972.

[283] Shankar, P., Ahuja, S. & Sriram, K. (2013). Non-nutritive sweeteners: review and update. Nutrition, 29(11–12), 1293–1299.

[284] Janakiram, C., Ceepan Kumar, C.V. & Joseph, J. (2017). Xylitol in preventing dental caries: A systematic review and meta-analyses. J Nat Sci Biol Med, 8(1), 16–21.

[285] Ruiz-Ojeda, F.J., Plaza-Díaz, J., Sáez-Lara, M.J. & Gil, A. (2019). Effects of Sweeteners on the Gut Microbiota: A Review of Experimental Studies and Clinical Trials. Adv Nutr, 10(1), 31–48.

[286] Ur-Rehman, S., Mushtaq, Z., Zahoor, T., Jamil, A. & Murtaza, M.A. (2015). Xylitol: a review on bioproduction, application, health benefits, and related safety issues. Crit Rev Food Sci Nutr, 55(11), 1514–1528.

[287] Deutsche Gesellschaft für Ernährung [German Nutrition Society], Österreichische Gesellschaft für Ernährung [Austrian Nutrition Society], Schweizerische Gesellschaft für Ernährung [Swiss Nutrition Society]. (2018). *Referenzwerte für die Nährstoffzufuhr [Reference values for nutrient intake]* (4th edition), Bonn: Neuer Umschau Verlag.

[288] Mariotti, F. (2018). Plant Protein, Animal Protein, and Protein Quality. In: Mariotti, F., Hrsg.: Vegetarian and Plant-Based Diets in Health and Disease Prevention. Cambridge: Academic Press, 621–637.

[289] Davis, B. C. & Kris-Etherton, P. M. (2003). Achieving optimal essential fatty acid status in vegetarians: current knowledge and practical implications. Am J Clin Nutr, 78(3), 640–646.

[290] Brown, M.J., Ferruzzi, M.G., Nguyen, M.L., Cooper, D.A., Eldridge, A.L., Schwartz, S.J. & White, W.S. (2004). Carotenoid bioavailability is higher from salads ingested with full-fat than with fat-reduced salad dressings as measured with electrochemical detection. Am J Clin Nutr, 80(2), 396–403.

[291] Gröber, U. & Holick, M. F. (2015). *Vitamin D – Die Heilkraft des Sonnenvitamins [Vitamin D – the healing power of the sunshine vitamin]* (3rd edition). Stuttgart: Wissenschaftliche Verlagsgesellschaft Stuttgart, 269.

[292] Ekwaru, J. P., Zwicker, J. D., Holick, M. F., Giovannucci, E. & Veugelers, P. J. (2014). The importance of body weight for the dose response relationship of oral vitamin D supplementation and serum 25-hydroxyvitamin D in healthy volunteers. PLoS One, 9(11), e111265.

[293] Bor, M. V., Lydeking-Olsen, E., Moller, J. & Nexo, E. (2006). A daily intake of approximately 6 microg vitamin B12 appears to saturate all the vitamin B12-related variables in Danish postmenopausal women. Am J Clin Nutr, 83, 52–58.

[294] The minimum dose of 250 µg/day for a once-a-day intake is calculated based on the limited absorption of roughly 1.5 µg and the passive diffusion of about 1% with a requirement of 4 µg/day. There is a detailed explanation of this on pages 111–113 of our previous book *Goodbye Vegan Cliché!*.

[295] Teas, J., Pino, S., Critchley, A. & Braverman, L.E. (2004). Variability of iodine content in common commercially available edible seaweeds. Thyroid, 14(10), 836–841.

[296] Ullmann, J. (2017). *Algen – Sonderdruck aus dem Handbuch*

Lebensmittelhygiene. [*Algae – Offprint from the Guide to Food Hygiene*] Hamburg: Behr's Verlag, 13.
[297] Parekha, P. P., Khana, A. R., Torresa, M. A. & Kittoa, M. E. (2008). Concentrations of selenium, barium, and radium in Brazil nuts. J Food Compost Anal, 21, 332–335.
[298] Deutsche Gesellschaft für Ernährung [German Nutrition Society], Österreichische Gesellschaft für Ernährung [Austrian Nutrition Society], Schweizerische Gesellschaft für Ernährung [Swiss Nutrition Society]. (2015). *Referenzwerte für die Nährstoffzufuhr – Selen* [*Reference values for nutrient intake – selenium*] (4th edition). Bonn: Neuer Umschau Verlag.
[299] Gröber, U. (2011). *Mikronährstoffe – Metabolic Tuning, Prävention, Therapie* [*Micronutrients – metabolic tuning, prevention, therapy*] (3rd edition). Stuttgart: Wissenschaftliche Verlagsgesellschaft Stuttgart.
[300] Biesalski, H.K. (2016). *Vitamine und Minerale – Indikation, Diagnostik, Therapie.* [*Vitamins and minerals – indication, diagnostics, treatment*] Stuttgart: Thieme.
[301] Aro, A., Alfthan, G. & Varo, P. (1995). Effects of supplementation of fertilizers on human selenium status in Finland. Analyst, 120(3), 841–843.
[302] Hahn, A., Ströhle, A. & Wolters, M. (2016). *Ernährung – Physiologische Grundlagen, Prävention, Therapie* [*Nutrition – physiological principles, prevention, therapy*] (3rd edition). Stuttgart: Wissenschaftliche Verlagsgesellschaft Stuttgart, 351.
[303] Fuhrman, J. (2014). *Eat to Live – Das wirkungsvolle nährstoffreiche Programm für schnelles und nachhaltiges Abnehmen* [*Eat to Live – The Amazing Nutrient-Rich Program for Fast and Sustained Weight Loss*] Kandern: Unimedica, 253f.
[304] Freeland-Graves, J.H. & Nitzke, S. (2013). Position of the academy of nutrition and dietetics: total diet approach to healthy eating. J Acad Nutr Diet, 113(2), 307–317.
[305] International Food Information Council. (2011). 2011 Food and Health Survey. Accessed on 01 June 2019. Available at https://bit.ly/2HX8yFh
[306] Academy of Nutrition and Dietetics. (2011). Nutrition and you: Trends 2011. Accessed on 01 June 2019. Available at https://bit.ly/2WHtckQ
[307] Zeevi, D., Korem, T., Zmora, N., Israeli, D., Rothschild, D., Weinberger, A. et al. (2015). Personalized Nutrition by Prediction of Glycemic Responses. Cell, 163(5), 1079–1094.
[308] Freeland-Graves, J.H. & Nitzke, S. (2013). Position of the academy of nutrition and dietetics: total diet approach to healthy eating. J Acad Nutr Diet, 113(2), 307–317.
[309] Eck, B. (2017). *Starkoch Stefan Marquard begeistert das Publikum.* [*Celebrity chef Stefan Marquard amazes the audience*] Accessed on 01 June 2019. Available at https://bit.ly/2lmXe43
[310] Wolever, T. M., Jenkins, D. J., Ocana, A. M., Rao, V. A. & Collier, G. R. (1988). Second-meal effect: low-glycemic-index foods eaten at dinner improve subsequent breakfast glycemic response. Am J Clin Nutr, 48(4), 1041–1047.
[311] Johnston, C.S. & Buller, A.J. (2005). Vinegar and peanut products as complementary foods to reduce postprandial glycemia. J Am Diet Assoc, 105(12), 1939–1942.
[312] Sugiyama, M., Tang, A.C., Wakaki, Y. & Koyama, W. (2003). Glycemic index of single and mixed meal foods among common Japanese foods with white rice as a reference food. Eur J Clin Nutr, 57(6), 743–752.
[313] Törrönen, R., Sarkkinen, E., Niskanen, T., Tapola, N., Kilpi, K. & Niskanen, L. (2012). Postprandial glucose, insulin and glucagon-like peptide 1 responses to sucrose ingested with berries in healthy subjects. Br J Nutr, 107(10), 1445–1451.
[314] Watzl, B. & Leitzmann, C. (2005). *Bioaktive Substanzen in Lebensmitteln* [*Bioactive substances in foods*] (3rd edition). Stuttgart: Hippokrates Verlag.
[315] McHill, A.W., Phillips, A.J., Czeisler, C.A., Keating, L., Yee, K., Barger, L.K., et al. (2017). Later circadian timing of food intake is associated with increased body fat. Am J Clin Nutr, 106(5), 1213–1219.
[316] Ganesan, K., Habboush, Y. & Sultan, S. (2018). Intermittent Fasting: The Choice for a Healthier Lifestyle. Cureus, 10(7), e2947.
[317] Rynders, C.A., Weltman, J.I., Jiang, B., Breton, M., Patrie, J., Barrett, E.J. & Weltman, A. (2014). Effects of Exercise Intensity on Postprandial Improvement in Glucose Disposal and Insulin Sensitivity in Prediabetic Adults. J Clin Endocrinol Metab, 99(1), 220–228.
[318] Freeland-Graves, J.H. & Nitzke, S. (2013). Position of the academy of nutrition and dietetics: total diet approach to healthy eating. J Acad Nutr Diet, 113(2), 307–317.
[319] Römer-Lüthi, C. & Theobald, S. (2015). *Ernährungstherapie – Ein evidenzbasiertes Kompaktlehrbuch* [*Nutritional therapy – an evidence-based, compact textbook*] Bern: Haupt Verlag.
[320] Pramuková, B., Szabadosová, V. & Šoltésová, A. (2011). Current knowledge about sports nutrition. Australas Med J, 4(3), 107–110.
[321] Beaton, G. H. (1981). Joint FAO/WHO/UNU Expert Consultation on Energy and Protein Requirements. Accessed on 01 June 2019. Available at https://bit.ly/2Gcfdr1
[322] Mariotti, F. (2018). Plant Protein, Animal Protein, and Protein Quality. In: Mariotti, F., Hrsg.: Vegetarian and Plant-Based Diets in Health and Disease Prevention. Cambridge: Academic Press, 621–637.
[323] Yáñez, E., Uauy, R., Zacarías, I. & Barrera, G. (1986). Long-term validation of 1g of protein per kilogram body weight from a predominantly vegetable mixed diet to meet the requirements of young adult males. J Nutr, 6 (5), 865–72.
[324] Liu, A.G., Ford, N.A., Hu, F.B., Zelman, K.M., Mozaffarian, D. & Kris-Etherton, P.M. (2017). A healthy approach to dietary fats: understanding the science and taking action to reduce consumer confusion. Nutr J, 16, 53.
[325] EFSA Panel on Dietetic Products, Nutrition, and Allergies. (2010). Scientific Opinion on Dietary Reference Values for carbohydrates and dietary fibre. EFSA Journal, 8 (3), 1462.
[326] World Health Organization (WHO) (2007). Protein and Amino Acid requirements in human nutrition. Report of a joint FAO/WHO/UNU expert consultation. WHO Technical Report Series 935, Geneva, 137.
[327] Davis, B. C. & Kris-Etherton, P. M. (2003). Achieving optimal essential fatty acid status in vegetarians: current knowledge and practical implications. Am J Clin Nutr, 78(3), 640–646.
[328] Pulde, A. & Lederman, M. (2014). *The Forks Over Knives Plan: A 4-Week Meal-By-Meal Makeover.* New York: Touch Stone, 33.
[329] Lang, F. & Lang, P. (2007). *Basiswissen Physiologie* [*Basic knowledge of physiology*] (2nd edition). Heidelberg: Springer, 155.
[330] Fuhrman, J., Sarter, B., Glaser, D. & Acocella, S. (2010). Changing perceptions of hunger on a high nutrient density diet. Nutr J, 9, 51.
[331] Wright, N., Wilson, L., Smith, M., Duncan, B. & McHugh, P. (2017). The BROAD study: A randomised controlled trial using a whole food plant-based diet in the community for obesity, ischaemic heart disease or diabetes. Nutrition & Diabetes, 7, e256.
[332] Heseker, H. & Heseker, B. (2016). *Die Nährwerttabelle* [*Nutritional table*] (4th edition). Neustadt an der Weinstrasse: Neuer Umschau Buchverlag.
[333] Wrangham, R. (2009). *Feuer Fangen – Wie uns das Kochen zum Menschen machte – eine neue Theorie der menschlichen Evolution* [*Catching Fire: How Cooking Made Us Human. A new theory of human evolution*] Munich: Deutsche Verlags-Anstalt, 20.
[334] Wholewheat pasta from Rapunzel, Bolognese sauce from Alnatura, Tuscan sauce from Rapunzel, Soya Bolognese from Rapunzel, Cashews from Alnatura, Yeast flakes from Alnatura.
[335] Souci, S. W., Fachmann, W. & Kraut, H. (2016). *Die Zusammensetzung der Lebensmittel – Nährwerttabellen* [*The composition of food – nutritional value tables*] (8th edition). Stuttgart: Wissenschaftliche Verlagsgesellschaft Stuttgart, 618–635.
[336] Ornish, D., Brown, S.E., Scherwitz, L.W., Billings, J.H., Armstrong, W.T., Ports, T.A. et al. (1990). Can lifestyle changes reverse coronary heart disease? The Lifestyle Heart Trial. Lancet, 336(8708), 129–133.
[337] Esselstyn, C.B. Jr., Ellis, S.G., Medendorp, S.V., Crowe, T.D. (1995). A strategy to arrest and reverse coronary artery disease: a 5-year longitudinal study of a single physician's practice. J Fam Pract, 41(6), 560–568.
[338] Barnard, N.D., Cohen, J., Jenkins, D.J., Turner-McGrievy, G., Gloede, L., Green, A. & Ferdowsian, H. (2009). A low-fat vegan diet and a conventional diabetes diet in the treatment of type 2 diabetes: a randomized, controlled, 74-wk clinical trial. Am J Clin Nutr, 89(5), 1588–1596.
[339] McDougall, J., Thomas, L.E., McDougall, C., Moloney, G., Saul, B., Finnell, J.S., Richardson, K. & Petersen, K.M. (2014). Effects of 7 days on an *ad libitum* low-fat vegan diet: the McDougall Program cohort. Nutr J, 13, 99.
[340] Jungvogel, A., Wendt, I., Schäbethal, K., Leschik-Bonnet, E. & Oberritter, H. (2013). *Überarbeitet: Die 10 Regeln der DGE* [*Revised: the German Nutrition Society's 10 rules*] Ernährungs Umschau, 11, 644–645.
[341] German Nutrition Society (Deutsche Gesellschaft für Ernährung). (2017). *Vollwertig essen und trinken nach den 10 Regeln der DGE.* [*Healthy eating and drinking following the German Nutrition Society's 10 rules*] Accessed on 01 June 2019. Available at https://bit.ly/2nZ7SSo
[342] Willett, W.C. & Leibel, R.L. (2002). Dietary fat is not a major determinant of body fat. Am J Med, 113(9), 47–59.
[343] Sacks, F.M., Lichtenstein, A.H., Wu, J.H.Y., Appel, L.J., Creager, M.A., Kris-Etherton, P.M., (2017). Dietary Fats and Cardiovascular Disease: A Presidential Advisory From the American Heart Association. Circulation, 136(3), e1-e23.
[344] World Health Organization. (2015). FACT SHEET N°394 – Healthy Diets. Accessed on 01 June 2019. Available at https://bit.ly/2Xa8Hxr
[345] Vannice, G. & Rasmussen, H. (2014). Position of the academy of nutrition and dietetics: dietary fatty acids for healthy adults. J Acad Nutr Diet, 114(1), 136–153.

[346] German Nutrition Society (Deutsche Gesellschaft für Ernährung). (no date). *Vollwertig essen und trinken nach den 10 Regeln der DGE [Healthy eating and drinking following the German Nutrition Society's 10 rules]* Accessed on 01 June 2019. Available at https://bit.ly/1BGSSy0
[347] Richling, C. (2016). New Scientifically Validated Guidelines: Nuts and Seeds. Accessed on 01 June 2018. Available at https://bit.ly/2DVzZtG
[348] Hahn, A., Ströhle, A. & Wolters, M. (2016). *Ernährung – Physiologische Grundlagen, Prävention, Therapie [Nutrition – physiological principles, prevention, therapy]* (3rd edition). Stuttgart: Wissenschaftliche Verlagsgesellschaft Stuttgart, 99.
[349] Simopoulos, A.P. (2002). The importance of the ratio of omega-6/omega-3 essential fatty acids. Biomed Pharmacother, 56(8), 365–379.
[350] Davis, B. C. & Kris-Etherton, P. M. (2003). Achieving optimal essential fatty acid status in vegetarians: current knowledge and practical implications. Am J Clin Nutr, 78(3), 640–646.
[351] Institute of Medicine Food and Nutrition Board. (2005). Dietary Reference Intakes for Energy, Carbohydrate, Fiber, Fat, Fatty Acids, Cholesterol, Protein, and Amino Acids. Washington: National Academy Press.
[352] Deutsche Gesellschaft für Ernährung [German Nutrition Society], Österreichische Gesellschaft für Ernährung [Austrian Nutrition Society], Schweizerische Gesellschaft für Ernährung [Swiss Nutrition Society]. (2015). *Referenzwerte für die Nährstoffzufuhr – Essenzielle Fettsäuren. [Reference values for nutrient intake – essential fatty acids]* (2nd edition). Bonn: Neuer Umschau Buchverlag.
[353] Institute of Medicine Food and Nutrition Board. (2005). *Dietary Reference Intakes for Energy, Carbohydrate, Fiber, Fat, Fatty Acids, Cholesterol, Protein, and Amino Acids.* Washington: National Academy Press.
[354] Brenna, J. T. (2002). Efficiency of conversion of alpha-linolenic acid to long chain n-3 fatty acids in man. Curr Opin Clin Nutr Metab Care, 5(2), 127–132.
[355] Simopoulos, A. P. (2002). The importance of the ratio of omega-6/ omega-3 essential fatty acids. Biomed Pharmacother, 56(8), 365–379.
[356] Brown, M.J., Ferruzzi, M.G., Nguyen, M.L., Cooper, D.A., Eldridge, A.L., Schwartz, S.J. & White, W.S. (2004). Carotenoid bioavailability is higher from salads ingested with full-fat than with fat-reduced salad dressings as measured with electrochemical detection. Am J Clin Nutr, 80(2), 396–403.
[357] Brown, M.J., Ferruzzi, M.G., Nguyen, M.L., Cooper, D.A., Eldridge, A.L., Schwartz, S.J. & White, W.S. (2004). Carotenoid bioavailability is higher from salads ingested with full-fat than with fat-reduced salad dressings as measured with electrochemical detection. Am J Clin Nutr, 80(2), 396–403.
[358] Cuomo, J. Appendino, G., Dern, A.S., Schneider, E., McKinnon, T.P., Brown, M.J., Togni, S. & Dixon, B.M. (2011). Comparative absorption of a standardized curcuminoid mixture and its lecithin formulation. J Nat Prod, 74(4), 664–669.
[359] Yuan, X., Liu, X., McClements, D.J., Cao, Y. & Xiao, H. (2018). Enhancement of phytochemical bioaccessibility from plant-based foods using excipient emulsions: impact of lipid type on carotenoid solubilization from spinach. Food Funct, 19(8), 4352–4365.
[360] Albahrani, A.A., & Greaves, R.F. (2016). Fat-Soluble Vitamins: Clinical Indications and Current Challenges for Chromatographic Measurement. The Clinical Biochemist Reviews, 37(1), 27–47.
[361] Dawson-Hughes, B., Harris, S.S., Lichtenstein, A.H., Dolnikowski, G., Palermo, N.J., Rasmussen, H. (2015). Dietary fat increases vitamin D-3 absorption. J Acad Nutr Diet. 115(2), 225–30.
[362] Jeanes, Y.M., Hall, W.L., Ellard, S., Lee, E. & Lodge, J.K. (2004). The absorption of vitamin E is influenced by the amount of fat in a meal and the food matrix. Br J Nutr, 92(4), 575–579.
[363] Institute of Medicine (2001). Panel on Micronutrients: Dietary Reference Intakes for Vitamin A, Vitamin K, Arsenic, Boron, Chromium, Copper, Iodine, Iron, Manganese, Molybdenum, Nickel, Silicon, Vanadium, and Zinc. Washington, DC: National Academies Press.
[364] Davidson, M.H., Johnson, J., Rooney, M.W., Kyle, M.L. & Kling, D.F. (2012). A novel omega-3 free fatty acid formulation has dramatically improved bioavailability during a low-fat diet compared with omega-3-acid ethyl esters: the ECLIPSE (Epanova(®) compared to Lovaza(®) in a pharmacokinetic single-dose evaluation) study. J Clin Lipidol. 6(6), 573–584.
[365] Richter, M., Boeing, H., Grünewald-Funk, D., Heseker, H., Kroke, A., Leschik-Bonnet, E., Oberritter, H., Strohm, D. & Watzl, B. (2016). Position der Deutschen Gesellschaft für Ernährung e. V. (DGE) – Vegane Ernährung. [Position of the German Nutrition Society – vegan diet] Ernährungs Umschau, 63(04), 92–102.
[366] Gupta, R. K., Gangoliya, S. S. & Singh, N. K. (2015). Reduction of phytic acid and enhancement of bioavailable micronutrients in food grains. J Food Sci Technol, 52(2), 676–684.
[367] Watzl, B. & Leitzmann, C. (2005). *Bioaktive Substanzen in Lebensmitteln [Bioactive substances in foods]* (3rd edition). Stuttgart: Hippokrates Verlag, 23.
[368] Schlemmer, U., Frølich, W., Prieto, R. M. & Grases, F. (2009). Phytate in foods and significance for humans: food sources, intake, processing, bioavailability, protective role and analysis. Mol Nutr Food Res, 53(2), 330–375.
[369] Gupta, R. K., Gangoliya, S. S. & Singh, N. K. (2013). Reduction of phytic acid and enhancement of bioavailable micronutrients in food grains. J Food Sci Technol, 52(2), 676–684.
[370] Fidler, M. C., Davidsson, L., Zeder, C. & Hurrell, R. F. (2004). Erythorbic acid is a potent enhancer of nonheme-iron absorption. Am J Clin Nutr, 79(1), 99–102.
[371] Souci, S. W., Fachmann, W. & Kraut, H. (2016). *Die Zusammensetzung der Lebensmittel Nährwerttabellen [The composition of food – nutritional tables]* (8th edition). Stuttgart: Wissenschaftliche Verlagsgesellschaft Stuttgart.
[372] Hallberg, L. (1981). Bioavailability of dietary iron in man. Annu Rev Nutr, 1, 123–147.
[373] Gibson, R.S., Perlas, L. & Hotz C. (2006). Improving the bioavailability of nutrients in plant foods at the household level. Proc Nutr Soc, 65(2), 160–168.
[374] Souci, S. W., Fachmann, W. & Kraut, H. (2016). *Die Zusammensetzung der Lebensmittel Nährwerttabellen [The composition of food – nutritional tables]* (8th edition). Stuttgart: Wissenschaftliche Verlagsgesellschaft Stuttgart.
[375] Souci, S. W., Fachmann, W. & Kraut, H. (2016). *Die Zusammensetzung der Lebensmittel Nährwerttabellen [The composition of food – nutritional tables]* (8th edition). Stuttgart: Wissenschaftliche Verlagsgesellschaft Stuttgart.
[376] Gillooly, M., Bothwell, T. H., Torrance, J. D., MacPhail, A. P., Derman, D. P., Bezwoda, W. R. et al. (1983). The effects of organic acids, phytates and polyphenols on the absorption of iron from vegetables. Br J Nutr, 49(3), 331–342.
[377] Baynes, R. D., Macfarlane, B. J., Bothwell, T. H., Siegenberg, D., Bezwoda, W. R., Schmidt, U., et al. (1990). The promotive effect of soy sauce on iron absorption in human subjects. Eur J Clin Nutr, 44(6), 419–424.
[378] García-Casal, M. N., Layrisse, M., Solano, L. & Tropper, E. (1998). Vitamin A and beta-carotene can improve nonheme iron absorption from rice, wheat and corn by humans. J Nutr, 128, 646–650.
[379] Layrisse, M., García-Casal, M. N., Solano, L., Barón, M. A., Arguello, F., Llovera, D. et al. (2000). New property of vitamin A and beta-carotene on human iron absorption: effect on phytate and polyphenols as inhibitors of iron absorption. Arch Latinoam Nutr, 50(3), 243–248.
[380] Gautam, S., Platel, K. & Srinivasan, K. (2010). Higher bioaccessibility of iron and zinc from food grains in the presence of garlic and onion. J Agric Food Chem, 58(14), 8426–8429.
[381] Sandström, B. & Cederblad, A. (1987). Effect of ascorbic acid on the absorption of zinc and calcium in man. Int J Vitam Nutr Res. 57(1), 87-90.
[382] Morcos, S.R., El-Shobaki, F.A., El-Hawary, Z. & Saleh, N. (1976). Effect of vitamin C and carotene on the absorption of calcium from the intestine. Z Ernahrungswiss, 15(4), 387–390.
[383] Aloia, J.F., Dhaliwal, R., Shieh, A., Mikhail, M., Fazzari, M., Ragolia, L. & Abrams, S.A. (2014). Vitamin D supplementation increases calcium absorption without a threshold effect. Am J Clin Nutr, 99(3), 624–631.
[384] Mangano, K.M., Sahni, S. & Kerstetter, K.E. (2014). Dietary protein is beneficial to bone health under conditions of adequate calcium intake: an update on clinical research. Curr Opin Clin Nutr Metab Care, 17(1), 69-74.
[385] Shiowatana, J., Purawatt, S., Sottimai, U., Taebunpakul, S. & Siripinyanond, A. (2006). Enhancement effect study of some organic acids on the calcium availability of vegetables: application of the dynamic in vitro simulated gastrointestinal digestion method with continuous-flow dialysis. J Agric Food Chem, 54(24), 9010–9016.
[386] Carlson, J.L., Erickson, J.M., Lloyd, B.B. & Slavin, J.L. (2018). Health Effects and Sources of Prebiotic Dietary Fiber. Curr Dev Nutr, 2(3), nzy005.
[387] Abrams, S.A., Hawthorne, K.M., Aliu, O., Hicks, P.D., Chen, Z. & Griffin, I.J. (2007). An inulin-type fructan enhances calcium absorption primarily via an effect on colonic absorption in humans. J Nutr, 137(10), 2208–2212.
[388] Roberfroid, M.B. (2007). Inulin-type fructans: functional food ingredients. J Nutr, 137(11), 2493–2502.
[389] Lönnerdal, B. (2000). Dietary factors influencing zinc absorption. J Nutr. 130(5), 1378S–83.
[390] Gautam, S., Platel, K. & Srinivasan, K. (2010). Higher bioaccessibility of iron and zinc from food grains in the presence of garlic and onion. J Agric Food Chem, 58(14), 8426–8429.
[391] Scholz-Ahrens, K.E., Schaafsma, G., van den Heuvel, E.G. & Schrezenmeir, J. (2001). Effects of prebiotics on mineral metabolism. Am J Clin Nutr, 73(2), 459-464.
[392] Sandström, B. & Cederblad, A. (1987). Effect of ascorbic acid on the absorption of zinc and calcium in man. Int J Vitam Nutr Res, 57(1), 87–90.
[393] Gupta, R. K., Gangoliya, S. S. & Singh, N. K. (2013). Reduction of phytic acid and enhancement of bioavailable micronutrients in food grains. J Food Sci Technol, 52(2), 676–684.

[394] Watzl, B. & Leitzmann, C. (2005). Bioaktive Substanzen in Lebensmitteln [Bioactive substances in foods] (3rd edition). Stuttgart: Hippokrates.
[395] German Nutrition Society (Deutsche Gesellschaft für Ernährung). (2015). *Sekundäre Pflanzenstoffe und ihre Wirkungen auf die Gesundheit: Farbenfrohe Vielfalt mit Potenzial. [Secondary plant substances and their impact on health: colourful variety with potential]* Accessed on 01 June 2019. Available at https://bit.ly/2MNqExB
[396] Craig, W.J. (1997). Phytochemicals: guardians of our health. J Am Diet Assoc, 10(2), 199–204.
[397] Watzl, B. & Leitzmann, C. (2005). *Bioaktive Substanzen in Lebensmitteln [Bioactive substances in foods]* (3rd edition). Stuttgart: Hippokrates, 15.
[398] Semler, E. (2013). *Sekundäre Pflanzenstoffe – Substanzen mit vielen Unbekannten. [Secondary plant substances – substances with plenty of unknowns]* UGB-Forum, 2, 58–61.
[399] Leopold A.C. & Ardrey, R. (1972). Toxic substances in plants and the food habits of early man. Science. 1972 May 5;176(4034), 512–514.
[400] Watzl, B. (2008). *Einfluss sekundärer Pflanzenstoffe auf die Gesundheit. [Influence of secondary plant substances on health]* In: German Nutrition Society (Deutsche Gesellschaft für Ernährung), Publ.: Ernährungsbericht 2008. [nutrition report] Bonn: DGE, 335–379.
[401] Watzl, B. & Leitzmann, C. (2005). *Bioaktive Substanzen in Lebensmitteln [Bioactive substances in foods]* (3rd edition). Stuttgart: Hippokrates, 15.
[402] Heber, D. (1997). The stinking rose: organosulfur compounds and cancer. Am J Clin Nutr, 66(2), 425–426.
[403] Steinmetz, K.A. & Potter, J.D. (1991). Vegetables, fruit, and cancer. I. Epidemiology. Cancer Causes Control, 2(5), 325–357.
[404] Leitzmann, C. (2016). Characteristics and Health Benefits of Phytochemicals. Forsch Komplementmed, 23(2), 69–74.
[405] Khoo, H.E., Azlan, A., Tang, S.T. & Li, S.M. (2017). Anthocyanidins and anthocyanins: colored pigments as food, pharmaceutical ingredients, and the potential health benefits. Food Nutr Res, 61(1), 1361779.
[406] Nagpal, M. & Sood, S. (2013). Role of curcumin in systemic and oral health: An overview. J Nat Sci Biol Med, 4(1), 3–7.
[407] Leitzmann, C. (2016). Characteristics and Health Benefits of Phytochemicals. Forsch Komplementmed, 23(2), 69-74.
[408] Stahl, W. & Sies, H. (1996). Lycopene: a biologically important carotenoid for humans? Arch Biochem Biophys, 336(1), 1–9.
[409] Paiva, S.A. & Russell, R.M. (1999). Beta-carotene and other carotenoids as antioxidants. J Am Coll Nutr, 18(5), 426–433.
[410] Leitzmann, C. (2016). Characteristics and Health Benefits of Phytochemicals. Forsch Komplementmed, 23(2), 69–74.
[411] Brown, M.J., Ferruzzi, M.G., Nguyen, M.L., Cooper, D.A., Eldridge, A.L., Schwartz, S.J. & White, W.S. (2004). Carotenoid bioavailability is higher from salads ingested with full-fat than with fat-reduced salad dressings as measured with electrochemical detection. Am J Clin Nutr, 80(2), 396–403.
[412] German Nutrition Society (*Deutsche Gesellschaft für Ernährung*). (2014). *Sekundäre Pflanzenstoffe und ihre Wirkung auf die Gesundheit – Eine Aktualisierung anhand des Ernährungsberichts 2012. [Secondary plant substances and their impact on health – an update based on the 2012 nutrition report]* DGEinfo, 12, 178–186.
[413] Wang, E. & Wink, M. (2016). Chlorophyll enhances oxidative stress tolerance in *Caenorhabditis elegans* and extends its lifespan. PeerJ, 4, e1879.
[414] Jubert, C., Mata, J., Bench, G., Dashwood, R., Pereira, C., Tracewell, W. et al. (2009). Effects of chlorophyll and chlorophyllin on low-dose aflatoxin B1 pharmacokinetics in human volunteers. Cancer Prev Res (Phila). 2(12), 1015–1022.
[415] He, F.J., Li, J. & Macgregor, G.A. (2013). Effect of longer term modest salt reduction on blood pressure: Cochrane systematic review and meta-analysis of randomised trials. BMJ, 346, 1325.
[416] Cook, N.R., Appel, L.J. & Whelton, P.K. (2014). Lower levels of sodium intake and reduced cardiovascular risk. Circulation. 129 (9), 981–9.
[417] Whelton, P.K., Appel, L.J., Sacco, R.L., Anderson, C.A., Antman, E.M., Campbell, N. et al. (2012). Sodium, blood pressure, and cardiovascular disease: further evidence supporting the American Heart Association sodium reduction recommendations. Circulation, 126 (24), 2880–9.
[418] D'Elia, L., Rossi, G., Ippolito, R., Cappuccio, F.P. & Strazzullo, P. (2012). Habitual salt intake and risk of gastric cancer: a meta-analysis of prospective studies. Clin Nutr, 31 (4), 489–98.
[419] German Nutrition Society (*Deutsche Gesellschaft für Ernährung*) e. V. (2016). *Ausgewählte Fragen und Antworten zu Speisesalz. [Selected questions and answers on table salt]* Accessed on 01 June 2019. Available at https://bit.ly/2F0TZAo
[420] Academy of Nutrition and Dietetics. (2017). Eating Right with Less Salt. Accessed on 01 June 2019. Available at https://bit.ly/2lMUMuo
[421] American Institute for Cancer Research. (2013). Nutrition for Healthy Aging. Accessed on 1 June 2019. Available at https://bit.ly/2F21C9S
[422] World Cancer Research Fund International. (2017). Cancer Prevention & Survival – Summary of global evidence on diet, weight, physical activity & what increases or decreases your risk of cancer. Accessed on 01 June 2019. Available at https://bit.ly/2sH1eE3
[423] American Heart Association. (2013). *Eat Less Salt: An Easy Action Plan for Finding and Reducing the Sodium Hidden in Your Diet*. New York: Harmony.
[424] Deutsche Herzstiftung. [German heart foundation] (2014). *Ernährung bei Herzschwäche. [Diet and cardiac insufficiency]* Accessed on 01 June 2019. Available at https://bit.ly/2FbwEeK
[425] Hahn, A., Ströhle, A. & Wolters, M. (2016). *Ernährung – Physiologische Grundlagen, Prävention, Therapie [Nutrition – physiological principles, prevention, therapy]* (3rd edition). Stuttgart: Wissenschaftliche Verlagsgesellschaft, 272.
[426] World Health Organization. (2012). Guideline: Sodium intake for adults and children. Accessed on 01 June 2019. Available at https://bit.ly/1gEfuyo
[427] American Heart Association. (2017). Why Should I Limit Sodium? Accessed on 01 June 2019. Available at https://bit.ly/1FdpqOL
[428] Deutsche Gesellschaft für Ernährung [German Nutrition Society], Österreichische Gesellschaft für Ernährung [Austrian Nutrition Society], Schweizerische Gesellschaft für Ernährung [Swiss Nutrition Society]. (2015). *Referenzwerte für die Nährstoffzufuhr – Natrium, Chlorid, Kalium [Reference values for nutrient intake – sodium, chloride, potassium]* (2nd edition). Bonn: Neuer Umschau Buchverlag.
[429] *Statista.* [German market research company] (2018). Proportion of the German population who exceed or consume less than the recommended daily requirement for salt. Accessed on 01 June 2019. Available at https://bit.ly/31Gen1p
[430] *Bundesministerium für Ernährung und Landwirtschaft. [German Federal Ministry for Food and Agriculture]* (no date) Results of the DEGS study [on adult health in Germany] Accessed on 01 June 2019. Available at https://bit.ly/2QzMcLM
[431] GBD 2017 Diet Collaborators. (2019). Health effects of dietary risks in 195 countries, 1990–2017: a systematic analysis for the Global Burden of Disease Study 2017. Lancet, 0140-6736(19), 30041–30048.
[432] www.food.gov.uk/research/national-diet-and-nutrition-survey-ndns/national-diet-and-nutrition-survey-ndns-assessment-of-dietary-sodium
[433] Blais, C.A., Pangborn, R.M., Borhani, N.O., Ferrell, M.F., Prineas, R.J. & Laing, B. (1986). Effect of dietary sodium restriction on taste responses to sodium chloride: a longitudinal study. Am J Clin Nutr, 44(2), 232–243.
[434] Blais, C.A., Pangborn, R.M., Borhani, N.O., Ferrell, M.F., Prineas, R.J. & Laing, B. (1986). Effect of dietary sodium restriction on taste responses to sodium chloride: a longitudinal study. Am J Clin Nutr, 44(2), 232–243.
[435] "Blood pressure salt" is sold in Germany by companies such as Dr. Jacob's® and Raab Vitalfood.
[436] Information taken from the product description for Dr. Jacob's® Blutdrucksalz [low-sodium salt]. Accessed on 01 June 2019. Available at https://www.zurrose.de/media/lmiv/07783169.pdf
[437] Salt-free vegetable and herb mixes are sold in Germany by companies such as Sonnentor and VeggiePur®.
[438] Hirayama, T. (1982). Relationship of soybean paste soup intake to gastric cancer risk. Nutr Cancer, 3(4), 223–233.
[439] Streppel, M.T., Arends, L.R., van't Veer, P., Grobbee, D.E. & Geleijnse, J.M. (2005). Dietary fiber and blood pressure: a meta-analysis of randomized placebo-controlled trials. Arch Intern Med, 165(2), 150–156.
[440] Geleijnse, J.M., Kok, F.J. & Grobbee, D.E. (2003). Blood pressure response to changes in sodium and potassium intake: a metaregression analysis of randomised trials. J Hum Hypertens, 17(7), 471–80.
[441] Gupta, C. & Prakash, D. (2014). Phytonutrients as therapeutic agents. J Complement Integr Med, 11(3), 151–169.
[442] Brown, L., Rosner, B., Willett, W.W., Sacks, F.M. (1999). Cholesterol-lowering effects of dietary fiber: a meta-analysis. Am J Clin Nutr. 69 (1), 30-42.
[443] Hahn, A., Ströhle, A. & Wolters, M. (2016). *Ernährung – Physiologische Grundlagen, Prävention, Therapie [Nutrition – physiological principles, prevention, therapy]* (3rd edition). Stuttgart: Wissenschaftliche Verlagsgesellschaft, 141.
[444] Peel, M. (1997). Hunger Strikes. BMJ, 315, 829.
[445] Deutsche Gesellschaft für Ernährung [German Nutrition Society], Österreichische Gesellschaft für Ernährung [Austrian Nutrition Society], Schweizerische Gesellschaft für Ernährung [Swiss Nutrition Society]. (Hrsg.) (2015). *Referenzwerte für die Nährstoffzufuhr – Wasser [Reference values for nutrient intake – water]* (2nd edition). Bonn: Neuer Umschau Buchverlag.

[446] Insel, P., Ross, D., McMahon, K., & Bernstein, M. (2017). *Nutrition* (6. Edition). Burlington: Jones & Bartlett Learning, 473.
[447] Pross, N., Demazières, A., Girard, N., Barnouin, R., Santoro, F., Chevillotte, E., Klein, A. & Le Bellego, L. (2013). Influence of progressive fluid restriction on mood and physiological markers of dehydration in women. Br J Nutr, 109(2), 313–321.
[448] Chan, J., Knutsen, S.F., Blix, G.G., Lee, J.W., Fraser, G.E. (2002). Water, other fluids, and fatal coronary heart disease: the Adventist Health Study. Am J Epidemiol, 155 (9), 827–33.
[449] Hahn, A., Ströhle, A. & Wolters, M. (2016). *Ernährung – Physiologische Grundlagen, Prävention, Therapie [Nutrition – physiological principles, prevention, therapy]* (3rd edition). Stuttgart: Wissenschaftliche Verlagsgesellschaft, 146.
[450] Hahn, A., Ströhle, A. & Wolters, M. (2016). *Ernährung – Physiologische Grundlagen, Prävention, Therapie [Nutrition – physiological principles, prevention, therapy]* (3rd edition). Stuttgart: Wissenschaftliche Verlagsgesellschaft, 146.
[451] Hahn, A., Ströhle, A. & Wolters, M. (2016). *Ernährung – Physiologische Grundlagen, Prävention, Therapie [Nutrition – physiological principles, prevention, therapy]* (3rd edition). Stuttgart: Wissenschaftliche Verlagsgesellschaft, 146.
[452] Popkin, B.M., D'Anci, K.E. & Rosenberg, I.H. (2010). Water, Hydration and Health. Nutr Rev, 68(8), 439–458.
[453] Köhnke, K. (2011). *Der Wasserhaushalt und die ernährungsphysiologische Bedeutung von Wasser und Getränken [Water balance and the nutritional significance of water and drinks]* Ernährungs Umschau, 2, 88–95.
[454] Köhnke, K. (2011). *Der Wasserhaushalt und die ernährungsphysiologische Bedeutung von Wasser und Getränken [Water balance and the nutritional significance of water and drinks]* Ernährungs Umschau, 2, 88–95.
[455] Deutsche Gesellschaft für Ernährung [German Nutrition Society], Österreichische Gesellschaft für Ernährung [Austrian Nutrition Society], Schweizerische Gesellschaft für Ernährung [Swiss Nutrition Society]. (Publ.) (2015). *Referenzwerte für die Nährstoffzufuhr – Wasser [Reference values for nutrient intake – water]* (2nd edition). Bonn: Neuer Umschau Buchverlag.
[456] Deutsche Gesellschaft für Ernährung [German Nutrition Society], Österreichische Gesellschaft für Ernährung [Austrian Nutrition Society], Schweizerische Gesellschaft für Ernährung [Swiss Nutrition Society]. (Publ.) (2015). *Referenzwerte für die Nährstoffzufuhr – Wasser [Reference values for nutrient intake – water]* (2nd edition). Bonn: Neuer Umschau Buchverlag.
[457] Popkin, B.M., Armstrong, L.E., Bray, G.M., Caballero, B., Frei, B. & Willett, W.C. (2006). A new proposed guidance system for beverage consumption in the United States. Am J Clin Nutr, 83(3), 529–542.
[458] Amy Pogue provides lots of inspirational ideas for different kinds of infused water free of charge at www.infusedwaters.com
[459] Onakpoya, I., Spencer, E., Heneghan, C. & Thompson M. (2014). The effect of green tea on blood pressure and lipid profile: a systematic review and meta-analysis of randomized clinical trials. Nutr Metab Cardiovasc Dis, 24 (8), 823–36.
[460] Khalesi, S., Sun, J., Buys, N., Jamshidi, A., Nikbakht-Nasrabadi, E. & Khosravi-Boroujeni H. (2014). Green tea catechins and blood pressure: a systematic review and meta-analysis of randomised controlled trials. Eur J Nutr. 53 (6), 1299–311.
[461] Liu, K., Zhou, R., Wang, B., Chen, K., Shi, LY., Zhu, J.D., Mi, M.T. (2013). Effect of green tea on glucose control and insulin sensitivity: a meta-analysis of 17 randomized controlled trials. Am J Clin Nutr, 98 (2), 340–348.
[462] Caldeira, D., Martins, C., Alves, L.B., Pereira, H., Ferreira, J.J. & Costa, J. (2013). Caffeine does not increase the risk of atrial fibrillation: a systematic review and meta-analysis of observational studies. Heart, 99(19), 1383–1389.
[463] Malerba, S., Turati, F., Galeone, C., Pelucchi, C., Verga, F., La Vecchia, C. & Tavani, A. (2013). A meta-analysis of prospective studies of coffee consumption and mortality for all causes, cancers and cardiovascular diseases. Eur J Epidemiol, 28(7), 527–539.
[464] Souci, S. W., Fachmann, W. & Kraut, H. (2016). *Die Zusammensetzung der Lebensmittel – Nährwerttabellen [The composition of food – nutritional tables]* (8th edition). Stuttgart: Wissenschaftliche Verlagsgesellschaft.
[465] EU Commission (2008). Commission Regulation (EC) No 889/2008. Official Journal of the European Union. Accessed on 1 June 2019. Available at http://bit.ly/2GzmzGm
[466] The article "Responsible Juicing", and other articles and recipes, can be found at www.juicingbook.com
[467] Stockwell, T., Zhao, J., Panwar, S., Roemer, A., Naimi, T. & Chikritzhs, T. (2016). Do 'Moderate' Drinkers Have Reduced Mortality Risk? A Systematic Review and Meta-Analysis of Alcohol Consumption and All-Cause Mortality. J Stud Alcohol Drugs, 77(2), 185–198.
[468] Maggs, J.L. & Staff, J. (2017). No Benefit of Light to Moderate Drinking for Mortality From Coronary Heart Disease When Better Comparison Groups and Controls Included: A Commentary on Zhao et al. (2017). J Stud Alcohol Drugs, 78(3), 387–388.
[469] Jiang, P. & Turek, F.W. (2017). Timing of meals: when is as critical as what and how much. Am J Physiol Endocrinol Metab, 312(5), 369–380.
[470] Hill, P. (1991). It is not what you eat, but how you eat it, digestion, life-style, nutrition. Nutrition, 7(6), 385–395.
[471] Vanderschelden, M. (2016). *The Scientific Approach to Intermittent Fasting*. USA: Dr. Michael Vanderschleden (Self Publishing), 21.
[472] Melkani, G.C. & Panda, S. (2017). Time-restricted feeding for prevention and treatment of cardiometabolic disorders. J Physiol, 595(12), 3691–3700.
[473] St-Onge, M.-P., Ard, J., Baskin, M.L., Chiuve, S.E., Johnson, H.E., Kris-Etherton, P. & Varady, K. (2017). Meal Timing and Frequency: Implications for Cardiovascular Disease Prevention: A Scientific Statement From the American Heart Association. Circulation, 135, e96–e121.
[474] Fung, J. & Moore, J. (2018). *Fasten – das große Handbuch. [Fasting – the big handbook]* Munich: Riva, 159.
[475] Kast, B. & Baur, M. (2019). *Der Ernährungskompass – Das Kochbuch. [The nutritional compass – the cookbook]* Munich: C. Bertelsmann, 34.
[476] Kessler, K., Hornemann, S., Petzke, K.J., Kemper, M., Kramer, A., Pfeiffer, A.F. et al. (2017). The effect of diurnal distribution of carbohydrates and fat on glycaemic control in humans: a randomized controlled trial. Sci Rep, 7, 44170.
[477] Fung, J. & Moore, J. (2018). *Fasten – das große Handbuch. [Fasting – the big handbook]* Munich: Riva, 159.
[478] Kast, B. & Baur, M. (2019). *Der Ernährungskompass – Das Kochbuch. [The nutritional compass – the cookbook]* Munich: C. Bertelsmann, 34.
[479] Kessler, K., Hornemann, S., Petzke, K.J., Kemper, M., Kramer, A., Pfeiffer, A.F. et al. (2017). The effect of diurnal distribution of carbohydrates and fat on glycaemic control in humans: a randomized controlled trial. Sci Rep, 7, 44170.
[480] Fung, J. & Moore, J. (2018). *Fasten – das große Handbuch. [Fasting – the big handbook]* Munich: Riva, 163.
[481] Sofer, S., Stark, A.H. & Madar, Z. (2015). Nutrition Targeting by Food Timing: Time-Related Dietary Approaches to Combat Obesity and Metabolic Syndrome. Adv Nutr, 6(2), 214–223.
[482] Arble, D.M., Bass, J., Laposky, A.D., Vitaterna, M.H. & Turek, F.W. (2009). Circadian timing of food intake contributes to weight gain. Obesity (Silver Spring), 7, 2100–2102.
[483] McHill, A.W., Phillips, A.J., Czeisler, C.A., Keating, L., Yee, K., Barger, L.K., Garaulet, M., Scheer, F.A. & Klerman, E.B. (2017). Later circadian timing of food intake is associated with increased body fat. Am J Clin Nutr, 106(5), 1213–1219.
[484] Ruddick-Collins, L.C., Johnston, J.D., Morgan, P.J. & Johnstone, A.M. (2018). The Big Breakfast Study: Chrono-nutrition influence on energy expenditure and bodyweight. Nutr Bull, 43(2), 174–183.
[485] Jakubowicz, D., Barnea, M., Wainstein, J. & Froy, O. (2013). High caloric intake at breakfast vs. dinner differentially influences weight loss of overweight and obese women. Obesity (Silver Spring), 21(12), 2504–2512.
[486] Huseinovic, E., Winkvist, A., Freisling, H., Slimani, N., Boeing, H. & Buckland, G. (2019). Timing of eating across ten European countries – results from the European Prospective Investigation into Cancer and Nutrition (EPIC) calibration study. Public Health Nutr, 22(2), 324–335.
[487] Van Cauter, E., Shapiro, E.T., Tilli, I. H. & Polonsky, K.S. (1992). Circadian modulation of glucose and insulin responses to meals: relationship to cortisol rhythm. Am J Physiol, 262(4), 467–475.
[488] Hutchison, A.T., Wittert, G.A. & Heilbronn, L.K. (2017). Matching Meals to Body Clocks – Impact on Weight and Glucose Metabolism. Nutrients, 9(3), 222.
[489] Kessler, K., Hornemann, S., Petzke, K.J., Kemper, M., Kramer, A., Pfeiffer, A.F., Pivovarova, O. & Rudovich, N. (2017). The effect of diurnal distribution of carbohydrates and fat on glycaemic control in humans: a randomized controlled trial. Sci Rep, 7, 44170.
[490] Borghouts, L.B. & Keizer, H.A. (2000). Exercise and insulin sensitivity: a review. Int J Sports Med, 21(1), 1–12.
[491] Gill, S. & Panda, S. (2015). A Smartphone App Reveals Erratic Diurnal Eating Patterns in Humans that Can Be Modulated for Health Benefits. Cell Metab, 22(5), 789–798.
[492] Lao, X.Q., Liu, X., Deng, H., Chan, T., Ho, K.F., Wang, F. et al. (2015). Sleep Quality, Sleep Duration, and the Risk of Coronary Heart Disease: A Prospective Cohort Study With 60,586 Adults. J Clin Sleep Med, 14(1), 109–117.
[493] Arora, T. & Taheri, S. (2015). Sleep Optimization and Diabetes Control: A Review of the Literature. Diabetes Ther, 6(4), 425–468.
[494] Sutton, E.F., Beyl, R., Early, K.S., Cefalu, W.T., Ravussin, E. & Peterson, C.M. (2018). Early Time-Restricted Feeding Improves Insulin Sensitivity, Blood

Pressure, and Oxidative Stress Even without Weight Loss in Men with Prediabetes. Cell Metab, 27(6), 1212–1221.
[495] Malinowski, B., Zalewska, K., Węsierska, A., Sokołowska, M.M., Socha, M., Liczner, G., Pawlak-Osińska, K. & Wiciński, M. (2019). Intermittent Fasting in Cardiovascular Disorders – An Overview. Nutrients, 11(3), 673.
[496] Gabel, K., Hoddy, K.K., Haggerty, N., Song, J., Kroeger, C.M., Trepanowski, J.F., Panda, S. & Varadya, K.A. (2018). Effects of 8-hour time restricted feeding on body weight and metabolic disease risk factors in obese adults: A pilot study. Nutr Healthy Aging, 4(4), 345–353.
[497] Cherif, A., Roelands, B., Meeusen, R. & Chamari, K. (2016). Effects of Intermittent Fasting, Caloric Restriction, and Ramadan Intermittent Fasting on Cognitive Performance at Rest and During Exercise in Adults. Sports Med, 46(1), 35–47.
[498] Mattson, M.P., Longo, V.D. & Harvied, M. (2017). Impact of intermittent fasting on health and disease processes. Ageing Res Rev, 39, 46–58.
[499] Antunes, F., Erustes, A.G., Costa, A.J., Nascimento, A.J., Bincoletto, C., Ureshino, R.P. et al. (2018). Autophagy and intermittent fasting: the connection for cancer therapy? Clinics (Sao Paulo), 73, e814.
[500] Longo, V.D. & Panda, S. (2016). Fasting, circadian rhythms, and time restricted feeding in healthy lifespan. Cell Metab, 23(6), 1048–1059.
[501] Rubinsztein, D.C., Mariño, G. & Kroemer, G. (2011). Autophagy and aging. Cell, 146(5), 682–695.
[502] Gröber, U. (2008). *Orthomolekulare Medizin: Ein Leitfaden für Apotheker und Ärzte*. [*Orthomolecular medicine: a guide for pharmacists and doctors*] (3rd edition). Stuttgart: Wissenschaftliche Verlagsgesellschaft.
[503] Guallar, E., Stranges, S., Mulrow, C., Appel, L.J. & Miller, E.R. (2013). Enough is enough: Stop wasting money on vitamin and mineral supplements. Ann Intern Med, 159(12), 850–851.
[504] Bjelakovic, G., Nikolova, D. & Gluud, C. (2013). Antioxidant supplements to prevent mortality. JAMA, 310(11), 1178–1179.
[505] Miller, E.R., Pastor-Barriuso, R., Dalal, D., Riemersma, R.A., Appel, L.J. & Guallar, E. (2005). Meta-analysis: high-dosage vitamin E supplementation may increase all-cause mortality, Ann Intern Med, 14237–14246.
[506] Max Rubner-Institut, *Bundesforschungsinstitut für Ernährung und Lebensmittel* [*Federal research institute for nutrition and food*] (2008). *Nationale Verzehrsstudie 2, Ergebnisbericht, Teil 2 – Die bundesweite Befragung zur Ernährung von Jugendlichen und Erwachsenen*. [*National consumption survey 2, report, part 2 – The German diet survey for young people and adults*] Accessed on 1 June 2019. Available at http://bit.ly/23d1feH
[507] Schüpbach, R., Wegmüller, R., Berguerand, C., Bui, M. & Herter-Aeberli, I. (2017). Micronutrient status and intake in omnivores, vegetarians and vegans in Switzerland. Eur J Nutr, 56(1),283–293.
[508] Craig, W.J. (2009). Health effects of vegan diets. Am J Clin Nutr, 89(5), 1627–1633.
[509] Schüpbach, R., Wegmüller, R., Berguerand, C., Bui, M. & Herter-Aeberli, I. (2017). Micronutrient status and intake in omnivores, vegetarians and vegans in Switzerland. Eur J Nutr, 56(1),283–293.
[510] Sobiecki, J.G., Appleby, P.N., Bradbury, K.E. & Keya, T.J. (2016). High compliance with dietary recommendations in a cohort of meat eaters, fish eaters, vegetarians, and vegans: results from the European Prospective Investigation into Cancer and Nutrition-Oxford study. Nutr Res, 36(5), 464–477.
[511] Biesalski, H.K. (2016). *Vitamine und Minerale – Indikation, Diagnostik, Therapie*. [*Vitamins and minerals – indication, diagnostics, treatment*] Stuttgart: Thieme.
[512] Gröber, U. (2011). *Mikronährstoffe – Metabolic Tuning, Prävention, Therapie* [*Micronutrients – metabolic tuning, prevention, therapy*] (3rd edition). Stuttgart: Wissenschaftliche Verlagsgesellschaft Stuttgart.
[513] Gröber, U. & Holick, M.F. (2015). *Vitamin D – Die Heilkraft des Sonnenvitamins* [*Vitamin D – the healing power of the sunshine vitamin*] (3rd edition). Stuttgart: Wissenschaftliche Verlagsgesellschaft Stuttgart.
[514] Nehls, M. (2018). *Algenöl – Die Ernährungsrevolution aus dem Meer*. [*Algae oil – the nutritional revolution from the sea*] Munich: Wilhelm Heyne Verlag.
[515] Murff, H.J. & Edwards, T.L. (2014). Endogenous Production of Long-Chain Polyunsaturated Fatty Acids and Metabolic Disease Risk. Curr Cardiovasc Risk Rep, 8(12), 418.
[516] Harris, W. S. (2008). The omega-3 index as a risk factor for coronary heart disease. Am J Clin Nutr, 87(6), 1997–2002.
[517] German Nutrition Society (Deutsche Gesellschaft für Ernährung). (2015). *Evidenzbasierte Leitlinie – Fettzufuhr und Prävention ausgewählter ernährungsmit- bedingter Krankheiten* [*Evidence-based guide – fat intake and the prevention of certain diet-related diseases*] (2nd Version). Accessed on 1 June 2019. Available at http://bit.ly/2HBYEFV
[518] Vannice, G. & Rasmussen, H. (2014). Position of the academy of nutrition and dietetics: dietary fatty acids for healthy adults. J Acad Nutr Diet, 114(1), 136–153.
[519] Geppert, J., Kraft, V., Demmelmair, H. & Koletzko, B. (2005). Docosahexaenoic acid supplementation in vegetarians effectively increases omega-3 index: a randomized trial. Lipids, 40(8), 807–814.
[520] Gu, Q., Zhang, C., Song, D., Li, P. & Zhu, X. (2015). Enhancing vitamin B12 content in soy-yogurt by *Lactobacillus reuteri*. Int J Food Microbiol, 206, 56–59.
[521] Watanabe, F., Yabuta, Y., Tanioka, Y. & Bito, T. (1988). Biologically active vitamin B12 compounds in foods for preventing deficiency among vegetarians and elderly subjects. Agric Food Chem, 61(28), 6769–6775.
[522] Croft, M. T., Lawrence, A. D., Raux-Deery, E., Warren, M. J. & Smith, A. G. (2005). Algae acquire vitamin B12 through a symbiotic relationship with bacteria. Nature, 438(7064), 90–93.
[523] Kumudha, A., Selvakumar, S., Dilshad, P., Vaidyanathan, G., Thakur, M. S. & Sarada, R. (2015). Methylcobalamin – a form of vitamin B12 identified and characterised in Chlorella vulgaris. Food Chem, 170, 316–320.
[524] O'Leary, F. & Samman, S. (2010). Vitamin B12 in Health and Disease. Nutrients, 2(3), 299–316.
[525] Bor, M. V., Lydeking-Olsen, E., Moller, J. & Nexo, E. (2006). A daily intake of approximately 6 microg vitamin B12 appears to saturate all the vitamin B12-related variables in Danish postmenopausal women. Am J Clin Nutr, 83, 52–58.
[526] Gropper, S. S., Smith, J. L. & Carr, T. P. (2017). *Advanced Nutrition and Human Metabolism* (7th edition). Boston: Cengage Learning, 354.
[527] Obeid, R., Fedosov, S. N. & Nexo, E. (2015). Cobalamin coenzyme forms are not likely to be superior to cyano- and hydroxyl-cobalamin in prevention or treatment of cobalamin deficiency. Mol Nutr Food Res, 59(7), 1364–1372.
[528] Freeman, A. G. (1996). Hydroxocobalamin versus cyanocobalamin. J R Soc Med, 89(11), 659.
[529] Koyama, K., Yoshida, A., Takeda, A., Morozumi, K., Fujinami, T. & Tanaka, N. (1997). Abnormal cyanide metabolism in uraemic patients. Nephrol Dial Transplant, 12(8), 1622–1628.
[530] Nexo, E., Hvas, A. M., Bleie, Ø. et al. (2002). Holo-transcobalamin is an early marker of changes in cobalamin homeostasis. A randomized placebo-controlled study. Clin Chem, 48(10),1768–1771.
[531] Lüthgens, K. J. & Müller, M. (o. D.). *Neuer Marker zur verbesserten Erkennung von Vitamin-B12-Mangelzuständen*. [*New marker for improved detection of vitamin B12 deficiency*] Accessed on 1 June 2019. Available at https://bit.ly/2JpXGIE
[532] Max-Rubner-Institut. (2008). *Nationale Verzehrsstudie II Ergebnisbericht, Teil 2*. [*National consumption study II report, part 2*] Accessed on 01 June 2018. Available at https://bit.ly/2C6k0It
[533] Gröber, U. & Holick, M. F. (2015). *Vitamin D – Die Heilkraft des Sonnenvitamins* [*Vitamin D – the healing power of the sunshine vitamin*] (3rd edition). Stuttgart: Wissenschaftliche Verlagsgesellschaft, 261.
[534] Vasquez, A., Manso, G. & Cannell, J. (2004). The clinical importance of vitamin D (cholecalciferol): a paradigm shift with implications for all healthcare providers. Altern Ther Health Med, 10(5), 28–36.
[535] www.nutrition.org.uk/nutritioninthenews/new-reports/983-newvitamind.html
[536] Gröber, U. & Holick, M. F. (2015). *Vitamin D – Die Heilkraft des Sonnenvitamins* [*Vitamin D – the healing power of the sunshine vitamin*] (3rd edition). Stuttgart: Wissenschaftliche Verlagsgesellschaft Stuttgart, 268.
[537] Richter, M., Boeing, H., Grünewald-Funk, D., Heseker, H., Kroke, A., Leschik-Bonnet, E., Oberritter, H., Strohm, D. & Watzl, B. (2016). *Position der Deutschen Gesellschaft für Ernährung e. V.* (DGE) – Vegane Ernährung. [*Position of the German Nutrition Society – vegan diet*] Ernährungs Umschau, 63(04), 92–102.
[538] Max Rubner-Institut. (2017). Bundeslebensmittelschlüssel [nutritional information database produced by the German Federal Ministry for Food and Agriculture] (Version 3.02). Accessed on 1 June 2019. Available at https://bit.ly/2dJwkCX
[539] Grune, T., Lietz, G., Palou, A., Ross, A. C., Stahl, W., Tang, G. et al. (2010). ß-Carotene Is an Important Vitamin A Source for Humans. J Nutr, 140(12), 2268–2285.
[540] www.nhs.uk/live-well/eat-well/the-vegan-diet/
[541] Tang, G. (2010). Bioconversion of dietary provitamin A carotenoids to vitamin A in humans. Am J Clin Nutr, 91(5), 1468–1473.
[542] Lemke, S.L., Dueker, S.R., Follett, J.R. et al. (2003). Absorption and retinol equivalence of ß-carotene in humans is influenced by dietary vitamin A intake. J Lipid Res, 44, 1591–1600.

[543] Brown, M.J., Ferruzzi, M.G., Nguyen, M.L., Cooper, D.A., Eldridge, A.L., Schwartz, S.J. & White, W.S. (2004). Carotenoid bioavailability is higher from salads ingested with full-fat than with fat-reduced salad dressings as measured with electrochemical detection. Am J Clin Nutr, 80(2), 396–403.
[544] Penniston, K.L. & Tanumihardjo, S.A. (2006). The acute and chronic toxic effects of vitamin A. Am J Clin Nutr. 83(2), 191–201.
[545] Gröber, U. (2011). *Mikronährstoffe: Metabolic Tuning – Prävention – Therapie [Micronutrients: metabolic tuning – prevention – therapy]* (3rd edition). Stuttgart: Wissenschaftliche Verlagsgesellschaft Stuttgart, 122.
[546] *Arbeitskreis Jodmangel*. [Working group on iodine deficiency] (2013). Jod: *Mangel und Versorgung in Deutschland – Aktuelles zum derzeitigen Versorgungsstand und Handlungsbedarf. [Iodine: deficiency and supply in Germany – latest information on current supply status and need for action]* Accessed on 1 June 2019. Available at https://bit.ly/2vPqltT
[547] Ullmann, J. (2017). *Algen – Sonderdruck aus dem Handbuch Lebensmittelhygiene. [Algae – Offprint from the Guide to Food Hygiene]* Hamburg: Behr's Verlag, 21.
[548] Teas, J., Pino, S., Critchley, A. & Braverman, L.E. (2004). Variability of iodine content in common commercially available edible seaweeds. Thyroid, 14(10), 836–841.
[549] Aslam, M. N., Kreider, J. M., Paruchuri, T., Bhagavathula, N., DaSilva, M., Zernicke, R. F. et al. (2010). A Mineral-Rich Extract from the Red Marine Algae Lithothamnion calcareum Preserves Bone Structure and Function in Female Mice on a Western-Style Diet. Calcif Tissue Int, 86(4), 313–324.
[550] Thamm, M., Ellert, U., Thierfelder, W., Liesenkötter, K.P. & Völzke, H. (2007). *Jodurie bei Kindern und Jugendlichen in Deutschland - Ergebnisse des Jodmonitorings im Kinder- und Jugendgesundheitssurvey* (KiGGS). *[Urinary iodine for children and young people in Germany – results of iodine monitoring from the KiGGS survey on children and young people's health]* Ernährung, 1(5), 220–224.
[551] Deutsche Gesellschaft für Ernährung [German Nutrition Society], Österreichische Gesellschaft für Ernährung [Austrian Nutrition Society], Schweizerische Gesellschaft für Ernährung [Swiss Nutrition Society]. (2015). *Referenzwerte für die Nährstoffzufuhr – Selen [Reference values for nutrient intake – selenium]* (4th edition). Bonn: Neuer Umschau Verlag.
[552] Aro, A., Alfthan, G. & Varo, P. (1995). Effects of supplementation of fertilizers on human selenium status in Finland. Analyst, 120(3), 841–843.
[553] European Commission (2004). List of the authorised additives in foodstuffs Accessed on 1 June 2019. Available at https://bit.ly/2vlakG9
[554] Thomson, C. D., Chisholm, A., McLachlan S. K. & Campbell, J. M. (2008). Brazil nuts: an effective way to improve selenium status. Am J Clin Nutr, 87(2), 379–384.
[555] Parekha, P. P., Khana, A. R., Torresa, M. A. & Kittoa, M. E. (2008). Concentrations of selenium, barium, and radium in Brazil nuts. J Food Compost Anal, 21, 332–335.
[556] Gröber, U. (2011). *Mikronährstoffe – Metabolic Tuning, Prävention, Therapie [Micronutrients – metabolic tuning, prevention, therapy]* (3rd edition). Stuttgart: Wissenschaftliche Verlagsgesellschaft Stuttgart.
[557] Gröber, U. (2011). *Mikronährstoffe – Metabolic Tuning, Prävention, Therapie [Micronutrients – metabolic tuning, prevention, therapy]* (3rd edition). Stuttgart: Wissenschaftliche Verlagsgesellschaft Stuttgart, 265.
[558] Gröber, U. (2011). *Mikronährstoffe – Metabolic Tuning, Prävention, Therapie [Micronutrients – metabolic tuning, prevention, therapy]* (3rd edition). Stuttgart: Wissenschaftliche Verlagsgesellschaft Stuttgart, 267f.
[559] Gröber, U. (2011). *Mikronährstoffe – Metabolic Tuning, Prävention, Therapie [Micronutrients – metabolic tuning, prevention, therapy]* (3rd edition). Stuttgart: Wissenschaftliche Verlagsgesellschaft Stuttgart, 275.

List of references: practical tips and recipe building blocks (pp.83–99)

[1] Finger, T.E. & Kinnamon, S.C. (2011). Taste isn't just for taste buds anymore. Biol Rep, 3, 20.
[2] Moss, M. (2014). *Salt Sugar Fat: How the Food Giants Hooked Us*. New York: Random House Trade Paperback.
[3] Berg, J.M., Tymoczko, J.L. & Stryer, L. (2002). *Biochemistry* (5th edition). New York: W H Freeman.
[4] Besnard, P., Passilly-Degrace, P. & Khan, N.A. (2016). Taste of Fat: A Sixth Taste Modality? Physiol Rev, 96(1), 151–176.
[5] Finger, T.E. & Kinnamon, S.C. (2011). Taste isn't just for taste buds anymore. Biol Rep, 3, 20.
[6] Lisle, D.J. & Goldhamer, A. (2006). *The Pleasure Trap: Mastering the Hidden Force that Undermines Health & Happiness*. Summertown: Healthy Living Publications.
[7] Institute for Quality and Efficiency in Health Care (2006). How does our sense of taste work? Accessed on 1 June 2019. Available at https://bit.ly/2WAkhm4
[8] Valussi, M. (2012). Functional foods with digestion-enhancing properties. Int J Food Sci Nutr, 63(1), 82–89.
[9] Drewnowski, A. & Gomez-Carneros, C. (2000). Bitter taste, phytonutrients, and the consumer: a review. Am J Clin Nutr, 72(6), 1424–1435.
[10] Cook, N.R., Appel, L.J. & Whelton, P.K. (2014). Lower levels of sodium intake and reduced cardiovascular risk. Circulation. 129 (9), 981–989.
[11] Stevens, R. (2014). Nutritonal [sic] Star: How celery can replace salt in your diet. Accessed on 1 June 2019. Available at https://bit.ly/2Wzk7LA
[12] Institute for Quality and Efficiency in Health Care (2006). How does our sense of taste work? Accessed on 1 June 2019. Available at https://bit.ly/2WAkhm4
[13] Berg, J.M., Tymoczko, J.L. & Stryer, L. (2002). *Biochemistry* (5th edition). New York: W H Freeman.
[14] Barclay, G.R., McKenzie, H., Pennington, J., Parratt, D. & Pennington, C.R. (1992). The effect of dietary yeast on the activity of stable chronic Crohn's disease. Scand J Gastroenterol, 27(3), 196–200.
[15] Henry, A. G., Brooks, A. S. & Pipernob, D. R. (2011). Microfossils in calculus demonstrate consumption of plants and cooked foods in Neanderthal diets (Shanidar III, Iraq; Spy I and II, Belgium). Proc Natl Acad Sci USA, 108(2), 486–491.
[16] Mercader, J. (2009). Mozambican grass seed consumption during the Middle Stone Age. Science, 326(5960), 1680–1683.
[17] Zanovec, M., O'Neil, C. E. & Nicklas, T. A. (2011). Comparison of Nutrient Density and Nutrient-to-Cost between Cooked and Canned Beans. Food and Nutrition Sciences, 2, 66–73.
[18] Lally, P., van Jaarsveld, C.H.M., Potts, H.W.W. & Wardle, J. (2010). How are habits formed: Modelling habit formation in the real world. Eur J Soc Psychol, 40(6), 998–1009.

Tables and list of figures

Figures:

Tables:

Index of recipes

Acknowledgments

DK would like to thank

John Friend for proofreading and Anna Sander for additional help with translation.

Julia Hildebrand thanks Motel A Miio, Rosenthal, and Serax for providing pottery, porcelain, and cooking utensils.

Picture credits

The publisher thanks the following individuals and organisations for their kind permission to print these photographs:

5 123RF.com: antimo andriani (pulses); handmadepictures (raspberries); tevarak11 (herbs); Rodica Ciorba (cauliflower); Brent Hofacker (grains, kale); iStockphoto.com: FotografiaBasica (apples). 13 Dreamstime.com: Goncharuk Maksym (cucumber). 14 Dreamstime.com: Tomboy2290 (lettuce). 59 Dreamstime.com: Goncharuk Maksym (cucumber). 75 123RF.com: Baiba Opule. 89 123RF.com: antimo andriani (pulses); Rodica Ciorba (cauliflower); Brent Hofacker (grains, kale); tevarak11 (herbs). 100 iStockphoto.com: FotografiaBasica. 132 123RF.com: Brent Hofacker. 152 123RF.com: Rodica Ciorba. 172 123RF.com: Brent Hofacker. 186 123RF.com: antimo andriani. 208 123RF.com: tevarak11. 222 123RF.com: handmadepictures.

Index of contents

About the authors

About Niko Rittenau:

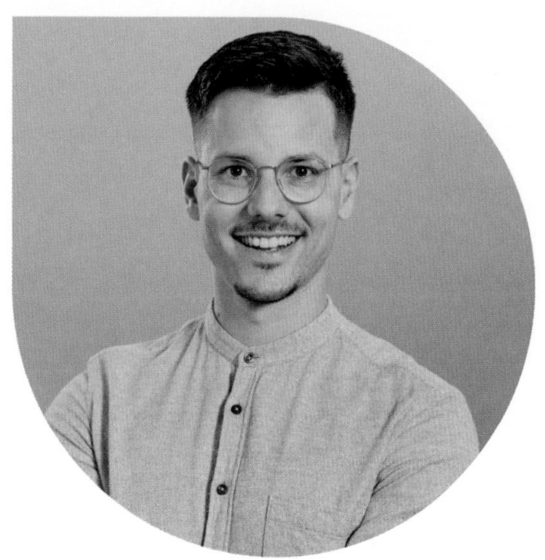

Niko Rittenau is a nutrition scientist specializing in plant-based diet. Born in Austria, he combines the culinary skills he acquired when he originally trained in the tourism industry with his academic nutritional expertise to create innovative food with an emphasis on great taste, health awareness, and sustainable consumption. Through his lectures and seminars, Niko presents his concept for the growing global population and he encourages an appreciation of high-quality food. Having completed both a bachelor's and master's degree in the field of nutrition science, he is currently writing his dissertation for his PhD.

About Sebastian Copien:

Sebastian Copien's ambition and purpose is to encourage others to incorporate the key features of exceptional vegan cuisine into everyday catering and domestic cooking. As a chef, author, surf instructor, and permaculture practitioner, this ethos is the basis for all the courses, seminars, and events he runs, through which he conveys the simplicity and joy of vegan cooking. He also hosts regular fine-dining evenings offering high-quality plant-based menus at his Munich kitchen. Sebastian is a co-founder and lecturer at the Plant Based Institute, which he runs with Niko Rittenau and Boris Lauser. Several times a year, this is the venue for training and development courses on vegan nutrition and cuisine. The Vegan Masterclass platform founded by Sebastian offers extensive remote-learning opportunities with all sorts of online courses for anyone interested in further training in vegan cuisine.

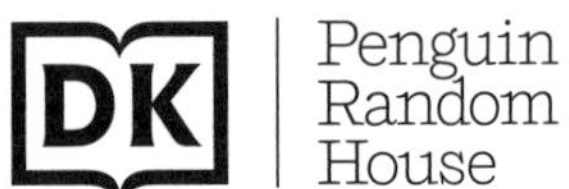

DK LONDON
Translator Alison Tunley
Editor Helena Caldon
Editorial Assistant Lucy Philpott
Designer Hannah Moore
Senior Designer Glenda Fisher
Managing Editor Ruth O'Rourke
Managing Art Editor Christine Keilty
Production Editor Heather Blagden
Production Controller Rebecca Parton
Jacket Designer Nicola Powling
Jacket Coordinator Lucy Philpott
Art Director Maxine Pedliham
Publishing Director Katie Cowan

DK DELHI
Assistant Editor Ankita Gupta
CTS Designer Umesh Singh Rawat
Pre-production Manager Sunil Sharma

DK GERMANY
Recipes Sebastian Copien
Text Niko Rittenau
Food photography Julia Hildebrand & Ingolf Hatz, www.augustundjuli.de
People photography and cover photo Ingolf Hatz, www.ingolfhatz.com
Food styling Margit Proebst, www.margit-proebst.de
Styling Julia Hildebrand
Editorial Cora Wetzstein
Internal design, graphics, implementation, cover design Jürgen Katzenberger
Programme management Monika Schlitzer
Editorial management Anne Heinel
Project support Jessica Kleppel
Production manager Dorothee Whittaker
Production controller Ksenia Lebedeva
Production Stefanie Staat

First published in Great Britain in 2021 by
Dorling Kindersley Limited
DK, One Embassy Gardens, 8 Viaduct Gardens,
London, SW11 7BW

The authorised representative in the EEA is
Dorling Kindersley Verlag GmbH. Arnulfstr. 124,
80636 Munich, Germany

10 9 8 7 6 5 4 3 2 1
001–322744–Jul/2021

A CIP catalogue record for this book is available from the British Library.
ISBN: 978-0-2414-8044-1

Printed and bound in China

For the curious

www.dk.com

Note
The information and suggestions in this book have been carefully considered and checked by the authors and publisher, however, no guarantee is assumed. Neither the authors nor the publisher and its representatives are liable for any personal, material, or financial damage.

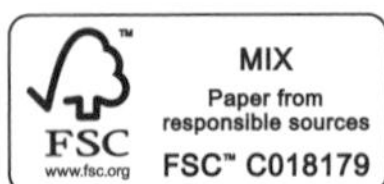

This book was made with Forest Stewardship Council ™ certified paper – one small step in DK's commitment to a sustainable future.
For more information go to
www.dk.com/our-green-pledge